D0327248

CLINICAL WORK WITH SUBSTANCE-ABUSING CLIENTS

THE GUILFORD SUBSTANCE ABUSE SERIES

Howard T. Blane and Thomas R. Kosten, Editors

Clinical Work with Substance-Abusing Clients

Second Edition

Edited by
Shulamith Lala Ashenberg Straussner

THE GUILFORD PRESS
New York   London

© 2004 The Guilford Press
A Division of Guilford Publications, Inc.
72 Spring Street, New York, NY 10012
www.guilford.com

All rights reserved

No part of this book may be reproduced, translated, stored in a
retrieval system, or transmitted, in any form or by any means,
electronic, mechanical, photocopying, microfilming, recording,
or otherwise, without written permission from the Publisher.

Printed in the United States of America

This book is printed on acid-free paper.

Last digit is print number: 9 8 7 6 5 4 3 2 1

Library of Congress Cataloging-in-Publication Data

Clinical work with substance-abusing clients / edited by Shulamith Lala
Ashenberg Straussner.—2nd ed.
     p. cm. — (The Guilford substance abuse series)
  Includes bibliographical references and index.
  ISBN 1-59385-067-0 (hard)
  1. Substance abuse—Treatment. 2. Social work with alcoholics. 3. Social
work with narcotics addicts. I. Straussner, Shulamith Lala Ashenberg.
II. Series.
  RC564.C57 2004
  616.86′06—dc22

                                     2004005221

About the Editor

Shulamith Lala Ashenberg Straussner, DSW, CSW, CEAP, BCD, CAS, is Professor at the Shirley M. Ehrenkranz School of Social Work at New York University and Director of their Post-Master's Program in the Treatment of Alcohol- and Drug-Abusing Clients. She was a Fulbright Senior Scholar to Israel in 2003; Distinguished Visiting Professor at Ben-Gurion University of the Negev in Beer-Sheva, Israel, in January 2002; and Visiting Professor at the Omsk State Pedagogical University in Siberia, Russia, in the spring of 2000.

Dr. Straussner has written numerous publications dealing with substance abuse. Among her 13 books are *International Aspects of Social Work Practice in the Addictions* (coedited with Larry Harrison; 2003, Haworth Press), *Understanding Mass Violence: A Social Work Perspective* (coedited with Norma Phillips; 2003, Allyn & Bacon), *The Handbook of Addiction Treatment for Women* (coedited with Stephanie Brown; 2002, Jossey-Bass), *Ethnocultural Factors in Substance Abuse Treatment* (2001, Guilford Press), and *Gender and Addictions: Men and Women in Treatment* (coedited with Elizabeth Zelvin; 1997, Jason Aronson). She also is the founding editor of the new *Journal of Social Work Practice in the Addictions.*

Dr. Straussner has served on the National Center on Substance Abuse Treatment panel on workforce issues and is a founding board member of the New York State Institute for Professional Development in Addictions. She serves as a consultant to various hospitals, agencies, and other organizations in New York and lectures on a variety of topics throughout the United States and abroad. She also has a private therapeutic and supervisory practice in New York City.

Contributors

Armin R. Baier, JD, CSW, Parallax Center, New York, New York

Insoo Kim Berg, MSSW, Brief Family Therapy Center, Milwaukee, Wisconsin

Edgar E. Coons, PhD, Department of Psychology, New York University, New York, New York

Jenna Davis, CSW, private practice, Newtown, Pennsylvania

Nabila El-Bassel, PhD, School of Social Work, Columbia University, New York, New York

Kathleen J. Farkas, PhD, LISW, ASCW, Mandel School of Applied Social Sciences, Case Western Reserve University, Cleveland, Ohio

Christine Huff Fewell, CSW, CASAC, Ehrenkranz School of Social Work, New York University, New York, New York

Audrey Freshman, CSW, CASAC, Tempo Group, Inc., Woodmere, New York, and Graduate Department of Family Studies, Hofstra University, Hempstead, New York

Ellen Grace Friedman, MSW, CSW, CASAC, Greenwich House, New York, New York, and Ehrenkranz School of Social Work, New York University, New York, New York

Larry M. Gant, CSW, PhD, School of Social Work, University of Michigan, Ann Arbor, Michigan

Sandy Gibson, PhD, private practice, Morrisville, Pennsylvania

Eda G. Goldstein, DSW, Ehrenkranz School of Social Work, New York University, New York, New York

Muriel Gray, PhD, School of Social Work, University of Maryland, Baltimore, Maryland

Meredith Hanson, DSW, Graduate School of Social Service, Fordham University, New York, New York

Roberta Markowitz, MSW, CSW, Oakwood Center, White Plains, New York

Jeffrey R. McIntyre, CADAC, CGP, LMHC, LMFT, Hawley–McIntyre Associates, Cambridge, Massachusetts

David Ockert, DSW, Parallax Center, New York, New York

Philip O'Dwyer, EdD, CSW, CAC, Brookfield Clinics, Garden City, Michigan

Margaret O'Neill, PhD, private practice, Riverdale, New York

Lois Orlin, CSW, CASAC, private practice, New York, New York

Patricia A. Pape, MSW, Pape & Associates, Wheaton, Illinois

Shelley Scheffler, PhD, CSW, University Behavioral Health Care, University of Medicine and Dentistry of New Jersey, Union City, New Jersey

Belinda Housenbold Seiger, CSW, Ehrenkranz School of Social Work, New York University, New York, New York

Evan Senreich, CSW, ACSW, CASAC, Ehrenkranz School of Social Work, New York University, New York, New York

Kathryn C. Shafer, PhD, LCSW, CAP, School of Social Work, University of South Florida, Tampa, Florida

Betsy Robin Spiegel, MSW, CSW, private practice, New York, New York

Diane Pincus Strom, MSW, ACSW, Department of Medicine and AIDS Program, Bronx Lebanon Hospital Center, Bronx, New York

Shulamith Lala Ashenberg Straussner, DSW, CAS, Ehrenkranz School of Social Work, New York University, New York, New York

Elena Vairo, CSW, New York City Department of Education and private practice, New York, New York

Robin Wilson, LCSW, CSW, ACSW, Addiction Treatment Services, Catholic Community Services/Behavioral Health, Union City, New Jersey

Elizabeth Zelvin, MSW, CSW-R, CASAC, LZcybershrink.com, New York, New York

Preface

Much has changed in the field of substance abuse (or addiction) since 1993, when the first edition of this book was published. As indicated in the final chapter of this book, the field is constantly evolving as new substances, new populations, and new treatment approaches develop within ever-changing political and organizational climates. This second edition is an attempt to cover the main issues in this changing field.

Like the previous edition, this book is organized into five main sections, with an additional chapter that takes a brief look at the future. However, updating the state of knowledge required a major reconceptualization of the organization of this book and the addition of a number of new chapters. Chapters on the motivation of substance-abusing clients, harm reduction, working with involuntary clients, and treatment of older adults and of gay and lesbian clients have been added, whereas others— intervention with substance abusers in medical settings, the workplace, and private clinical settings, and on the use of family "intervention"—had to be eliminated due to space limitation. When possible, many of the core issues of the omitted chapters have been incorporated into other chapters. Additional important topics, in particular, ethnocultural issues, have been omitted because they are addressed elsewhere (see *Ethnocultural Factors in Substance Abuse Treatment* [Straussner, 2001]).

As was true in the first edition, this book is aimed at both beginning and experienced clinicians, and all of the chapters are written by people who have front-line experience working with the substance-abusing population.

Part I provides an overview of the impact of alcohol and other drugs on individuals and discusses basic clinical practice issues.

Part II offers varying perspectives on intervention with substance abusers and includes chapters on motivational interviewing, the practice of harm reduction, the use of a solution-focused approach with involuntary clients, helping clients with coexisting major psychiatric and substance-related disorders, the use of 12-step programs, and relapse prevention.

Part III considers intervention with individuals dependent on different substances: alcohol, opiates, and stimulants.

Part IV deals with assessment and intervention issues with families of substance abusers, including partners and children.

Part V examines the unique treatment issues for such populations as adolescents, older adults, women, those with borderline personality disorders, gay and lesbian clients, homeless persons, and those impacted by HIV/AIDS.

The final chapter provides a brief discussion of future practice and policy issues.

This edition took much longer than expected. Personal, professional, and social issues—particularly the impact of September 11, 2001, on my life—played a large role in the delay of this publication. The fact that it has been completed at all is due to the tremendous support of many people: my family—my children, both "old" and "new," Adam, Sarina, and Allie; my sister Lusia; my wonderful friends Richard, Norma, Betsy, Audrey, Christine, Eileen, and Stanton, who provided encouragement, as well as critical nudging and feedback when I needed it; my friends from the monthly "West 79th Street Salon," Liz, Rita, Val, and Ita; and my colleagues from NYU, in particular, Dean Suzanne England. I want to thank my editor, Jim Nageotte, of The Guilford Press for not giving up on me. Most important, I want to thank all the contributors who waited, some more patiently than others, to see this book in print.

Here it is.

SHULAMITH LALA ASHENBERG STRAUSSNER

REFERENCE

Straussner, S. L. A. (Ed.). (2001). *Ethnocultural factors in substance abuse treatment.* New York: Guilford Press.

Contents

CLINICAL WORK WITH SUBSTANCE-ABUSING CLIENTS

PART I

An Introduction to Clinical Practice with Substance-Abusing Clients

CHAPTER 1

Assessment and Treatment of Clients with Alcohol and Other Drug Abuse Problems

An Overview

Shulamith Lala Ashenberg Straussner

The courage to be is rooted in the God who appears when God has disappeared in the anxiety of doubt.
—PAUL TILLICH, *The Courage to Be*

From the infant born to a woman addicted to crack cocaine to the older alcoholic man who needs nursing home care, the abuse of alcohol and other drugs is a major health and social problem affecting every segment of our society. The direct or indirect impact of substance abuse and dependence is experienced by social workers and other clinicians in all types of settings and requires each worker to have some familiarity with the various substances and the assessment and treatment needs of those abusing them. The purpose of this chapter is to provide an overview of the impact of alcohol and other drugs on individuals and to discuss the issues related to clinical assessment and intervention with drug- or alcohol-abusing clients and their families.

DEFINITION OF TERMS

Every day millions of Americans use alcohol and other psychoactive substances; however, not everyone experiences a problem due to such use. It is therefore helpful to conceptualize alcohol and other drug (AOD) use as ranging on a continuum from non-problematic experimental and social *use* to substance *misuse* (such as using pain medication to get high) to *abuse* (excessive use of a substance that results in a negative impact on the life of the individual and those around him or her), and finally, to AOD *dependence* or *addiction* (which may require physical detoxification and/or formal treatment).

The potential for addiction of different substances varies greatly; for example, narcotics or crack cocaine have a much higher potential for addiction than alcohol or marijuana. The terms *alcoholism* and *drug addiction* both imply a progressive deterioration of the individual's social, physical, and mental status, best exemplified in the well-known Jellinek chart, named after the man who first described the various symptoms and the downhill progression of the typical alcoholic (Jellinek, 1952).

Although, technically, alcohol is classified as a mood-altering drug or chemical compound (Levin, 1990), traditionally, alcohol abuse and alcoholism were viewed as distinct from, and more acceptable than, abuse of and addiction to other drugs (due to a combination of political, historical, economic, and possibly racial factors). During the 1970s, however, clinicians treating patients with alcoholism became aware that many people, especially women and younger men, tended to abuse and become dependent not only on alcohol (in addition to caffeine and nicotine) but also other sedative–hypnotics, such as minor tranquilizers and sleeping medications. Thus the term *chemical dependency* was coined to indicate the harmful use of alcohol and other sedative–hypnotics, and terms such as *drug abuse, substance abuse,* and *addiction* were relegated to illicit substances such as heroin, amphetamines, and marijuana.

The growing use of cocaine during the early 1980s changed the clinical picture as well as the vocabulary in the field. Due to a lack of treatment facilities, numerous middle-class cocaine abusers, who also tended to use alcohol to cope with the side effects of cocaine, were referred to alcoholism treatment facilities (Washton & Gold, 1987). Moreover, methadone patients, who tended to increase their drinking as they gave up heroin, were also coming to these facilities. Thus, in spite of the omission of alcohol from most "war on drugs" legislation and the separate federal funding streams for alcohol and drug programs, the line separating "alcoholism/chemical dependency" from "drug abuse" had started to erode, and the treatment for people in both groups began to converge. According to the National Survey of Substance Abuse Treatment Services, by 2002 nearly half of all 1.1 million people receiving substance abuse treatment were in treatment for *both* drug and alcohol problems (Substance Abuse and Mental Health Services Administration [SAMHSA], 2003).

The change in client population led to a change in nomenclature. By the end of the 1980s, the Division of Communication programs in the federal Office of Substance Abuse Prevention (currently referred to as the Center for Substance Abuse Prevention, or CSAP) recommended the use of the terms *alcohol and other drug use* and *abuse,* whereas the American Psychiatric Association (APA) used the category of *psychoactive substance use disorders* (SUD) as a catchall term for the dysfunctional use of all mood-altering chemicals.

Currently, the APA's *Diagnostic and Statistical Manual of Mental Disorders* (DSM) uses the term *substance-related disorders* (SRD) to classify all disorders related to the problematic consequences of substance use. The SRD category is further divided into *substance use disorders* (SUD), which includes the criteria for diagnosing *substance abuse* and *substance dependence* (discussed in more detail below), and *substance-induced disorders* (SID), which contains 11 disorders. As the term implies, SID includes those disorders that are caused or induced by the use of a substance; these range from substance intoxication or withdrawal symptoms to substance-induced mood, anxiety, psychotic, or sleeping disorders. It is assumed that once a person stops his or her abuse of or dependence on a substance, these SID will disappear within a relatively short time. Individuals whose psychiatric symptoms do not disappear over time are likely to receive additional diagnoses, variously referred to as coexisting, co-occurring, or comorbid disorders, or, most commonly, as MICA—individuals who are both *mentally ill* and abusing *chemicals* (or substances).

The Use of DSM Criteria

According to the latest edition of the APA manual (DSM-IV-TR; APA, 2000, pp. 198–199), *substance abuse* is defined as "a maladaptive pattern of substance use leading to clinically significant impairment or distress" in *one or more* of the following: the continued use of psychoactive substances despite experiencing social, occupational, psychological, or physical problems; inability to fulfill "major role obligations at work, school, or home"; recurrent use in situations in which use is physically hazardous, such as driving while intoxicated; and/or recurrent legal problems related to the use of a substance. These symptoms must occur within a 12-month time frame. DSM-IV-TR further differentiates substance *abuse* from substance *dependence,* which it defines as the existence of *at least three* of the following seven symptoms within a 12- month period (American Psychiatric Association, 2000, p. 197):

1. Tolerance, as defined by either a need for increased amounts of a substance to achieve a desired effect or diminished effect with use of the same quantity of substances.
2. Withdrawal, as characterized by specific withdrawal syndromes defined for each substance, or using a substance in order to relieve or avoid withdrawal symptoms.
3. Taking the substance in larger amounts or over a longer period than was intended.
4. A persistent desire or unsuccessful efforts to reduce or control use.
5. A great deal of time spent obtaining, using and recovering from substance abuse.
6. Important social, occupational, or recreational activities are given up or reduced because of the substance use.
7. The substance continues to be used despite knowledge of resulting serious physical or psychological problems.

In essence, substance dependence refers to compulsive and continued use of AOD despite adverse consequences. The terms *alcoholism* and *drug addiction* are synonymous with *substance dependence*. Once an individual has been diagnosed with substance dependence, he or she will never be diagnosed with the less severe diagnosis of substance abuse. At the same time, the term *substance abuse* is often used as the catchall term for substance use disorders—and it is only the context in which the term is used that differentiates its meaning. This chapter follows conventions and uses this term in both of its meanings.

The DSM diagnosis of substance abuse or dependence also calls for one of six "course specifiers" delineating the longer-term outcome of these disorders. These specifiers can only be given *after* the individual has stopped using a given substance for at least *1 month*. They include *early full remission*, defined as being substance-free for more than 1 month but less than 12 months; *early partial remission*, whereby the individual resumes some use of a substance (sometimes referred to as having a "slip") and subsequently meets at least one criterion of abuse or dependence within the first year of recovery; *sustained full remission*, defined as being totally substance-free for more than 1 year; and *sustained partial remission*, in which the individual resumes substance use after 12 months of not having any symptoms, and then meets at least one criterion related to substance abuse or dependence. The two final specifiers are *on agonist therapy*, which refers to the use of agonist or antagonist medication to treat the substance of choice, such as using methadone as a replacement for the use of opiates; and *in a controlled environment*, indicating that the individual is not using a substance because of living in a substance-free environment, such as a therapeutic community or a federal prison.

THE SCOPE AND IMPACT OF SUBSTANCE ABUSE

An estimated 22 million Americans (9.4% of the total population), age 12 or older in 2002, were classified as abusing or being dependent on a substance (SAMHSA, 2003). The abuse of alcohol and other drugs affects individuals, families, communities, and society as a whole. Substance abuse causes more deaths, illnesses, accidents, and disabilities than any other preventable health problem today (Horgan, 1995; Robert Wood Johnson Foundation, 2001). At the end of the 20th century at least half of all adults arrested for major crimes, such as homicide, theft, and assault, tested positive for alcohol or other drugs at the time of arrest (U.S. Department of Health and Human Services, 2000a, 2000b).

Despite the government and media focus on users of illicit drugs, clinically it is important to note that there are approximately *4 million* individuals with a drug use disorder, compared to close to *18 million* with alcohol use disorder. Unfortunately, only 18% of the federal drug control budget is devoted to treatment, whereas 60% is spent on the criminal justice system and interdiction. Most tragically, fewer than one-fourth of those individuals who need help for their abuse or dependence on alcohol or other drugs ever get treatment (Robert Wood Johnson Foundation, 2001).

Below is a brief overview of the scope and impact of substance abuse as it relates to clinical practice.

Scope of Alcohol-Related Problems

Although figures vary, there are approximately 11 million adults suffering from alcohol dependence and an additional 7 million alcohol-abusing individuals in the United States (Grant et al., 1994; SAMHSA, 2003).

Alcohol abuse is associated with a wide variety of illnesses and social problems: A minimum of three out of every 100 deaths is attributed to alcohol-related causes, including liver and pancreas diseases, cancer, and cardiovascular problems (Horgan, 1995; Williams, Grant, Hartford, & Noble, 1989). Nearly half of all violent deaths (accidents, suicides, and homicides), particularly of men below age 34, are alcohol related, and alcohol has been found to be a consistent factor in reports of child physical and sexual abuse, including incest, and in cases of rape and domestic violence (Robert Wood Johnson Foundation, 2001). Up to 60% of sexual offenders drink at the time of the offense, and more than 75% of female victims of nonfatal domestic violence reports that the assailant was drinking or using drugs (Robert Wood Johnson Foundation, 2001).

Alcohol abuse and dependence vary according to age and gender as well as ethnic and racial factors (for fuller discussion of ethnocultural and gender issues, see Straussner, 1985, 2001b; Straussner & Brown, 2002; Straussner & Zelvin, 1997). Males are more than four times as likely as fe-

males to be alcohol abusers, although the ratio of men to women with alcohol dependence is lower (Grant et al., 1994). Women at highest risk for
alcohol abuse and dependence are usually (1) in their 20s or 30s, (2) are
unmarried but living with a partner, (3) are in a relationship with an alcohol-
abusing man (U.S. Department of Health and Human Services, 2000b).

Among young adults (ages 18–29), white males have the highest risk
for alcohol problems, whereas black men and women have the highest
rates among the middle-aged and older population and are at higher risk
for alcohol-related diseases as well as personal and social problems (Grant
et al., 1994; U.S. Department of Health and Human Services, 1989). Socioeconomic factors also correlate with race and gender: Limited education
and poverty are related to alcohol dependence in black males but not in
white males (Robert Wood Johnson Foundation, 2001). Among Hispanic
men, the rate of alcohol abuse increases sharply for men in their 30s but
declines thereafter, with Mexican American men and women having higher
rates of both abstention and alcohol abuse when compared to men and
women of Puerto Rican or Cuban origin (U.S. Department of Health and
Human Services, 2000a). American Indian and Alaska Native groups, as a
whole, have very high rates of alcohol abuse and dependence (SAMHSA,
2003), whereas Asian Americans (a term that encompasses an extremely
diverse population) have a lower level of alcohol abuse and dependence
than other racial and ethnic groups, a finding accounted for by their physiological sensitivity to the effects of alcohol, the so-called flushing response
(SAMHSA, 2003; Sue, 1987).

Scope of Problems Related to Other Drugs

Government data indicate that an estimated 14 million Americans, or
6.3% of the population 12 years and older, were using illicit drugs during
the 2000 calendar year. Of those, an estimate 2.8 million individuals were
dependent on drugs, with an additional 1.5 million individuals considered
to be drug abusers (2002 National Drug Control Strategy National Priorities II: Healing America's Drug Users, *www.whitehousedrugpolicy.gov/
publications/policy/03ndcs/2priorities.html*, retrieved June, 10, 2003).

The 2000 National Household Survey on Drug Abuse (NHSDA)
found that men have a higher rate of current illicit drug use than women
(7.7% vs. 5.0%) and are twice as likely to use marijuana heavily. However,
the rates of nonmedical use of psychotherapeutic drugs (pain relievers,
tranquilizers, stimulants, and sedatives) were similar for both males (1.8%)
and females (1.7%) (Robert Wood Johnson Foundation, 2001).

One of the most tragic consequences of drug abuse, particularly injected drugs, is the possible transmission of HIV/AIDS. This drug–AIDS
connection is especially detrimental to communities of color. During
1997, AIDS was the leading cause of death among African American in-

dividuals between the ages of 25 and 44, with over 60% of these deaths related to drug injection: "Among those who inject drugs, African Americans are five times as likely as whites to get AIDS" (Day, 1999, p. 1). AIDS was the second leading cause of death for Hispanic individuals in the same age group, with over half of the deaths related to drug injection, compared with less than a quarter for white individuals. Both African American and Hispanic women suffer disproportionately from this epidemic: African American women account for over half of all injection-related AIDS cases among women, while representing only 12% of the population, and Hispanic women, who represent 10% of the female population in the United States, account for 20% of all injection-related AIDS cases (Day, 1999).

In addition to AIDS, the use of dirty, shared, and reused needles results in various systemic infections. Illnesses such as anemia, tuberculosis, heart disease, diabetes, pneumonia, and hepatitis are also common among heroin abusers, and cocaine use affects the cardiovascular system, resulting in blockages in blood circulation, abnormal heart rhythms, and strokes. Prostitution, a frequent means of support for drug-dependent women, leads to a high incidence of sexually transmitted diseases (O'Connor, Esherick, & Vieten, 2002).

Prenatal Impact of Alcohol and Other Drugs

A unique issue among women who abuse alcohol and/or drugs is the prenatal impact of these substances upon their children. The degree of impact on the fetus due to exposure to alcohol or other drugs is determined by many factors, including the type of substance, the gestation age of the fetus, the route and duration of exposure, the dosage and frequency of drug intake, other substances consumed simultaneously, and environmental factors (Nadel, 1985). Substances used by the mother are transmitted to the fetus during pregnancy and may result in the birth of an addicted baby or a baby with permanent physiological and brain damage, depending on the substance used and the timing of use (Azmitia, 2001; Straussner, 1989).

Although the impact of paternal drug and alcohol use has not been widely researched, authorities have taken a harsh view of the damages caused to the fetus and the newborn due to maternal abuse of drugs and alcohol. In many states, children who are born addicted or test positive to illicit substances are legally viewed as abused, and hospital workers are required to report such cases to local child welfare agencies (Straussner & Attia, 2002). Among the consequences to the mother are imprisonment or mandatory treatment and foster care placement of the child after birth. There is abundant evidence that the laws requiring mandatory reporting are applied unfairly toward women of low socioeconomic class, particularly to women of color. For example, a Florida study demonstrated that despite equal percentages of black and white mothers testing positive for cocaine in obstetrical offices, black women were 10 times more likely to be reported to state officials than were white women (Gustavsson & MacEachron, 1997). Unfortunately, treatment of substance-abusing mothers is not always required or readily available.

Substance Abuse by Young People

Unlike the relatively constant rate of alcohol and drug abuse by adults over the years, the use of substances by young people tends to fluctuate over time. Such fluctuation reflects the availability of particular substances, their popularity among certain subgroups, and the nature of governmental data collection.

After a relatively high use of illicit substances by young people in the 1960s and 1970s, the proportion of high school and college students using any illicit drug dropped steadily throughout the 1980s (Johnston, O'Malley, & Bachman, 1988), only to rise once again during the early and mid-1990s. Following a slight decrease at the end of 20th century, the use of illicit drugs (and tobacco) seems to be on the increase. In particular, there has been a growing use of (1) marijuana, (2) the so-called club drugs, such as Ecstasy, and (3) the nonmedical painkillers, such as OxyContin (SAMHSA, 2003).

The heavy use of alcohol among young people is often viewed as a "gateway" to other drugs; research studies have shown that among youths who drink heavily, 66% were also current illicit drug users, compared to only 4.2% of nondrinkers who were current illicit drug users (Robert Wood Johnson Foundation, 2001).

What is important to note is that despite these upward and downward trends, "this nation's high school students and other young adults show a level of involvement with illicit drugs which is greater than can be found in any other industrialized nation in the world" (Johnston et al., 1988, p. 14). More significantly, young people are experimenting with drugs, alcohol, and tobacco at earlier ages.

> The younger use begins, the more likely the users are to have substance abuse problems later in life. More than 40% of those who started drinking at age 14 or younger developed alcohol dependence, compared with 10% of those who began drinking at age 20 or older. High school students who use illicit drugs are also more likely to experience difficulties in school, in their personal relationships, and in their mental and physical health. (Robert Wood Johnson Foundation, 2001).

Such findings resulted in the rapid growth of prevention programs whose aim is to postpone the age of initiation into drug use.

THEORIES OF ADDICTION

Research and clinical data reveal no single etiological factor that accounts for why some people become dependent on a substance and others do not. Some of the factors frequently cited are discussed below.

Biochemical and Genetic Factors

Studies on twins, half-siblings, and adopted children of alcoholics (Goodwin, 1984) as well as newer research on markers of inherited susceptibility (Begleiter & Kissen, 1995; Tabakoff et al., 1988) point to the presence of a genetic factor in the intergenerational transmission of alcoholism, especially in males, whereas neurochemical studies point to the importance of biochemical factors in narcotic and cocaine abuse (U.S. Department of Health and Human Services, 1991b).

Familial Factors

Studies of the backgrounds of people with alcoholism or opiate addictions in treatment indicate that they are more likely to have experienced early separation from one or both parents and tended to receive inadequate care during childhood (Kaufman, 1985). Many were physically or sexually abused during childhood (Roberts, Nishimoto, & Kirk, 2003) and/or grew up in families with high incidences of multigenerational abuse of alcohol or other drugs. Substance abuse also has been viewed as serving as an important stabilizing force in dysfunctional families (Alexander & Dibb, 1975; Steinglass, Weiner, & Mendelson, 1971).

Psychological Factors

Psychological explanations of substance abuse encompass various perspectives, including classical and modern psychoanalytic theory, developmental and personality theories, and behavioral, conditioning, and cognitive theories.

According to the classical psychoanalytic view, the individual uses a substance as a defense against unacceptable sexual and aggressive drives. In a letter to his friend Wilhelm Fleiss, Freud described addictions to "alcohol, morphine, tobacco, etc." as a "substitute and replacement" for the "primal addiction," masturbation (Freud, 1897/1954), and in his description of the case of Dr. Schreber, Freud (1911/1958) posited alcoholism as a defense against homosexuality. Other early psychoanalysts viewed alcoholism as the result of a fixation in and regression to the oral stage of development (Abraham, 1908/1979), as a response to underlying neurotic conflict between dependence and anger (Fenichel, 1945), and/or as a slow form of suicide (Menninger, 1938).

Modern psychoanalysts, focusing on object relations, ego, and self psychology theories, view the abuse of alcohol and other drugs as (1) an attempt to deal with poor ego development (Khantzian, 1981; Wurmser, 1978), (2) regression to or fixation at the stage of pathological narcissism (Kernberg, 1975), or (3) an effort to overcome a deficiency in the sense of self (Kohut, 1971, 1977; Levin, 1987). According to this view, alcohol and other drugs provide a "sense of internal homeostasis which substitutes for the basic lack of a sense of integration of self" (Kaufman, 1985, p. 14).

Other psychological perspectives view the abuse of alcohol and other drugs as:

- Attempts to "medicate" preexisting emotional problems, such as mood or anxiety disorders, as well as to cope with borderline, narcissistic, or antisocial personality disorders and psychosis (Khantzian, 1981; Waldinger, 1986).
- Efforts to diminish anxieties about self-assertion and to obliterate unacceptable feelings of anger and hostility (Kaufman, 1985).
- Ways of expressing unacceptable dependency needs (McCord & McCord, 1960).
- Efforts to compensate for feelings of inferiority or powerlessness (McClelland, Davis, Kalin, & Wanner, 1972).
- Ways of coping with situational stress (Peele, 1998).
- Related to personality characteristics such as novelty seeking, field dependence, low frustration tolerance, high impulsivity, or inability to endure anxiety or tension (Leonard & Blane, 1999; Vaillant, 1983).

According to learning and behavioral theories, substance abuse is a conditioned behavioral response that results from positive reinforcement following initial alcohol or other drug use. Although drug use originally may have been motivated by a desire for the pleasurable effects, the aversive consequence of taking a substance may be equally as reinforcing under certain environmental conditions (Littrell, 2001). Moreover, withdrawal signs could be conditioned to specific environmental cues. Expectancy, modeling, imitation, and identification also may play a role in substance abuse (Marlatt, Baer, Donovan, & Kivlahan, 1988).

Cognitive-behavioral theorists such as Albert Ellis (Ellis, McInterney, DiGiuseppe, & Yaeger, 1988) and Aaron Beck (Beck, Wright, Newman, & Liese, 1993) focus on the mental schemas or distorted cognitive beliefs about self and others. Such distorted or irrational beliefs make it difficult for the individual to respond appropriately to certain triggers; absence of the ability to respond appropriately, in turn, leads to a chain of negative behaviors and consequences including substance abuse.

Environmental and Sociocultural Factors

Numerous environmental, social, cultural, and economic factors have been linked to substance use and abuse, including the increasing availability of various substances; exposure opportunity (Wagner & Anthony, 2002), whereby young people who are using one substance, such as marijuana, are shown to be more likely to expose themselves to more harmful drugs; a paucity of alternatives to a meaningful life or source of income, particularly among minority populations in inner-city communities; the influence of peer groups and the mass media (Robert Wood Johnson Foundation, 2001); and social acceptance, even cultural idealization, of various substances (Kaufman, 1985).

Studies of female substance abusers, particularly those in lower socioeconomic classes, show a high correlation between substance abuse by women *and* their spouses or boyfriends, suggesting women's emotional as well as economic dependence on men as a factor in substance abuse (Straussner & Attia, 2002; Straussner, Kitman, Straussner, & Demos, 1980).

Multifactorial Perspective

Each theory of substance abuse has implications for both prevention and treatment; however, the etiology of alcohol and other drug abuse remains debatable. Most likely, substance abuse and dependence result from a combination of factors, including biochemical, genetic, familial, environmental, and cultural ones, as well as personality dynamics. Therefore, as pointed out by Pattison and Kaufman (1982), it may be best to view substance abuse as a multivariate syndrome, in which multiple patterns of dysfunctional substance abuse occur in various types of people with multiple prognoses requiring a variety of interventions.

PSYCHOPHARMACOLOGY

Every individual who takes a mind-altering substance in sufficient quantity will experience a physiological reaction or a state of intoxication. Moreover, many substances, if taken in large doses over a long period of time, lead to addiction or physiological dependence, regardless of the individual's predisposing characteristics. Thus it is important to understand the physiological impact of drugs on the human brain and body. Of the various ways of categorizing the numerous substances available today, the most useful classification is based on their effect on the central nervous system.

Central Nervous System Depressants

This category includes alcoholic beverages, barbiturates, and nonbarbiturate sedative–hypnotics (antianxiety and sleeping medications) such as Amytal, Luminal, Tuinal, Doriden, Quaalude, Placidyl, Noludar, Nembutal, and Seconal; benzodiazepines (minor tranquilizers) such as Miltown, Librium, Valium, Xanax, Ativan, Restoril, Tranxene, Dalmane, and Serax; anesthetics such as chloroform, ether, and nitrous oxide; volatile solvents such as toluene, xylene, and benzene; and low doses of cannabinoids such as marijuana and hashish. These drugs slow down, or sedate, the excitable brain tissues. Such sedation affects the brain centers that control speech, vision, coordination, and social judgment. The individual also experiences increased agitation and excitability when coming off these drugs—a withdrawal effect commonly known as a hangover.

Individuals under the influence of alcohol or other central nervous system (CNS) depressants are likely to have poor judgment, which is often manifested in inappropriate and even destructive behavior. Whereas low doses of a CNS depressant, particularly alcohol, block the usual inhibitions, making the person appear to be relaxed or unreserved, high doses slow down the heart rate and respiration, produce lethargy and stupor, and may result in death. Numerous descriptions of deaths among young people resulting from ingestion of massive amounts of alcohol in short periods of time have been reported in the popular press.

Another dangerous situation arises from the potentiating effect of combining two or more substances within this category. Thus a combination of alcohol with Valium or any other sedative–hypnotic is a common cause of purposeful or accidental overdose, particularly among women (Straussner et al., 1980).

Central Nervous System Stimulants

This category includes amphetamines and methamphetamine (known variously as Speed, Ice, Chalk, Meth, Crystal Crank, Fire, Glass), cocaine and crack, prescription drugs such as Dexedrine and Ritalin, and caffeine and nicotine. In varying degrees, these drugs increase or speed up the function of excitable brain tissues, resulting in energized muscles, increased heart rate and blood pressure, and decreased appetite.

Low doses of amphetamines are commonly used by people wishing to stay awake, such as students and truck drivers; however, when coming off these drugs, users experience exhaustion and "crash" or fall asleep. Large doses of such stimulants as amphetamines and cocaine can produce acute delirium and psychosis. At times, the psychotic symptoms can be difficult to distinguish from schizophrenia and may include hallucinations, paranoia, and hypersexuality. The abuse of cocaine also may lead to a variety of other toxic effects, including severe feelings of depression and sudden heart attacks. Suicidal and violent behavior under the influence of amphetamines and the more potent forms of cocaine, such as crack, have been noted by researchers and clinicians (Wetli, 1987).

Narcotics or Opiates

These drugs decrease pain by binding to specific receptors in the brain. This category includes opium and its derivatives, such as morphine, heroin, codeine, and paragoric, as well as synthetic drugs such as methadone (Dolophine), Demerol, Darvon, Prinadol, Lomotil, Talwin, Percodan, Percocet, OxyContin, and Vicodin, which tend to serve as narcotic analgesics.

The use of opiates generally tends to have a sedative and tranquilizing effect. However, unlike the users of sedative substances, narcotic users do not usually experience poor motor coordination or loss of consciousness. The opiate-using individual is likely to experience a state of stuporous inactivity and dwell in daydreaming fantasies. Due to the physical agitation caused by withdrawal and the psychological panic related to anticipation of withdrawal symptoms, antisocial behaviors may occur during drug-seeking behavior or actual withdrawal.

Psychedelics/Hallucinogens

These drugs produce gross distortions of thinking and sensory processes, thereby inducing a psychosis-like state that often includes visual hallucinations. Included in this category are the "alphabet drugs," such as LSD, PCP, DOM, or STP, mescaline, psilocybin, and large or highly potent doses of cannabinoids or marijuana.

Psychedelics are less physiologically addictive than other substances; however, they may precipitate psychosis in vulnerable individuals. They also result in feelings of extreme anxiety and misperception of reality, particularly for users of phencyclidine (PCP, also known as "angel dust"), who frequently experience distorted body image, depersonalization, depression, and hostility that may be expressed through violence (Waldinger, 1986).

It is important to note that the marijuana used today is much more potent than that used during the 1960s and 1970s. Frequent use of marijuana by adolescents and young adults has been correlated with the development of the so-called amotivational syndrome, characterized by passivity and lack of ambition leading to poor school and work performance and personality deterioration (Alexander, 2003).

Designer and Club Drugs

Also commonly used by young people are the so-called designer, or lookalike, drugs, such as MPTP and China White, which are synthesized in clandestine laboratories and resemble highly potent doses of amphetamines or narcotics in their impact. Currently, one of the most widely used club drugs is MDMA or Ecstasy (also known as XTC, X, Adam, or Lover's Speed). Other club drugs include GHB (Grievous Bodily Harm, G, Liquid Ecstasy, Georgia Home Boy), Rohypnol (Roofies, Rophies, Roche, Forget-me Pill), and Ketamine (Special K, K, Vitamin K, Cat Valiums).

The chemicals found in club drugs vary widely, depending on manufacturing sources. Such contaminants have resulted in negative physical and psychological reactions in some young people. Moreover, since these substances tend to be colorless, tasteless, and odorless, there have been numerous reports of club drugs, particularly Rohypnol, being added unknowingly to beverages of individuals who then become victims of sexual assaults (see *www.clubdrugs.org* for a fuller discussion).

Combinations of Drugs

Various combinations of drugs—such as heroin and cocaine (commonly referred to as *speedball*), cocaine and alcohol or marijuana, cocaine and PCP, methadone and alcohol or cocaine, tranquilizers and alcohol, and so forth—are frequently used to counteract the side effects of any one drug or to synergistically increase the impact of the drugs.

As can be seen from the above discussion, the various substances have a differential impact on a person's mood and behavior, regardless of his or her premorbid personality. Thus familiarity with the impact of the various substances on behavior and thinking processes is a crucial aspect of clinical assessment and treatment.

CLINICAL INTERVENTIONS

Although fewer than one-fourth of those individuals who need help for their substance abuse or dependence ever get treatment, those who do obtain treatment do get better (Robert Wood Johnson Foundation, 2001). According to Horgan, "The improvement rate for people completing substance abuse treatment is comparable to that of people treated for asthma and other chronic, relapsing health conditions" (1995, p. 3).

Clinical interventions with substance abusers, as with all clients, begins with a comprehensive assessment followed by appropriate intervention approaches that include some or all of the following:

- Identifying the kinds of substances being abused and the degree of physical and psychological dependence.
- Assessing the degree to which these substances interfere with daily life.
- Identifying appropriate community resources.
- Motivating the abuser to obtain appropriate treatment.
- Helping the abuser achieve recovery.
- Monitoring ongoing recovery.
- Helping family members and significant others understand substance abuse and its impact on them.

Screening and Assessment

Screening attempts to identify people whose substance abuse problems are not clearly evident, whereas *assessment* is undertaken once a problem is more apparent. Assessment is an ongoing, interactive process comprised of several important tasks, including (1) determining a formal diagnosis, (2) ascertaining the severity and impact of substance abuse on the user and those around him or her, (3) establishing a baseline of the patient's condition for future comparison, (4) providing a guide to treatment planning and the patient's progress in treatment, and (5) evaluating the impact of environmental influences and appropriate preventive efforts. A comprehensive assessment may include a medical examination, clinical interviews, collateral information, and data obtained through a variety of formal instruments (U.S. Department of Health and Human Services, 1991a).

The first task in screening and assessing people who abuse drugs or alcohol is to avoid stereotyping them. As noted, there are tremendous variations in the background and characteristics of substance abusers, in the kinds of substances being abused, and in the impact of these chemicals on the users and their significant others. Nonetheless, there are certain characteristics and behavioral patterns that *are* common to many substance abusers and provide basic assessment clues.

All clients whose behavior is highly volatile and unpredictable or whose history indicates interpersonal, occupational, financial, and/or legal problems should be questioned about possible substance abuse. Whereas some individuals may readily admit to their substance abuse, others may not. It is often helpful to obtain factual information from family members or other relevant sources, to conduct urine or other screenings, as well as to rely on behavioral clues such as a runny nose, the wearing of long sleeves in the summer to cover up needle marks, or the smell of alcohol on the breath (especially, early in the day).

Due to the biopsychosocial impact of substance abuse, alcohol and other drug abusers tend to rely excessively on such defense mechanisms as denial, projection, and rationalization (Griffin, 1991). Because defense mechanisms are unconscious, substance abusers are often unaware of the full impact of the substance abuse on their lives. Thus it is up to the worker to ask the "right" questions in order to form an appropriate assessment.

Given that most people in this society drink, it is less threatening to start with questions about alcohol consumption before gathering data about illicit drugs. It is also important to obtain information about the onset of substance use. Clinically, it is helpful to conceptualize the person as developmentally arrested at the age at which the substance abuse (not just use) first began, regardless of current chronological age, because there are profound developmental differences between an individual who started abusing alcohol and/or smoking marijuana heavily at age 13 and one who did so at age 23.

The following set of questions can be used as part of an initial assessment (Straussner, 1989):

1. "What do you usually drink?"
2. "How much do you drink a day/week?"
3. "How old were you when you had your first drink?"
4. "How old were you when you started drinking on a regular basis?"
5. "Are you now drinking more/less than a year ago [testing for increase/decrease in tolerance]?"
6. "Have you ever used [insert a–j]? How much? How often? When did you start? Date of last use? Source of supply? Method of use [i.e., smoking, injecting, etc.]?"
   a. marijuana
   b. heroin
   c. methadone
   d. cocaine/crack
   e. amphetamines/uppers
   f. sleeping medication (what kind?)
   g. tranquilizers/downers (what kind?)
   h. club drugs (what kind?)
   i. other medication/drugs obtained from family/friends or on the street
   j. other medication/drugs obtained from a doctor

7. "Have you ever tried to stop your alcohol/drug use? What happened?"
8. "Have you ever been in treatment for substance abuse? Where? When? For how long? What happened?"
9. "Have you ever attended an AA or NA meeting (or any other self-help group)? How did you feel there?"
10. "Does/did your mother/father drink too much?"

11. "Does/did your mother/father use drugs? What kind?"
12. "Does your spouse/boyfriend/girlfriend drink a lot/use drugs? What kind?"
13. "Has anyone ever complained about your use of alcohol/drugs?"
14. "Have you ever been in any kind of legal trouble because of your use of alcohol/drugs?"
15. "Do you think that you have a problem with drugs/alcohol?"

Answers to the above questions can provide a rough assessment of substance abuse. A growing number of clinicians is also using standardized screening and assessment instruments (King & Bordnick, 2002). Among the most frequently used instruments are various versions of the CAGE for assessing alcohol problems, and the CAGE-AID (which also includes other drugs; Brown & Rounds, 1995; Mayfield, McLeod, & Hall, 1974), the SASSI (Substance Abuse Subtle Screening Inventory; Miller, 1997), the MAST (Michigan Alcohol Screening Test; Selzer, 1971), the AUDIT (Alcohol Use Disorders Identification Test; Babor et al., 1992), the DAST (Drug Abuse Screening Test; Maisto, Carey, Carey, Gordon, & Gleason, 2000; Skinner, 1982), the CRAFT (for assessing adolescents; Knight et al., 1999), and the ASI (Addiction Severity Instrument; McLellan et al., 1992).

It is crucial that all assessment questions be asked in a nonjudgmental manner. The clinician needs to remember that once individuals start abusing substances such as alcohol, opiates, or cocaine, they often become addicted to them. They cannot just stop using the drug or drugs through willpower alone. They should not be condemned or made to feel guilty for their dependence on a chemical any more than a client would be condemned for having an uncontrolled medical condition. It is also essential for the clinician to be attuned to perceiving the severe feelings of worthlessness and self-hate and the expectations of scorn and rejection that often lie beneath the grandiose self-presentation of many substance abusers.

Also important in assessment is the differential biopsychosocial effects of various substances. The use of an illicit substance such as crack, with its 30-second high and immediately recurring craving, will have different emotional, legal, financial, and social sequelae than the drinking of a legally obtained bottle of Scotch (Straussner, 1994).

Lastly, it is important to be cognizant of the fact that substance abuse is a "family disease" (Straussner, Weinstein, & Hernandez, 1979)—that although a client may not be the one who abuses alcohol or other drugs, he or she may be the spouse or child of a substance abuser and thus a part of a substance-abusing family system. Assessing the impact of familial substance abuse on mental health and daily functioning is an important intervention with all clients, regardless of their presenting problems.

Clinicians unsure about their assessment regarding substance abuse should refer the client to an appropriate community agency, such as the local alcoholism council or a substance abuse clinic. Just as clinicians may refer a client to a physician for an assessment of a possible physical problem, they need to feel comfortable making referrals for assessment of a substance abuse problem. It is a proper professional response for a worker in a non-substance-abuse setting to tell a client that "I am concerned about your use of _____ (alcohol, drugs, etc.) and want you to go to _____ for an evaluation [or checkup]" or "Although I believe you when you tell me that you do not have a problem with drugs/alcohol, it is still important for you to go to _____ for an evaluation before we can make any further plans regarding your treatment."

An important assessment area is differentiating between substance abuse and other psychopathology. Individuals with a diagnosis of "substance use disorder" also may be diagnosed with a comorbid major psychiatric (Axis I on DSM-IV-TR) condition and/or have an underlying personality disorder (Axis II), necessitating a comprehensive psychiatric assessment in addition to assessment of their substance abuse. (For further discussion of dual diagnoses, see Orlin, O'Neill, & Davis, Chapter 5, and Goldstein, Chapter 17, this volume).

Motivation for Treatment

A comprehensive assessment must include an exploration of the client's motivation for treatment. As a rule, substance abusers do not enter treatment voluntarily. Due to the effects of alcohol and other drugs on the brain and the extensive use of denial and other defenses, substance abusers usually need to be pushed into treatment. Although a highly motivated client is generally more likely to make better use of treatment, recovery from substance abuse is not always dependent upon whether or not the initial contact with treatment was voluntary. In fact, studies show that some individuals who are coerced into treatment may have an even better recovery rate than those who enter voluntarily (Lawental, McLellan, Grissom, Brill, & O'Brien, 1996; Mark, 1988).

The use of coercion in the form of instrumental (e.g., legal authority) or affective authority (e.g., loving family members) to get a substance abuser into treatment has been found to be of value to individuals of all socioeconomic levels and ethnic backgrounds. It is the basis for the use of the family intervention approach (see McIntyre, Chapter 11, this volume), for student (Griffin & Svendsen, 1986) and employee assistance programs (Trice & Beyer, 1984), for drunk-driving programs, and for various legal and professional diversion programs, such as those for impaired physicians and lawyers. Although the use of coercion does raise some ethical dilemmas, it is important to keep in mind that individuals who are addicted to a substance are unable to exercise freedom of choice in their decision-making process (King, 1986). At the same time, it is essential to note the growing literature describing the use of the more supportive, motivational interviewing approaches.

Miller and Rollnick's (1991) five principles of motivational interviewing provide a useful framework that helps motivate clients to move from one stage of change to another. The five general principles are (1) expressing empathy, (2) developing discrepancy, (3) avoiding argumentation, (4) rolling with resistance, and (5) supporting self-efficacy. The goal of motivational interviewing is to ignite motivation for change, despite the fact that a client may enter treatment due to external pressures. It is the job of the clinician to provide feedback to the client that illustrates the discrepancy between his or her ability to achieve the desired goals and the client's continuing use of substances. To be effective, such feedback must be given within an emphatic environment that avoids argumentation or direct confrontation of resistance, and one that supports self-efficacy (i.e., the client's belief in his or her own ability to make changes; Straussner & Attia, 2001).

TREATMENT FACILITIES AND APPROACHES

An important task for social workers is to determine appropriate forms of treatment for clients with substance abuse problems. Workers need to be aware of the various treatment options available for these clients in their community. The most important of these are discussed in the following sections.

Detoxification

Detoxification is the first step in the treatment of patients who are physically addicted to opioids, alcohol, barbiturates or other sedative–hypnotics, and amphetamines. It is not required for cocaine/crack abusers or for marijuana smokers. Physical dependence or addiction is defined primarily by signs of withdrawal: the presence of symptoms that appear when the intake of a given substance is terminated. Frequently, these symptoms are the opposite of the signs of acute intoxication. The withdrawal symptoms from stimulants such as amphetamines include severe depression; symptoms of withdrawal from sedative–hypnotics such as alcohol, which occur 6–48 hours after cessation of alcohol consumption, may include sweating, anxiety, and agitation. Alcohol withdrawal abates after 2–5 days; however, it may be complicated by grand mal seizures and progress to delirium (known as delirium tremens, or DTs).

Although withdrawal from opiates has been given much publicity, it is not life threatening, as it can be from severe alcohol, Xanax, or barbiturate addiction. Opiate withdrawal has been compared to "a one-week bout with influenza" (Waldinger, 1986, p. 315).

Traditionally, detoxification has been conducted on medical or psychiatric inpatient units to allow for careful monitoring of physical status and to prevent potentially lethal withdrawal reactions. Inpatient detoxification treatment also increases the likelihood that the patient will undergo a comprehensive assessment and develop a greater acceptance of further treatment. Managed care has promoted an increasing use of detoxification that is provided in outpatient settings or by physicians in private practice. Heroin addicts can be detoxified on an outpatient basis with the help of chemicals such as clonodine or decreasing doses of methadone.

Rehabilitation Treatment Programs

Detoxification is usually only the beginning of a long and difficult course of recovery. When substance abusers give up their chemicals, they may experience a prolonged period of physiological and psychological withdrawal. Moreover, the lives of many substance abusers revolve around the process of obtaining drugs or alcohol; this focus provides a daily routine as well as relationships with other substance abusers, both of which must be replaced if the individual is to maintain a drug-free existence. Furthermore, since substance abusers often medicate unpleasant feelings such as anxiety or depression, these feelings are likely to surface or worsen when the substance is removed.

To address these challenges, short- and long-term inpatient and outpatient rehabilitation programs and drug-free residential therapeutic communities are invaluable. In these structured settings, substance abusers can examine the impact of alcohol and/or other drugs on their lives, their ability to relate to other people, and the necessary changes they must make in their lifestyle if they want to recover from substance abuse. Although cocaine and crack users do not require detoxification, they do require ongoing outpatient counseling and, at times, antidepressants or other medications. Currently, much of the treatment is provided via intensive outpatient rehabilitation programs.

Also available in some communities are day treatment programs and part-time residential facilities such as halfway and quarter-way houses and substance-free housing. Such programs and facilities are of particular value to those who have limited social and vocational supports, such as a young-adult crack or heroin addict or an older person with alcoholism.

The Use of Chemical and Nonchemical Substitutes: Methadone, Naltrexone, Antabuse, Buprenorphine, and Acupuncture

The utilization of methadone maintenance programs as a substitute for narcotics can lead to better prognosis for rehabilitation and allow narcotic addicts to avail themselves of such services as individual or group counseling and educational or vocational training; it can also help them improve the overall quality of their lives once the daily concern about obtaining drugs is alleviated. Moreover, the potential for becoming infected with HIV is an important factor in referring intravenous narcotic users clients to methadone maintenance programs (Friedman & Wilson, Chapter 9, this volume). However, it is crucial to note that methadone is more addictive and more difficult to withdraw from than heroin, and that methadone maintenance programs vary greatly in their provision of supportive and social services. Therefore, it is important to help clients determine whether a particular program is likely to be effective in meeting their needs.

Although less extensively used than methadone, opioid antagonists such as naltrexone, which prevent addicts from experiencing the effects of narcotics, have been utilized by a growing number of treatment facilities. Unlike methadone, naltrexone has no narcotic effect of its own and is not physiologically addictive. Under the brand name of ReVia, it also is being used for people with alcohol dependence. Other medications, such as Acamprosate (for alcohol dependence) and buprenorphine (for opioid dependence), have increased in popularity (Erickson & Wilcox, 2001).

A chemical that is sometimes used to help alcoholics is disulfiram, commonly known as Antabuse. It is a medication that blocks the normal oxidation of alcohol so that acetaldehyde, a by-product of alcohol, accumulates in the bloodstream and causes unpleasant, and at times even life-threatening, symptoms, such as rapid pulse and vomiting. These distressing symptoms serve as a conscious deterrent to drinking while the person is using Antabuse.

The value of long-term utilization of any one of these chemical substitutes is still a matter of debate. By and large, they should be viewed as useful adjuncts to other forms of treatment, but not as a total treatment by themselves.

A number of substance abuse settings have incorporated acupuncture treatment into the withdrawal process and the early phase of rehabilitation treatment. Other commonly used nontraditional treatment supplements include yoga and meditation.

Outpatient Individual Therapy or Counseling

Generally, outpatient psychodynamically oriented individual psychotherapy is not recommended until the person is secure in his or her abstinence from chemicals, because the anxiety aroused during treatment may lead to the resumption of alcohol or drug use. Moreover, conducting individual counseling or therapy with an active substance abuser is questionable, due to the impact of the chemicals on the brain and the possibility of blackouts (i.e., memory loss while intoxicated). However, if a client has stopped using substances or is making serious efforts to diminish their drug and alcohol use, ego-supportive counseling (Goldstein, 1995) or a self psychological approach (Levin, 1987) can be particularly useful.

Because chronic substance abusers usually substitute a chemical for human contact, a crucial part of treatment is the establishment of a nonthreatening relationship with a caring and consistently reliable individual. The goal of individual treatment is to enhance patients' self-image and provide needed ego support so that they can begin to examine their use of chemicals and their current feelings and behavior.

The view of substance abuse as a disease is invaluable in helping drug and alcohol abusers to alleviate frequently extreme feelings of guilt without absolving them from responsibility for their future behavior. This perspective also diminishes the usually negative countertransference reactions of workers.

Motivational interviewing, mentioned earlier, is both an interviewing technique and a treatment approach (Miller, 1999; Miller & Rollnick, 1991). The client's motivation for change is assessed and encouraged, while the therapist builds a strong and trusting relationship. Stage of change theory (Prochaska, DiClemente, & Norcross, 1992) can guide the clinician in assessing a client's current level of awareness regarding his or her problem. The stages of change include precontemplation, contemplation, determination, action, and maintenance. Relapse can occur at any stage in the process. This perspective has been found effective in keeping clients in treatment and supporting his or her efforts toward recovery (see Hanson & El-Bassel, Chapter 2, this volume).

Another alternative to the mainstream addictive/disease approach is solution-focused therapy. Specific techniques might involve (1) asking for exceptions to the problem ("When is the last period of time you were not drinking? What was different about that time?"), (2) use of scaling questions ("On a scale of 1–10, with 10 being the most motivated, where would you rate your motivation to change your marijuana use patterns?"), and (3) use of coping questions ("How did you manage to get your children dressed and to school yesterday, after all you've told me about your difficulties?"). This approach focuses on the client's strengths and past successes in dealing with problems and on the acceptance of the client's definition of the problem and immediate goals (see Berg & Shafer, Chapter 4, this volume, for a fuller discussion).

Group Interventions

Group counseling and group activities appear to be the treatment of choice for many substance abusers. Group therapy with fellow recovering substance abusers provides helpful peer interaction and support as well as useful confrontations of substance-abusing patients with the consequences of their attitudes and behavior (Straussner, 1997). The value of separate groups for substance-abusing women has been noted by many clinicians (Beyer & Carnabucci, 2002).

Activity groups focused around cooking, program planning, sports, art, and so forth, allow for social interaction, the development of a variety of essential life skills, and sublimation of self- and other-destructive feelings (Brandler & Roman, 1999). Psychodrama groups are particularly helpful for patients because they provide a forum in which repressed feelings can be concretized and expressed and "unfinished business" resolved (Buchbinder, 1986).

Self-help "12-step" programs, such as Alcoholics Anonymous (AA), Narcotics Anonymous (NA), Pills Anonymous (PA), and Cocaine Anonymous (CA), have proven to be particularly helpful and are free and available in every community. These groups provide continuously available support and help to replace drinking and drugging companions with a new group of peers with whom the substance abuser can identify. Self-help groups allow members not only to receive help but also to give help to others, thereby enhancing self-esteem (Straussner & Spiegel, 1996; see also Spiegel & Fewell, Chapter 6, this volume).

It is strongly recommended that all clinicians attend a few "open" meetings of the various self-help groups, especially AA. At times, it may be helpful to escort a substance-abusing patient to a meeting or to encourage the client to call, in the presence of the worker, the main number of the self-help group and ask for help. Workers also can request a 12-step group to conduct an institutional meeting for clients at the worker's agency.

In addition to 12-step groups, other self-help groups for substance abusers can be utilized when appropriate; these include Women for Sobriety, Rational Recovery, SMART groups, Social Workers Helping Social Workers, and Double Trouble/Recovery groups for those with dual diagnoses.

Psychoeducational Approaches

Didactic education is an effective strategy in the treatment of substance abuse. Lectures and discussion on such topics as the signs and symptoms of substance abuse and addiction, the addiction cycle for specific substances (such as cocaine, with its euphoric binges and depressive crashes), relapse prevention, the impact of substance abuse on the family, effective communication skills, coping with stress, human sexuality, and assertiveness training provide cognitive, non-ego-threatening understanding of the dynamics of substance abuse and practical information about how the individual and the family can help themselves. Such a psychoeducational approach also can be provided in settings that are not specifically connected to substance abuse treatment and can include individual, group, or family treatment modalities.

Social Supports

Substance-abusing patients usually experience various social problems. Thus the provision of financial and social supports—including adequate housing, vocational rehabilitation programs, and legal assistance—is an essential aspect of helping this population.

STAGES OF TREATMENT

As is the case with any other client population, treatment of clients with substance-abuse problems is an ongoing process that can be conceptualized as having a beginning, a middle or working phase, and an ending or termination stage.

The beginning phase consists of assessing current substance use, focusing on the steps needed to achieve abstinence, and establishing a working relationship. Like all people, these clients need acceptance and support. As pointed out by Washton (1991), the strong confrontational style that has been institutionalized and traditionally encouraged in the addiction treatment field tends to drive away the less motivated patient. Treatment studies show that although "patient characteristics did not differentiate between dropouts and treatment completers, clinicians with high dropout rates were characteristically more aggressive, controlling and critical while those with low dropouts tended to be more introspective, accepting and nurturing" (p. 8).

In addition to acceptance and nurturing, clinicians treating substance abusers may need to "lend their ego" to these clients, whose judgment and reality testing have been impaired by the use of chemicals as well as dysfunctional maturation. Direct advice giving and limit setting may be crucial during this stage, as is the use of collaterals, such as family members or friends, to obtain information and to provide emotional and economic support for the client.

An important aspect of the beginning phase of treatment is educating clients about the psychophysiological impact of various substances so that they can, for example, differentiate between a depression caused by withdrawal from a stimulant and one due to unexpressed rage at a loved one. Workers also need to help clients make proper use of self-help groups, because these groups can provide advice and support between sessions and/or upon termination of treatment. The beginning stage of treatment also may require extensive interdisciplinary collaborations and referrals. Finally, the worker must pay close attention to the use of self and transferential and countertransferential reactions. Interventions should be guided by clients' needs and abilities, not by workers' needs to rescue clients or by their anger at clients for not living up to workers' expectations.

Once a client is able to achieve abstinence, the work, with the same or a different clinician, moves into middle phase of treatment. During this stage issues such as unresolved grief over loss of loved ones, depression, guilt, shame, psychological mourning for the lost substance, and a sense of loss over wasted years need to be addressed (Brown, 1985). For some, the middle phase may involve dealing with early life traumas, including physical and sexual abuse; confusion about sexuality and role identity; examining and modifying dysfunctional patterns of defense and coping mechanisms; and improving interpersonal relationships. During this phase, clients need to learn how to both accept and prevent slips (relapse prevention; see Gray & Gibson, Chapter 7, this volume), as well as how to develop the ego function of adoptive regression—that is, how to relax, play, and have fun without alcohol or other drugs. Lastly, they need help in learning how to forgive themselves and others.

The final phase of treatment, the process of termination, may require helping patients cope with the separation and loss of the treatment relationship without regressing to the use of substances.

SPECIAL TREATMENT ISSUES AND SPECIAL POPULATIONS

Space limitations preclude a comprehensive discussion of the numerous treatment issues and the unique treatment needs of various substance-abusing populations. For example, clinicians need to take into account the life-cycle stages of clients (Carter & McGoldrick, 1999) and to realize that both assessment and intervention with an alcohol-abusing 17-year-old male will differ from that with a 67-year-old alcohol-abusing man (see Freshman, Chapter 14, and Farkas, Chapter 15, this volume). The issue of gender also has to be addressed differentially (see Pape, Chapter 16, this volume), as does that of patients with dual disorders (see Orlin, O'Neill, and Davis, Chapter 5, this volume).

Treatment of minorities, particularly African American clients, needs to take into account that "to survive in a brutalizing, inhospitable world, minorities have a higher tolerance for emotional pain. So they become an enabling community that tolerates addiction" (O'Connell, 1991, p. 13). Minorities are more likely to enter treatment through the courts than through formal intervention processes or 12-step programs, and they are more likely to access treatment much later and thus have a more difficult recovery process (O'Connell, 1991).

Ethnocultural norms and values need to be taken into account in treatment planning and relapse prevention with each client (see Straussner, 2001a), as do issues of sexual identity and sexual behavior, including the need for safe sex. The special needs of substance-abusing gay and lesbian clients need to be addressed (see Senreich & Vairo, Chapter 18, this volume). Lastly, we need to remember that substance abuse, "like many other medical problems, is a chronic disorder in which recurrences are common and repeated periods of treatment are frequently required" (U.S. Department of Health and Human Services, 1991b, p. 4).

IMPACT OF SUBSTANCE ABUSE ON THE FAMILY

Life with a substance-abusing family member is typically full of inconsistency and unpredictability, resulting in a chronic state of crisis. Legal and financial problems, serious illnesses, and various accidents are common occurrences that intrude on family life. When the substance abuser is a parent, dysfunctional cross-generational alliance and role reversal (i.e., children assume parental roles and responsibilities) are frequently seen (Straussner, 1994). Child neglect and, in more disturbed families, violence between parents, child abuse, and incest are some of the consequences and correlates of substance abuse; indeed, substance abuse is present in at least two-thirds of the families known to public child welfare agencies (Hampton, Senatore, & Gullotta, 1998). Studies highlight the need to address the intergenerational cycle of substance abuse and child abuse if effective progress is to be made on either problem.

The impact of substance abuse on the family has additional intergenerational repercussions: The sons of alcoholic fathers are four times more likely to become alcoholics, and the daughters of alcoholic parents are three times more likely to become alcoholics. Moreover, the daughters of alcoholic fathers are also more likely to marry alcoholic men (Straussner, 1985). Intergenerational repercussions also exist for families with parental opiate and other drug addiction.

Intervention with Family Members

Couple and family therapy, including multifamily groups (Kaufman, 1985), are effective treatment modalities for families with substance abusers who are already chemically free or are working on their recovery. A research-based, family-oriented treatment approach called CRAFT—Community Reinforcement and Family Training (Miller, Meyers, & Tonigan, 1999)—involves the following eight components:

1. Increasing family members' own motivation to change via the use of such techniques as questioning them about how their lives have changed for the worse due to the addicted member's substance abuse.
2. Teaching communications skills that allow the nonusing member

to give nonantagonistic feedback and encouragement to the substance abuser.

3. Increasing the couple's/family's positive interactions.
4. Focusing on the nonreinforcement of drug use by teaching the family member to ignore the addict when he or she is using.
5. Initiating activities that interfere and compete with addicted member's substance use.
6. Developing outside activities and reinforcement for the addicted person.
7. Making plans for escaping possibly dangerous situations, such as those with potential for violence.
8. Helping family members plan to introduce the idea of treatment at the right moment.

It is also beneficial to refer family members to self-help groups such as Al-Anon, Pill-Anon, Co-Anon, or Nar-Anon. These groups help adult family members examine their own role in "enabling" or perpetuating the behavior of the addicted person (Levinson & Straussner, 1978) and obtain support from others in the same circumstances. These groups are particularly useful for parents and spouses of substance abusers.

Adolescent children of alcohol- and narcotic-abusing parents may benefit from self-help groups such as Alateen and Narateen. Adult Children of Alcoholics (ACOA) groups are extremely helpful for mature adolescents and adult children of alcoholics, as are the Codependency Anonymous (CODA) groups that help people identify and work on their unmet dependency needs.

Intervention with latency-aged and adolescent children of substance abusers must focus not only on how to say "no" to their own substance use and abuse but also on helping the children recognize and understand familial substance abuse and its impact on them and other family members. Extensive literature, written specifically for children and adolescents, can be obtained from Al-Anon and Nar-Anon and is extremely valuable in helping children begin to understand what has happened to them and, hopefully, preventing the pattern from repeating itself in the next generation.

Clinicians also must be aware of their own countertransferential reactions to families of substance abusers, particularly in view of the fact that many in the helping professions are themselves affected by familial substance abuse (Straussner, 1987).

CONCLUSION

Helping substance-abusing clients and their families is a difficult, challenging, yet highly rewarding task. It is a task that requires a variety of treatment modalities and intervention approaches and calls upon the worker to be an astute diagnostician, a therapist, educator, advocate, and educated consumer of never-ending research data. Most of all, it requires a clinician who is sensitive to the impact of substance abuse on these individuals and those close to them, who can appreciate the strengths and the courage that these clients present, and who can provide hope for a better tomorrow.

REFERENCES

Abraham, K. (1979). The psychological relations between sexuality and alcoholism. In *Selected papers on psychoanalysis* (pp. 80–89). New York: Brunner/Mazel. (Original work published 1908).

Alexander, B. K., & Dibb, G. S. (1975). Opiate addicts and their parents. *Family Process, 14*, 499–514.

Alexander, D. (2003). A review of marijuana assessment dilemmas: Time for marijuana specific screening methods? *Journal of Social Work Practice in the Addictions, 3*(4), 5–28.

American Psychiatric Association. (2000). *Diagnostic and statistical manual of mental disorders* (4th ed., text rev.). Washington, DC: Author.

Azmitia, E. C. (2001). Impact of drugs and alcohol on the brain through the life cycle: Knowledge for social workers. *Journal of Social Work Practice in the Addictions, 1*(3), 41–63.

Babor, T. F, de la Fuente, J. R., Saunders, J., & Grant, M. (1992). *AUDIT: The Alcohol Use Disorders Identification Tests: Guidelines for use in primary health care.* Geneva, Switzerland: World Health Organization.

Beck, A. T., Wright, F. D., Newman, C. F., & Liese, B. S. (1993). *Cognitive therapy of substance abuse.* New York: Guilford Press.

Begleiter, H., & Kissen, B. (Eds.). (1995). *The genetics of alcoholism.* New York: Oxford University Press.

Beyer, E. P., & Carnabucci, K. (2002). Group treatment of substance-abusing women. In S. L. A. Straussner & S. Brown (Eds.), *The handbook of addiction treatment for women* (pp. 515–538). San Francisco: Jossey-Bass.

Brandler, S., & Roman, C. P. (1999). *Group work: Skills and strategies for effective interventions* (2nd ed.). New York: Haworth Press.

Brown, R. L., & Rounds, L. A. (1995). Conjoint screening questionnaires for alcohol and drug abuse. *Wisconsin Medical Journal, 94*, 135–140.

Brown, S. (1985). *Treating the alcoholic: A developmental model of recovery.* New York: Wiley.

Buchbinder, J. (1986). Gestalt therapy and its application to alcoholism treatment. *Alcoholism Treatment Quarterly, 13*(2), 49–67.

Carter, E. A., & McGoldrick, M. (1999). *The expanded family life cycle: Individual, family, and social perspectives* (3rd ed.). Boston: Allyn & Bacon.

Day, D. (1999). *Health emergency 1999: The spread of drug related AIDS and other deadly diseases among African Americans and Latinos.* Princeton, NJ: Dogwood Center.

Ellis, A., McInterney, J. F., DiGiuseppe, R., & Yeager, R. J. (1988). *Rational emotive therapy with alcoholics and substance abusers.* New York: Pergamon Press.

Erickson, C. K., & Wilcox, R. E. (2001). Neurobiological causes of addictions. *Journal of Social Work Practice in the Addictions, 1*(3), 7–22.

Fenichel, O. (1945). *The psychoanalytic theory of neurosis.* New York: Norton.

Freud, S. (1954). Letter 79, December 22, 1897. In M. Bonaparte, A. Freud, & E. Kris (Eds.) and E. Mosbacher & J. Strachey (Trans.), *The origins of psycho-analysis: Letters to Wilhelm Fliess, drafts and notes: 1887–1902.* London: Imago. (Original work published 1897)

Freud, S. (1958). Psycho-analytic notes on an autobiographical account of a case of paranoia. In K. Strachey (Ed. & Trans.), *The standard edition of the complete psychological works of Sigmund Freud* (Vol. 12, pp. 1–82). London: Hogarth Press. (Original work published 1911)

Goldstein, E. G. (1995). *Ego psychology and social work practice* (2nd ed). New York: Free Press.

Goodwin, D. W. (1984). Studies of familial alcoholism: A review. *Journal of Clinical Psychiatry, 45*(2), 14–17.

Grant, B., Harford, T. C., Deborah, A., Dawson, D. A., Chou, P., Dufour, M., & Pickering, R. (1994). Epidemiologic Bulletin No. 35: Prevalence of DSM-IV alcohol abuse and dependence, United States 1992. *Alcohol Health and Research World, 18*(3), 243–248.

Griffin, R. E. (1991). Assessing the drug-involved client. *Families in Society: Journal of Contemporary Human Services, 72*(2), 87–94.

Griffin, T., & Svendsen, R. (1986). *Student assistance program.* Minneapolis, MN: Hazelden Foundation.

Gustavsson, N.S., & MacEachron, A. E. (1997). Criminalizing women's behavior. *Journal of Drug Issues, 27,* 673–687.

Hampton, R. L., Senatore, V., & Gullotta, T. P. (1998). *Substance abuse, family violence, and child welfare: Bridging perspectives.* Thousand Oaks, CA: Sage.

Horgan, C. M. (1995, Spring). Cost of untreated substance abuse to society. *The Communique.* Rockville, MD: Center for Substance Abuse Treatment.

Jellinek, E. M. (1952). Phases of alcohol addiction. *Quarterly Journal of Studies on Alcohol, 13,* 673–684.

Johnston, L., O'Malley, P., & Bachman, J. (1988). *Illicit drug use, smoking and drinking by America's high school students, college students and young adults: 1975–1987.* Rockville, MD: National Institute on Drug Abuse.

Kaufman, E. (1985). *Substance abuse and family therapy.* New York: Grune & Stratton.

Kernberg, O. (1975). *Borderline conditions and pathological narcissism.* New York: Aronson.

Khantzian, E. J. (1981). Some treatment implications of the ego and self-disturbances in alcoholism. In M. H. Bean, E. J. Khantzian, J. E. Mack, G. E. Vaillant, & N. E. Zimberg (Eds.), *Dynamic approaches to the understanding and treatment of alcoholism* (pp. 163–188). New York: Free Press.

King, B. (1986). Decision making in the intervention process. *Alcoholism Treatment Quarterly, 3*(3), 5–22.

King, M. E., & Bordnick, P. S. (2002). Alcohol use disorders: A social worker's guide to clinical assessment. *Journal of Social Work Practice in the Addictions, 2*(1), 3–32.

Knight, J. R., Shrier, L. A., Bravender, T. D., Farrel, L. M., Vander Bilt, J., & Shaffer, H. J. (1999). A new brief screen for adolescent substance abuse. *Archives of Pediatric Adolescent Medicine, 153,* 591–596.

Kohut, H. (1971). *The analysis of the self: A systematic approach to the psychoanalytic treatment of narcissistic personality disorders.* New York: International Universities Press.

Kohut, H. (1977). Preface. In *Psychodynamics of drug dependence* (NIDA Research Monograph No. 12). Washington, DC: U.S. Government Printing Office.

Lawental, E., McLellan, A. T., Grissom, G. R., Brill, P., & O'Brien, C. (1996). Coerced treatment for substance abuse problems detected through workplace urine surveillance: Is it effective? *Journal of Substance Abuse, 8*(1), 115–128.

Leonard, K. E., & Blane, H. T. (Eds.). (1999). *Psychological theories of drinking and alcoholism* (2nd ed.). New York: Guilford Press.

Levin, J. D. (1987). *Treatment of alcoholism and other addictions: A self-psychology approach.* Northvale, NJ: Aronson.

Levin, J. D. (1990). *Alcoholism: A bio-psycho-social approach.* New York: Hemisphere.

Levinson, V., & Straussner, S. L. A. (1978). Social workers as "enablers" in the treatment of alcoholics. *Social Casework, 59*(1), 14–20.

Littrell, J. (2001). What neurobiology has to say about why people abuse alcohol and other drugs. *Journal of Social Work Practice in the Addictions, 1*(3), 23–40.

Maisto, S. A., Carey, M. P., Carey, K. B., Gordon, C. M., & Gleason, J. R. (2000). Use of the AUDIT and the DAST-10 to identify alcohol and drug use disorders among adults with a severe and persistent mental illness. *Psychological Assessment, 12*(2), 186–192.

Mark, F. (1988). Does coercion work? The role of referral source in motivating alcoholics in treatment. *Alcoholism Treatment Quarterly, 5*(3), 5–22.

Marlatt, G. A., Baer, J. S., Donovan, D. M., & Kivlahan, D. R. (1988). Addictive behaviors: Etiology and treatment. *Annual Review of Psychology, 39,* 223–252.

Mayfield, D., McLeod, G. N., & Hall, P. (1974). The CAGE questionnaire: Validation of a new alcoholism screening instrument. *American Journal of Psychiatry, 131*(10), 1121–1123.

McClelland, D. C., Davis, W., Kalin, R., & Wanner, E. (1972). *The drinking man: Alcohol and human motivation.* New York: Free Press.

McCord, W., & McCord, J. (1960). *Origins of alcoholism.* Stanford, CA: Stanford University Press.

McLellan, A. T., Kushner, H., Peters, F., Smith, I., Corse, S. J., & Alterman, A. I. (1992). The Addiction Severity Index ten years later. *Journal of Substance Abuse Treatment, 9,* 199–213.

Menninger, K. (1938). *Man against himself.* New York: Harcourt Brace.

Miller, F. G. (1997). SASSI: Application and assessment for substance-related problems. *Journal of Substance Misuse, 2,* 163–166.

Miller, W. R. (Chair). (1999). *Enhancing motivation for change in substance abuse treatment* (Treatment Improvement Protocol Series [TIPS] 35; DHHS Publication No. [SMA] 99–3354). Rockville, MD: Center for Substance Abuse Treatment.

Miller, W. R., Meyers. R. J., & Tonigan, J. S. (1999). Engaging the unmotivated in treatment for alcohol problems: A comparison of three strategies for intervention through family members. *Journal of Consulting and Clinical Psychology* 67, 688–697.

Miller, W. R., & Rollnick, S. (1991). *Motivational interviewing: Preparing people to change addictive behavior.* New York: Guilford Press.

Nadel, M. (1985). Offspring with fetal alcohol effects: Identification and intervention. In D. Cook, S. L. A. Straussner, & C. Fewell (Eds.), *Psychosocial issues in the treatment of alcoholism* (pp. 105–116). New York: Haworth Press.

O'Connell, T. (1991). Treatment of minorities. *Drug and Alcohol Dependence, 15*(10), 13.

O'Connor, L. E., Esherick, M., & Vieten, C. (2002). Drug- and alcohol-abusing women. In S. L. A. Straussner & S. Brown (Eds.), *The handbook of addictions treatment for women* (pp. 75–98). San Francisco: Jossey-Bass.

Pattison, E. M., & Kaufman, E. (1982). Alcoholism syndrome: Definition and models. In E. M. Pattison & E. Kaufman (Eds.), *Encyclopedic handbook of alcoholism* (pp. 3–30). New York: Gardner.

Peele, S. (1998). *The meaning of addiction* (2nd ed.). San Francisco: Jossey-Bass.

Prochaska, J. C., DiClemente, C. C., & Norcross, J. C. (1992). In search of how people change: Applications to addictive behaviors. *American Psychologist, 47,* 1102–1114.

Robert Wood Johnson Foundation. (2001, March 9). *Substance abuse: The nation's number one health problem.* Princeton, NJ: Robert Wood Johnson Foundation, Substance Abuse Resource Center.

Roberts, A. C., Nishimoto, R., & Kirk, R. S. (2003). Cocaine abusing women who report sexual abuse: Implications for treatment. *Journal of Social Work Practice in the Addictions, 3*(1), 5–24.

Schuckit, M., Goodwin, D. W., & Winokur, G. (1972). A study of alcoholism in half-siblings. *American Journal of Psychiatry, 128,* 1132–1136.

Selzer, M. L. (1971). The Michigan Alcoholism Screening Test: The quest for a new diagnostic instrument. *American Journal of Psychiatry, 127,* 1653–1658.

Skinner, H. A. (1982). The drug abuse screening test. *Addictive Behaviors, 7*(4), 363–371.

Steinglass, P., Weiner, S., & Mendelson, H. (1971). A systems approach to alcoholism: A model and its clinical application. *Archives of General Psychiatry, 24,* 401–408.

Straussner, S. L. A. (1985). Alcoholism in women: Current knowledge and implications for treatment. In D. Cook, S. L. A. Straussner, & C. Fewell (Eds.), *Psychosocial issues in the treatment of alcoholism* (pp. 61–77). New York: Haworth Press.

Straussner, S. L. A. (1987). *Substance abuse training for MSW students: Survey findings.* Unpublished study.

Straussner, S. L. A. (1989). Intervention with maltreating parents who are drug and alcohol abusers. In S. Ehrenkranz, E. Goldstein, L. Goodman, & J. Seinfeld (Eds.), *Clinical social work with maltreated children and their families: An introduction to practice* (pp. 149–177). New York: New York University Press.

Straussner, S. L. A. (1994). The impact of alcohol and other drug abuse on the American family. *Drug and Alcohol Review, 13,* 393–399.

Straussner, S. L. A. (1997). Group treatment with substance abusing clients: A model of treatment during the early phases of outpatient group therapy. *Journal of Chemical Dependency Treatment, 7*(1/2), 67–80.

Straussner, S. L. A. (Ed). (2001). *Ethnocultural factors in substance abuse treatment.* New York: Guilford Press.

Straussner. S. L. A., & Attia, P. R. (2001). Short-term treatment of substance abusers. In B. Dane, C. Tosone, & A. Wolson (Eds.), *Doing more with less: Using long-term skills in short-term treatment* (pp. 119–143). Northvale, NJ: Jason Aronson.

Straussner, S. L. A., & Attia, P. R. (2002). Women's addiction and treatment through a historical lens. In S. L. A. Straussner & S. Brown (Eds.), *The handbook of addictions treatment for women* (pp. 3–25). San Francisco: Jossey-Bass.

Straussner, S. L. A., & Brown, S. (Eds.). (2002). *The handbook of addictions treatment for women.* San Francisco: Jossey Bass.

Straussner, S. L. A., Kitman, C., Straussner, J. H., & Demos, E. (1980). The alcoholic housewife: A psychosocial analysis. *Focus on Women, 1*(1), 15–32.

Straussner, S. L. A., & Spiegel, B. R. (1996). An analysis of 12–step programs for substance abusers from a developmental perspective. *Clinical Social Work, 24*(3), 299–309.

Straussner, S. L. A., Weinstein, D. L., & Hernandez, R. (1979). The effects of alcoholism on the family system. *Health and Social Work, 4*(4), 11–27.

Straussner, S. L. A., & Zelvin, E. (Eds.). (1997). *Gender and addictions: Men and women in treatment.* Northvale, NJ: Aronson.

Substance Abuse and Mental Health Services Administration (SAMHSA). (2003). *Results from the 2002 National Survey on Drug Use and Health: National Findings* (Office of Applied Studies, NHSDA Series H-22, DHHS Publication No. SMA 03–3836). Rockville, MD: Author.

Sue, D. (1987). Use and abuse of alcohol by Asian Americans. *Journal of Psychoactive Drugs, 19*(1), 57–66.

Tabakoff, B., Hoffman, P. L., Lee, J. M., Saito, T., Willard, B., & De Leon-Jones, F. (1988). Differences in platelet enzyme activity between alcoholics and controls. *New England Journal of Medicine, 318,* 134–139.

Tillich, P. (1952). *The courage to be.* New Haven, CT: Yale University Press.

Trice, H. M., & Beyer, J. M. (1984). Work related outcomes of the constructive–confrontation strategy in a job based alcoholism program. *Journal of Studies on Alcohol, 45,* 393–404.

U.S. Department of Health and Human Services. (1989). *Substance abuse among blacks in the U.S.* (NIDA capsules). Washington, DC: U.S. Government Printing Office.

U.S. Department of Health and Human Services. (1991a). Assessing alcoholism (Alcohol Alert, NIAAA No. 12 PH 294). Washington, DC: U.S. Government Printing Office.

U.S. Department of Health and Human Services. (1991b). *Drug abuse and drug abuse research: The third triennial report to Congress from the Secretary, Department of Health and Human Services.* Washington, DC: U.S. Government Printing Office.

U.S. Department of Health and Human Services. (2000a). *Substance Abuse and Mental Health Services Administration (SAMHSA) 2000 National Household*

Survey on Drug Abuse (NHSDA). Washington, DC: U.S. Government Printing Office.

U.S. Department of Health and Human Services. (2000b). *Tenth special report to the U.S. Congress on alcohol and health*. Washington, DC: U.S. Government Printing Office.

Vaillant, G. E. (1983). *The natural history of alcoholism: Causes, patterns, and paths to recovery*. Cambridge, MA: Harvard University Press.

Wagner, F. A., & Anthony, J. C. (2002). Into the world of illegal drug use: Exposure opportunity and other mechanisms linking the use of alcohol, tobacco, marijuana, and cocaine. *American Journal of Epidemiology, 155*, 918–925.

Waldinger, R. J. (1986). *Fundamentals of psychiatry*. Washington, DC: American Psychiatric Press.

Washton, A. M. (1991). Attitudes shape treatment. *Drug and Alcohol Dependence, 15*(8), 8.

Washton, A. M., & Gold, M. S. (1987). Recent trend in cocaine abuse as seen from the "800-Cocaine" hotline. In A. M. Washton & M. S. Gold (Eds.), *Cocaine: A clinician's handbook* (pp. 10–22). New York: Guilford Press.

Wetli, C. V. (1987) Fatal reactions to cocaine. In A. M. Washton & M. S. Gold (Eds.), *Cocaine: A clinician's handbook* (pp. 33–54). New York: Guilford Press.

Williams, G. D., Grant, B. F., Hartford, T. C., & Noble, J. (1989). Population projections using DSM III criteria: Alcohol abuse and dependence 1990–2000. *Alcohol Health and Research World, 13*(4), 366–370.

Wurmser, L. (1978). *The hidden dimension: Psychodynamics in compulsive drug use*. New York: Aronson.

PART II

Varying Perspectives on Intervention with Substance Abusers

The six chapters in this section describe a variety of approaches to helping people with substance abuse problems and reinforce the growing awareness that there is no single "correct" model of intervention.

In the first chapter in Part II, the authors explore the concept of motivation for treatment and apply the notion of motivational interviewing to working with substance-abusing clients. Recognition of the fact that clients come to, or are referred for, treatment with different levels of motivation helps clinicians adapt their interventions to the needs of individual clients, thereby moving beyond the uniform treatment approach that we know does not work for many, if not most, of our clients.

In Chapter 3 the author explores the still controversial practice of harm reduction and shows its compatibility with traditional social work interventions. Here again clinicians are helped to recognize that clients have different needs and that interventions can take many different forms in many different places.

The next two chapters provide important tools for working with what have been termed "the difficult clients": those who are involuntarily mandated to treatment and those with coexisting psychiatric disabilities. The authors provide concrete and effective examples of helping such clients.

The authors of Chapter 6 explore the therapeutic nature of the well-known 12-step programs by identifying the psychodynamic principles underlying the so-called self-help groups. Although not all people can, or wish to, use a 12-step program, for those who do, the psychological benefits can be great. The final chapter in this part examines the concept of relapse prevention and provides the specific tools and approaches for helping clients deal with the possibility of having a lifelong disorder that has an ever-present danger of relapse.

CHAPTER 2

Motivating Substance-Abusing Clients through the Helping Process

Meredith Hanson
Nabila El-Bassel

The concept of motivation, especially as it relates to an individual's capacity to engage in and profit from treatment, has a long history within and outside the addictions field (Applebaum, 1972; Miller, 1985; Ripple, Alexander, & Polemis, 1964; Sterne & Pittman, 1965). Historically, discussions of motivation often were framed by an assumption that clients must desire help and want change *before* treatment can begin (Oxley, 1966). More recently, clinicians have begun to treat clients' motivation as an appropriate target for clinical work and an area of clinical practice that is essential to include in the recovery process (Higgins & Silverman, 1999; White & Wright, 1998). The purpose of this chapter is to review the evolution of the motivation concept in the addictions field and to identify empirically supported "best practices" that clinicians can use to increase clients' motivation and commitment to the therapeutic process.

UNDERSTANDING THE CONCEPT OF "MOTIVATION"

Motivation has been defined in many ways. Traditionally, many authors have asserted that motivation is a character trait (or individual attribute) of biopsychological origin that clients either do or do not possess (Gold, 1990). Moreover, the phrase "poor motivation" has been used interchangeably with "resistance" (Miller, Duncan, & Hubble, 1997). Poor motivation has been conceptualized further as both a manifestation of such defense mechanisms as denial (DiCicco, Unterberger, & Mack, 1978) and the result of constitutional factors that allegedly make it impossible for some people to control alcohol and other drug use (Milam & Ketcham, 1981). Sterne and Pittman (1965) caution, however, that many clinicians who view motivation in this manner use it as a "homologue" for will-power and place "complete responsibility for recovery" on the client (p. 48). William Miller (1985) adds that "this conception of motivation [can become] a thinly veiled resurrection of the much older moral-blame model of [addiction]: that clients could overcome the problem if they really wanted to and tried hard enough" (p. 85).

Over the years, as many clinicians became dissatisfied with trait-based models of motivation, other conceptualizations emerged (see Gold, 1990, and Miller, 1985, for critical reviews of different conceptualizations of motivation). Social work researchers expanded on trait-based views and suggested that motivation in combination with an individual's capacities (personal strengths and limitations) and opportunities (environmental resources and deficits) could explain disruptions in normal coping abilities, the persistence of problematic behavioral patterns, and responses to therapeutic interventions (Ripple et al., 1964).

Helen Harris Perlman drew on the work of Ripple and others (e.g., White, 1959) to produce a problem-solving model of clinical practice that directly addressed a client's motivational level (Goldstein, 1995). According to Perlman (1979),

> two conditions must hold for the sustainment of responsible willingness to work at problem-solving: discomfort and hope. . . . Discomfort without hope spells resignation, apathy, fixation. . . . Hopefulness without discomfort . . . is the mark of the immature, wishful person . . . who depends on others or on circumstances to work for his interests. (pp. 186–187)

Within this clinical model two critical components of clients' motivation to participate in treatment and to work on behavioral change are "arousal" (the push of discomfort) and "direction" (the pull of hope; see Ripple et al., 1964).

MOTIVATION IN THE ADDICTIONS FIELD

Some of the earliest references to motivation in the addictions field are found in the literature on the birth of Alcoholics Anonymous (AA, 1957). Henry Tiebout, a psychiatrist who treated Bill Wilson for depression at the time Wilson was founding AA with Dr. Bob Smith, asserted that a radical "ego deflation" was a necessary first step in the recovery process. Ego deflation was believed to counter alcoholic grandiosity and denial, trigger "surrender," and ultimately promote an identity transformation that would lead to personal growth and recovery (Levin, 1991; Tiebout, 1957; Whitfield, 1984).

The phrase "hitting bottom" was substituted for "ego deflation" in AA's parlance (Kurtz, 1991). To "hit bottom" meant coming to the realization that one's drinking was out of control. It signified more than the loss of family, home, job, or health. To hit bottom was to feel "licked," alone, hopeless, and in despair. According to Ernest Kurtz (1991), Bill Wilson believed that the experience of hitting bottom was essential to understand the AA approach, and a "common explanation offered for anyone's failure to grasp the program of Alcoholics Anonymous ran, 'He hasn't reached bottom yet' " (p. 115).

As the AA membership changed to include more people who were not as deteriorated as those who had comprised the fellowship's original cohort, the notion of hitting bottom remained. However, *bottom* was redefined to include "high bottoms" (low points in which a person encounters problems associated with drinking that do not include major devastation such as loss of family, job, and health) and "low bottoms" (points of utter devastation, such as institutionalization or financial or social ruin; Keller, McCormick, & Efron, 1982). According to Wilson, with the membership change "we began to develop a conscious technique of 'raising the bottom' [raising awareness to create a crisis] and hitting them with it" (Alcoholics Anonymous, 1957, p. 199).

The more aggressive confrontative strategies that characterized "raising the bottom" dominated the addictions field until quite recently. Classic examples of aggressive (hard) confrontation can be seen in the "chairing" techniques and "haircuts" of the original therapeutic communities (Yablonsky, 1967). Less harsh but still aggressive confrontations are apparent in some family interventions (Johnson, 1986) and "constructive confrontations" in the workplace (Roman, 1981). All three strategies attempt to mobilize substance-abusing persons to change addictive lifestyles by making them more aware of the negative consequences of substance use and thereby creating a personal crisis. The latter two strategies try to couple the confrontation with specific options for relieving the crisis.

For the most part, there is little inherent in these approaches to justify the punitive, authoritarian, and coercive tactics that appear in the counseling styles of some clinicians. Nevertheless, misguided beliefs that drug- and alcohol-involved persons have unusually strong and primitive defenses and distorted thinking patterns (DiCicco et al., 1978) have led to a greater reliance on negative, "pathologically" focused confrontative tactics than the conceptual and empirical literature supports (Miller, 1995; Miller & Rollnick, 2002).

Morris Chafetz's (1967) ideas about motivation for recovery from alcoholism presage some current views of motivation in the addictions field. According to Chafetz, clinicians must consider three aspects of motivation: (1) clients' internal motivations, which derive from their strengths and achievements; (2) the immediate environment's influence (i.e., contextual factors such as the availability of resources and interpersonal supports); and (3) the influence of the caretaking community (i.e., clinicians and other mental health professionals). In Chafetz's view, motivation is strongly linked to factors that strengthen people's positive qualities and minimize negative ones. He believes that the caretaking community is, potentially, "the main motivating force for recovery" (p. 114).

William Miller and Stephen Rollnick (2002) took a tact similar to Chafetz's when they developed their approach to motivational interviewing (discussed later in this chapter). According to Miller (1985), motivation is a dynamic state characterized by an eagerness or readiness to change. Pragmatically, it is "doing something to get better" (Miller, 1998a, p. 122). As a dynamic state, a client's motivational level is highly responsive to clinical influence (Miller, Benefield, & Tonigan, 1993).

Taken together, the many conceptualizations of motivation underscore the fact that motivation levels fluctuate over time and across situations. Motivation for change is affected by (1) the level of clients' distress, (2) clients' goals and their value to them, (3) outcome expectancies (i.e., clients' beliefs that goals are reachable), (4) perceived self-efficacy (i.e., beliefs that one can comply with the tasks and achieve the goals of treatment; Marlatt, Baer, & Quigley, 1995), (5) environmental resources and barriers, including social networks that support change, and (6) personal skill repertoires, such as having a capacity to resist pressures to use drugs.

MOTIVATIONAL READINESS TO CHANGE

James Prochaska, Carlo DiClemente, and associates developed a particularly informative and integrative model that differentiates two facets of a motivational readiness for change: *intention* and *action* (Connors, Donovan, & DiClemente, 2001; Prochaska & DiClemente, 1982; Prochaska, DiClemente, & Norcross, 1992; Velasquez, Maurer, Crouch, & DiClemente, 2001). The model, which is based on a rich body of empirical research, predicts that as individuals recognize the adverse consequences of addictive lifestyles, take steps to correct their behaviors, relapse, and begin the process over again, they move through five motivational stages in a cyclical fashion: precontemplation, contemplation, preparation, action, and maintenance (see Table 2.1).

TABLE 2.1. Motivational Readiness to Change

Stage of change	Client characteristics
Precontemplation	• No intention of changing targeted behavior (i.e., intravenous drug use). • No *action* toward change. • Engages in the targeted behavior freely. • Does not connect life difficulties to the behavior.
Contemplation	• Highly ambivalent. • Wavers considerably; ponders change and then rejects it. • "Yes-but" rationalizations. • *Low intention* to change and *no sustained action*.
Preparation	• *Serious intention* to change. • *More action*, but still not sustained. • Recognizes that change must occur, but not sure how. • May not believe change must be permanent.
Action	• Takes clearly identifiable steps toward change. • Efforts are sustained despite setbacks.
Maintenance	• Maintains change for a significant time period (e.g., 6 months). • Focuses efforts on preventing relapse and developing the capacity to live a sober lifestyle.

The Process of Change

Typically, the process of intentional change begins with *precontemplation*. In this stage, individuals have not identified their substance use as a problem, and they have no conscious intention to change their behaviors. Although they may acknowledge personal and social difficulties, they tend not to link those difficulties to substance use. Clinicians are not likely to see clients in this stage of change, unless they are seeking help for difficulties other than substance abuse or they have entered treatment involuntarily (Barber, 1995). According to Scott Miller and colleagues (1997), metaphorically, clients in this stage of change have not invited clinicians into their homes. Thus, although clinicians "may have many useful suggestions for arranging the clients' furniture . . ., such considerations are secondary to gaining admittance" (p. 92). Even when they gain entry, clinicians may find that precontemplative clients are "surprised" to learn that anyone thinks they have a "drug problem." Generally, they are highly reluctant to engage in treatment and may pay "lip service" to therapeutic suggestions that do not take into consideration their limited awareness of any serious substance use problem (Barber, 1995). If clients in this stage feel pressured to change, they may focus their energies on negating the clinician's views. Even when they make token changes to appease others, they often resume alcohol and other drug use when the pressure is removed.

The *contemplation* stage of change is marked by a high degree of ambivalence. It is at this stage that people begin to think more deliberately about negative aspects of their substance use. Although they may be laboring to come to grips with their drug-related difficulties and may be considering the advantages of sobriety, they usually have made no firm commitment to change. Their thinking and actions tend to be dominated by "yes-but" rationalizations in which ideas about change waffle back and forth with questions about whether change is necessary or worth the time and effort (Prochaska et al., 1992). Clients may stay in the contemplation stage for as long as 2 years. Although they are more receptive to feedback about their substance use and suggestions for change, they remain stuck due to doubts about their abilities to effect change as well as fear of the unknown (Hohman, 1998).

Miller (1998a) points out that "contemplative" ambivalence is a normal part of change. If clinicians try to challenge it too aggressively by taking one side of the clients' "inner arguments," they put the clients in a position where they are likely to argue the other side. The more clinicians press their views, the more vigorously clients defend themselves to minimize stress and to maintain some sense of balance. As a result, what essentially should be an inner struggle, in which clients, themselves, challenge their own actions and beliefs with the aid of their therapists, becomes an external struggle pitting clients against therapists and inadvertently forcing clients into more recalcitrant positions (Miller, 1983). Arguments between clients and therapists over whether or not one is an "alcoholic" typify the type of self-defeating exchanges that can occur when therapists challenge ambivalence prematurely and too forcefully.

Individuals in the *preparation* stage have made a decision or commitment to change but have not yet engaged in any sustained action. In this stage *intention* to change must be followed by an identification of criteria that indicate change (Prochaska et al., 1992). According to Miller and colleagues (1997), "by the time clients reach this stage they have crossed the Rubicon of change. . . . There is little question that change will occur, [thus] the main focus [should be on] identifying the criteria and strategies for success" (pp. 100–101). Many clients who are preparing to change have already taken preliminary steps (e.g., reducing their drug intake) and have made plans to take more definitive action in the near future (e.g., attending an NA meeting). They may still waver, however, about whether these changes must be permanent or if any additional steps toward recovery are warranted. Although clients in the preparation stage still resist accepting therapeutic directives, they are generally more willing to explore and consider a range of alternative goals and action plans.

During the *action* stage, which begins in the preparation stage and can last up to 6 months, clients take more decisive steps to modify their addictive behaviors and environments. Individuals in the action stage typically make behavioral and lifestyle changes and establish goals that are more obvious and acceptable to others. For example, problem drinkers may establish "action" goals that include abstaining from all alcoholic beverages for at least 30 days and keeping all medical and group therapy appointments during that time period. Heroin users may commit to entering a detoxification facility or apply to a methadone maintenance treatment program.

During the *maintenance* stage, which begins after individuals have sustained behavioral change for around 6 months, clients begin to focus on strengthening the change, consolidating gains, preventing relapse, and sustaining a sober lifestyle. The maintenance stage may be the most challenging. Since recovery is a lifelong process, there is no clear-cut endpoint to this stage. Only when they are maintaining therapeutic gains can clients be considered "survivors" who have liberated themselves from the throes of active addiction. They now can prevent future difficulties by living vigilantly—that is, by anticipating any possible threats to sobriety and handling them before they relapse.

For most drug- and alcohol-involved clients, recovery is a cyclical process in which there is a great deal of movement back and forth across stages of change. Relapse is not uncommon, and when it occurs, individuals may return to any of the earlier stages before eventually establishing lifelong sobriety.

The research of Prochaska and colleagues (1992) indicates that clients' willingness to participate in treatment and the change processes they use vary across the stages of change. Thus, clinicians must match therapeutic interventions to clients' stages of change. Clients in the precontemplation stage benefit from clinical strategies designed to provide information, raise doubt about current lifestyles, and permit emotional release. As they move toward contemplation, clients must be helped to identify reasons to change; they must become more consciously aware of the risks associated with *not* changing addictive behaviors. They also must be helped to develop confidence in their ability to alter old habits and adopt new ones. Individuals who are in the preparation stage, while still needing information and emotional support, require more active assistance in making treatment decisions and developing a clear plan for change. Finally, in the action and maintenance stages, clients benefit from interventions that help them to acquire additional coping skills and mobilize environmental resources that can prevent relapse.

To have optimal impact, clinicians must be prepared to begin treatment before clients are "ready" to change (as demonstrated by their entry into the preparation stage), and they must match their therapeutic tactics to the clients' stages of change. If they wait until clients are ready to change, or if their therapeutic efforts are mismatched to the stage of change, therapists will miss many opportunities to aid persons who could benefit from professional assistance.

DEVELOPING A THERAPEUTIC ALLIANCE AND PROMOTING CHANGE

Given that clients respond differently and use different change processes at different stages of change, and that clinicians must tailor their interventions to match clients' stages of change, a logical question is: What should clinicians do to motivate their clients and to form a therapeutic alliance? To answer this question, we must consider the tasks of engagement in therapy. During the initial phases of treatment, clinicians must accomplish three objectives:

1. They must create a "safe space" so that clients *can* talk with them.
2. They must establish a collaborative partnership so clients *will* talk to them.
3. They must reach a preliminary agreement that a problem exists so that clients have a *reason* to talk with them.

Although they need not convince their clients that change is necessary, they must gain agreement that continued therapeutic contact is worthwhile.

Core Features of Treatment

Research on effective brief therapies for problem drinkers has identified six core features of treatment that are applicable to forming therapeutic alliances with drug-involved clients and enhancing their motivation to change (Bien, Miller, & Tonigan, 1993). These core elements are summarized by the acronym FRAMES: *f*eedback, *r*esponsibility, *a*dvice, *m*enu of options, *e*mpathy, and *s*elf-efficacy (Hester & Bien, 1995; see Table 2.2).

Feedback

Most successful brief interventions are fairly structured and require more activity by clinicians. Most also include some form of systematic assessment and feedback about the nature of a client's substance-related difficulties. Unlike standardized substance abuse educational lectures and films that offer general information and which have little evidence of effectiveness (see Miller, Andrews, Wilbourne, & Bennett, 1998), feedback in effective brief interventions is *personalized* and directed specifically to a particular client's experiences.

TABLE 2.2. Core Components of Effective Brief Therapies for Problem Drinkers

Component	Description
Feedback	Therapist provides personalized feedback about client's current circumstances (e.g., health status, social consequences of drug use).
Responsibility	Therapist stresses that, ultimately, responsibility for change rests with the client (therapist may encourage clients to involve family members and others in this decision, especially when social and cultural norms support such involvement).
Advice	Therapist offers clear and specific advice about the advantages of changing addictive patterns as well as the different ways that change can occur.
Menu	Therapist provides a range of viable alternative strategies for changing addictive behaviors.
Empathy	Therapist demonstrates concern for clients and affirms their experiences while supporting the changes they make.
Self-efficacy	Therapist expresses confidence and nurtures clients' beliefs that they can carry out therapeutic tasks.

Feedback consists of information that is extracted from assessment interviews and clients' physical examinations (e.g., consumption levels, blood-screening levels, patterns of drug use). This information is compared to national norms and to information derived from samples of individuals in treatment, in an attempt to create a dialogue with new clients. For example, to counter a 21-year-old drinker's faulty assumptions that he did not consume much alcohol, and that he drank only to "chill out," his clinician pointed out that his consumption level placed him in the top 1% of drinkers nationwide. She also drew his attention to elevated liver enzymes that indicated alcohol-related tissue damage. In addition, she "wondered" whether the frequent fist fights that he tended to get into after he drank also indicated that his drinking was not as harmless as he believed. By inviting this young man to consider the old information of his drinking pattern in light of this new information, the clinician helped him to reexamine his behavior from a fresh perspective. This was a first step in establishing an open and critical dialogue about drinking and change.

Responsibility

Most effective substance abuse interventions are collaborative in nature, that is, they emphasize a client's role in the therapeutic process. Although clients may not be responsible (i.e., blamed) for becoming addicted, they are helped to understand that they have responsibility for continuing or changing current patterns (Miller, 1999). To avoid power struggles that emerge when they try to make decisions for clients, clinicians must "appreciate" the clients' definitions of their life situations (Matza, 1969). Clinicians need to convey to them that, ultimately, they (the clients) must decide whether they want to continue current patterns of drug use or make changes. Clients must "hear" from clinicians, and accept, that they are "experts" in their own lives and that they can develop viable solutions that meet their needs. Consistent with this view, clinicians do not impose their views on clients. When clients realize they have choices and the power to choose, their resistance tends to diminish and they become more persistent and committed to change efforts. Instead of arguing with therapists about different courses of action, clients become more likely to choose strategies and try to implement them with their therapist's help. In cases where clients decide that they do not want to change, they are more likely to leave the therapeutic encounter on a positive note, knowing that they can return if they change their mind.

Advice

Although successful practitioners of brief therapy do not insist that they have the "right" answers, they do let their clients know that they have expertise and knowledge. Thus, they offer clear and specific *advice* about the need to change dysfunctional and destructive drug-use patterns, as well as the ways in which change can take place. They create participatory dialogues in which the advantages and disadvantages of different treatment options are weighed openly and without threat. The research literature shows that when advice is offered in this manner, it is more likely to motivate individuals to take action toward changing addictive behavior (Bien et al., 1993; Miller, 1995).

Menu

Paired with the offer of advice is a menu of options for changing addictive patterns. This menu should include a range of treatment modalities and treatment settings. By informing a client about treatment alternatives, a clinician reinforces the client's choice in the change process. Actively involving clients in the decision-making process not only increases retention in treatment, but it also counters clients' tendencies to react against authority and resist control (Barber, 1994).

When developing menus of treatment options, clinicians should help clients generate ideas. Treatment in which clinicians control how and when clients participate is not collaborative and may lead, ultimately, to greater client resistance and poorer therapeutic outcomes (Breton, 1994).

Empathy

As is the case in other forms of therapy, brief interventions are empathic and affirming; they validate clients' experiences and help them to accept those experiences, while encouraging them to take action to change (Marlatt, 1994). An empathic, supportive clinical style is associated with client compliance and positive therapeutic outcomes for a wide variety of clinical concerns (Patterson & Forgatch, 1985). The beneficial impact of a therapist's strong interpersonal skills, in fact, is among the most robust findings in all research on the effectiveness of psychotherapy (Najavits & Weiss, 1994; Wright & Davis, 1994). In research on brief, self-control training with problem drinkers, for example, it was discovered that counselors' ranking on empathic understanding—a crude measure of their ability to listen reflectively—was a significant predictor of successful outcomes for all study participants (Miller & Baca, 1983; Miller, Taylor, & West, 1980). In contrast, a hostile, confrontational approach to treatment has been shown to lead to increased resistance, higher dropout rates, and poorer therapeutic outcomes (Miller et al., 1993).

Self-Efficacy

The sixth core component of effective brief interventions is a focus on (and support of) client self-efficacy (Bandura, 1997). Perceived self-efficacy is a belief that one is capable of carrying out actions necessary to attain a desired goal. Several types of efficacy self-appraisals have been identified. Of particular relevance to effective substance abuse treatment are (1) treatment self-efficacy, which is related to people's beliefs that they can perform tasks required in therapy; (2) resistance self-efficacy, which pertains to clients' confidence that they can avoid alcohol and other drug use in the future; (3) recovery self-efficacy, which focuses on clients' beliefs that they can rebound from slips and relapses; and (4) action self-efficacy, which addresses clients' beliefs in their abilities to achieve therapeutic goals (DiClemente, Fairhurst, & Piotrowski, 1995; Marlatt et al., 1995).

As observed earlier, "the pull of hope" is a key element in motivation. Clinicians must instill hope and communicate confidence in clients' ability to change in order to strengthen their commitment to the change process. If clients believe that their therapists are concerned about them, are motivated to help them, are committed to the therapeutic process, and are confident in their capacity to change, they are more likely to engage fully in therapy, persist with therapeutic tasks, and eliminate addictive behaviors (Miller, 1995; Thomas, Polansky, & Kounin, 1967).

MOTIVATIONAL INTERVIEWING

William Miller developed the core elements of motivational interviewing in 1982 (Miller, 1996, p. 835). Compelled by the questions raised by his supervisees to make explicit the practice approach he had learned from his clients, he devised a clinical approach that not only addressed a client's motivational readiness to change, but also integrated the core therapeutic elements of effective brief therapies. His efforts led to the first concept paper on motivational interviewing: "Motivational Interviewing with Problem Drinkers" (Miller, 1983).

Motivational interviewing is a brief, focused, directive, and client-centered clinical approach designed to elicit behavior change by helping alcohol- and drug-involved individuals (and their significant others) identify, explore, and resolve ambivalence (Rollnick & Miller, 1995). It is both a *collaborative style of helping* that utilizes a clinician's capacity to be warm, empathic, and genuine, and a set of *specific therapeutic techniques* (Miller, 1996). In broad terms, motivational interviewing synthesizes a nondirective, therapeutic approach with principles from motivational psychology and change theory (Schilling, El-Bassel, Finch, Roman, & Hanson, 2002).

According to Miller, "Motivational interviewing is a narrative process of evoking from the client reasons for and commitment to change" (1998b, p. 169). It consists of two phases: phase one, in which motivation for change is cultivated and phase two, in which commitment to change is strengthened. Motivational interviewers facilitate change by creating a supportive therapeutic environment in which they can develop discrepancies or cognitive dissonance (usually) between current problem behavior (e.g., excessive drinking) and a client's self-image, aspirations, or perceptions (Cox, Klinger, & Blount, 1991). By avoiding argumentation, acknowledging doubt, and selectively applying motivational interviewing tactics, clinicians help clients recognize the adverse consequences of their addictive behaviors and take action to address their dysfunctional patterns that are contributing to the addictive cycles.

Although motivational interviewing does not use the aggressive, confrontative tactics found in some traditional addiction counseling approaches, it *is* confrontational in nature. To confront clients is to help them "face" reality and become aware of inconsistencies and conflicts in their lives. Motivational interviewing attempts to do this. Sound therapeutic confrontation is a "goal," not a "means," of treatment (Miller & Rollnick, 2002). Motivational interviewing tactics are designed to reach this goal in an efficient, effective manner that will increase a client's active involvement in treatment, encourage a sense of responsibility for the work of therapy, and elicit self-generated reasons for change.

Motivational Interviewing Strategies

The foundation of motivational interviewing consists of four nondirective, client-centered counseling skills: asking open-ended questions, listening reflectively, affirming, and summarizing (Rollnick & Morgan, 1995).

Use of Open-Ended Questions

Open-ended questions encourage clients to elaborate on their concerns and to tell their story as they see it. By helping clients do most of the talking early in treatment, clinicians create an accepting atmosphere that supports openness. Miller and Rollnick (2002) suggest that if clinicians know in advance that clients have particular concerns about their drug use, they can draw attention to those concerns by asking questions such as "What brought you here today?" "How can I be of help?" or "When you called, you said you have been injecting heroin for a long time. Why don't you fill me in and start from the beginning: When did you begin using drugs and when did you become concerned about that drug use?"

When clients are ambivalent about their drug use, clinicians will find it helpful to ask questions that reflect both sides of the issue. For example: "What can you tell me about smoking marijuana? What do you like about it? On the other hand, what worries you about it?" or "Tell me what changes you have noticed in your drinking over the years. What have you noticed that concerns you or others?" (Miller & Rollnick, 2002, p. 66). When clinicians meet with involuntary clients, open-ended questions can be posed to help them tell their side of the story. For example: "Your boss called me and said that she sent you here because she thought your drinking was interfering with your work performance. I'd like to hear your views." This type of opening can be followed by questions about the client's drinking that attempt to clarify how the client perceives the situation. When questioning a reluctant client, it is important for clinicians to remain nonjudgmental while communicating both curiosity and concern about what is happening.

Reflective Listening

As clients begin sharing information and concerns about their drinking and drug use, clinicians may be tempted to give advice prematurely, analyze what clients are experiencing, or be overly reassuring. These responses are examples of "roadblocks" that divert the therapeutic process: Clinicians who use them are not truly listening. Instead, they are biding their time long enough to think of their own response to give a client (Miller & Rollnick, 2002, p. 68). Instead of responding in this manner, clinicians should *listen reflectively*. They should try to understand what the client *means* and then voice their impression in the form of a statement or conjecture that allows the client to confirm or correct it and to develop it in greater depth. Simple reflection involves repeating a few words from a client's statements. More complex reflections insert new words or add feelings to what a client says (Shea, 1998). By judiciously combining open-ended questions with reflective listening, therapists avoid creating an adversarial climate in which questions are followed by more questions and clients feel pressured to tell more and more—to "come clean."

Affirming Clients' Concerns

As they encourage clients to tell their stories and express their concerns, clinicians must be supportive and affirmative. Support is a necessary condition for change to occur (Nelsen, 1980). Through support, clinicians communicate acceptance. With affirmation they encourage clients to continue to explore aspects of substance use that are highly troubling to them. Affirmation in the form of a statement such as "I appreciate the effort it took to come in today and I want to thank you" can disarm a client who was "forced" by others to visit a therapist and who therefore feels angry and reluctant.

Summarizing

Summarization, the fourth fundamental therapeutic tactic in motivational interviewing, is particularly useful for tying together a client's statements and verifying the accuracy of the clinician's impressions. Summary statements—for example, "So, let me see if I understand what you've told me so far . . . "—demonstrate that the clinician has been listening and help the client move on to the next topic. These statements also draw attention to ambivalent and conflicting thoughts and feelings the client might hold. Lastly, they can bring a session to a close and pave the way for future meetings.

Eliciting Self-Motivational Statements

Besides the four nondirective counseling skills, a fifth core strategy—eliciting self-motivational statements—helps clients move beyond ambivalence. Self-motivational statements give direction and purpose to an interview, help clients examine their ambivalence, and encourage them to expand upon their concerns (Rollnick & Morgan, 1995). Self-motivating statements are comments elicited from clients that express reasons for change. Making these statements, clients hear themselves talk and discover what they feel. These statements generally fall into four categories: (1) recognition that a drug-use pattern and its consequences are problematic, (2) expressions of concern about the current situation, (3) indications of an intention or desire to change, and (4) words of hope and optimism about change (Miller & Rollnick, 2002). Examples include "I'm worried because I can't drink as much as I used to"; "If I drank less, I'd probably fight less with my children and they'd worry less about me"; "I notice that when I stop snorting cocaine for a while, I actually feel more alert and less irritable"; "I took the first step by coming in today—I really think I'll follow through this time."

Clinicians can use nondirective counseling skills to elicit self-motivational statements. Through evocative, open-ended questions they can explore areas that are likely to produce self-motivational statements. For example:

> "What concerns do you or other people have about your drinking?"
> "What do you think will happen with your health if you continue to use heroin as you have been?"
> "In what other ways have you made changes in your life?"

Therapists also can help clients explore what they like and dislike about their current drug-use patterns, as well as alternatives to drug use. Once clients make self-motivational statements, clinicians should continue to use nondirective interviewing to encourage them to elaborate. By taking an affirmative and inquisitive "What else?" or "Tell me more" approach, clinicians encourage clients to examine and clarify ambivalent conflicts. By reflecting clients' self-motivational statements back to them, clinicians help them to become more aware of their views and doubts, thereby increasing their motivation for change (Miller & Rollnick, 2002).

Phase-Specific Motivational Interviewing

When clinicians determine that clients are unready to change, or discover that clients doubt their abilities to change addictive behaviors, their clinical strategies need to focus on building motivation for change. Table 2.3 lists the possible strategies discussed in the following material.

Phase 1: Enhancing Motivation for Change

As indicated earlier, clinicians can enhance motivation for change by creating a facilitative, affirming context in which personalized feedback is provided, ambivalence and doubt are examined, and self-motivational state-

TABLE 2.3. Phase-Specific Motivational Interviewing:
Practical Strategies

Phase I: Enhancing motivation for change
- Empathic listening
- Open-ended questioning
- Personalized feedback
- Responding to resistance
- Reframing
- Eliciting self-motivational statements
- Summarization

Phase II: Strengthening commitment for change
- Acknowledging readiness to change
- Discussing a precise plan for change
- Stressing choice
- Reviewing the consequences of action and inaction
- Offering information and advice
- Stressing abstinence
- Developing a Change Plan Worksheet (contract)
- Handling doubt and reluctance
- Reviewing and recapitulating
- Seeking commitment

Note. Adapted from Miller, Zweben, DiClemente, and Rychtarik (1992).

ments are explored. Resistance to change should not be challenged aggressively. Rather, clinicians should realize that clients are likely protecting themselves from fear and conflict through their resistant actions. When clients display resistance (e.g., by arguing, changing topics, or interrupting the therapist), clinicians should recognize their own contributions to the intensity of a client's response (e.g., by acting as if a client is ready for change, when he or she is not).

Clinicians can handle resistance by "rolling with it" and reflecting it back to clients. Particularly useful with highly ambivalent clients are "double-sided reflections" in which clinicians state both sides of a conflict (Miller & Rollnick, 2002). For example, a clinician might say to a teenager who smokes marijuana, "So, on the one hand, you enjoy smoking pot because you like the feeling and many of your friends smoke. But, on the other hand, you're worried because you've been having trouble concentrating and your grades are slipping. That's quite a dilemma." This type of comment brings into sharp relief a client's struggle; hearing it stated clearly and nonjudgmentally can encourage him or her to explore the struggle without "demanding" that the client take one side or another.

Another way to handle resistance is to reframe it (Miller & Rollnick, 2002). When reframing, the clinician accepts a client's observations but reinterprets them. In the case of a young woman who blames her family for her drug use, the therapist might reinterpret the family's behavior: "You feel like your family nags you, and that nagging causes you to smoke crack more. I wonder if they are concerned about you but don't know how to express it. . . . Do you think we can help them to understand what you are going through and learn how to express their worries another way?" To a middle-aged man who feels hopeless and defeated in a detoxification ward, the clinician might say: "You feel pretty discouraged because you've relapsed and have gone through detox so often. The fact that you've tried so hard is hopeful, though. Like others, you've discovered a lot of ways that don't work. Why don't we use your strength and courage to identify other ways that can work for you?"

During phase 1 of motivational interviewing, clinicians try to create a dialogue in which information is shared freely. Because clients are still not committed to changing addictive behaviors, it is important to help them explore both the risks and the benefits of maintaining their addictive lifestyles. Drug use is continued, in part, because of its adaptive consequences—its benefits. By exploring the pros as well as the cons of drug use, clinicians increase their credibility (by recognizing that clients get something positive out of drug use) as they help clients to specify those benefits, determine whether they are worth the cost, and consider other ways to gain the ends they are seeking through drug use.

A useful decision-making tool that can be employed to raise a client's consciousness and to promote problem solving is the Decisional Balance Worksheet. This tool helps clients consider, in cognitive and rational terms, the positive and negative aspects of continuing (or changing) current actions (Janis & Mann, 1977; Scott, 1989).

Figure 2.1 contains a sample Decisional Balance Worksheet in which a client has identified the advantages and disadvantages of maintaining her current pattern of drug use. In this case example, the three preschool-age children of Mary Davis, a 25-year-old single mother, were removed from her custody because of child neglect. Neighbors reported that the children were often dirty and hungry, and that Ms. Davis was seen smoking crack with neighborhood "junkies." The child welfare agency removed the children and mandated that, among other things, Ms. Davis seek treatment for crack abuse before it would consider returning the children to her.

During meetings with a clinical social worker at a substance abuse facility, Ms. Davis insisted that she rarely smoked crack and that it was "no big deal." In the clinician's assessment, Ms. Davis was wavering between the precontemplation and contemplation stages of change. She determined that in order for Ms. Davis to benefit from treatment, her motivation had to increase and she had to decide that the consequences of drug use outweighed the benefits. By using open-ended questions and double-sided reflections, the clinician helped the client become more aware of both the "costs" and the "benefits" of smoking crack. For example, when Ms. Davis said, "I like getting high. It's a good feeling and I forget my problems," the clinician responded, "You like getting high. It feels good to you." When Ms. Davis nodded in agreement, the clinician asked, "What

	If I continue smoking crack . . .	If I stop smoking crack . . .
Benefits for me . . .	• I like getting high. • I have friends to hang out with. • I forget my problems.	• I won't lose custody of my children. • I'll feel less paranoid. • I'll have more money to spend. • I'll feel proud.
Benefits for people important to me . . .	• My friends will have an easy "mark" for money.	• I'll be a better mother. • I can buy my children the things they need.
Costs for me . . .	• I might lose my job. • I'll lose my children. • I'll keep losing weight. • I'll feel like a failure.	• I'll feel more nervous around people. • I'll lose some friends.
Costs for people important to me . . .	• My children will have a bad role model. • My children will be in foster care.	• I may be more short-tempered. • I'll be harder to get along with for a while.

FIGURE 2.1. Decisional Balance Worksheet.

concerns do you have about smoking crack?" The client replied that she occasionally worried about losing her job and that she would feel awful if she lost custody of her children. The clinician reflected both of Ms. Davis's thoughts back to her and added that it was important for her to be a good mother: "So, on the one hand, you enjoy smoking crack. But, on the other, it has caused you problems at work and with your children. It's very important to you to be a responsible parent." Ms. Davis picked up on this statement and made a stronger self-motivational statement: "Yes. I *must* be a good parent. I owe it to my children." Later, after reflecting further on her statements, she said, "I guess I have to do something, if I don't want to lose my children. I don't want to ruin their lives." Although she was still hesitant to commit to change, she weighed the possibility of making changes more openly. This exchange shows that by focusing on a client's primary concerns and helping him or her identify negative consequences of drug use, a clinician can promote a dialogue that enhances the client's motivational readiness to change.

As the interview continued, Ms. Davis wavered from anger to remorse, minimizing her crack use and expressing feelings of hopelessness. Through affirmation, empathic comments, and the use of other client-centered tactics, the clinician avoided "confrontation–denial" arguments (Miller & Rollnick, 2002). She used Ms. Davis's own words and concerns to help her build the case for staying in treatment and considering change. She also communicated an appreciation of the difficulty Ms. Davis was experiencing as well as her optimism that with treatment, the client would be able to decide what was best for her and her children. The clinician never used the label "drug addict." Instead, she relied on the stressful consequences of crack use and the potential benefits of change that the client, herself, identified to build motivation for change.

Phase 2: Strengthening Commitment for Change

Once the client passed through a "decision gate" (Rollnick & Morgan, 1995) and was more able to consider change (i.e., she was in the preparation stage of change), phase 2 of motivational interviewing could begin. As indicated in Table 2.3, during this phase, commitment to change is strengthened by examining different treatment options, creating precise plans, communicating free choice, developing a specific contract, and seeking verbal commitment.

Figure 2.2 shows a change plan that was developed with Ms. Davis. The plan makes explicit the basic elements of a therapeutic contract. The target problem is specified (Ms. Davis wants to stop using crack, and she wants to avoid situations that place her at risk). Motivators and incentives are identified (e.g., she wants to be a good parent who feels that she is in charge of her life). Action steps (e.g., attending a support group) and resource people (supporters) are identified (e.g., parents, clinician). Criteria for measuring success are pinpointed (e.g., remaining drug free, regaining child custody). Potential barriers to problem resolution and goal attainment are specified (e.g., contact with drug-using acquaintances, feeling discouraged).

Action plans represent sequential and incremental treatment contracts. Clients are encouraged to focus on areas that are the most important to them, the most crucial to recovery, and the most doable. As goals are accomplished, or if plans fail, new action plans are negotiated. Central to the process is a clinician's ability to help clients focus on areas that are likely to increase commitment to change. Clinicians repeatedly "check in" with clients to ensure that the plan is important and relevant, and they seek clients' feedback that reinforces their willingness to persist with their problem-solving efforts and move toward goal attainment.

INVOLVING FAMILY AND OTHER
SUPPORT NETWORK MEMBERS

Motivational interviewing focuses primarily on individual clients and underscores their responsibility and capacity for change. However, clinicians and researchers (O'Farrell, 1993) who study motivational interviewing rec-

The changes I want to make are:
I want to stop smoking crack, I want to learn how to resist the urges to smoke crack, and I want to stay away from people and places where I am tempted to smoke crack.

The most important reasons I want to make these changes are:
I want to be a good mother for my children. I want them to be proud of me. I want to feel like I can be in charge of my life.

The specific steps I plan to take are:
I will attend Cocaine Anonymous meetings every week.
I will join a support group at the clinic for women who are mothers and who have problems with drugs.
I will attend regular meetings with my therapist in which we will discuss my recovery, the problems I face, and my plans for handling those problems.

The ways others can help me are:

Person:	Possible ways to help:
My therapist	Meeting with me; helping me decide what to do
My parents	Giving me support and encouragement
CA members	Reminding me where I am and keeping me focused

Some things that could interfere with my plan are:
My former drug-using associates whom I have to avoid.
I need to stay confident and not get discouraged.

I will know if my plan is working if:
I stay drug free, I feel good about myself, and I am able to get my children back.

Client's Signature _____ Date: _____

Client's Signature _____ Date: _____

FIGURE 2.2. Change Plan Worksheet. Adapted from Riedel and Hanson (1998) and Miller, Zweben, DiClemente, and Rychtarik (1992).

ognize that its utility can be greatly enhanced by involving persons who are important to a client and supportive of recovery.

When exploring with clients whether or not to involve family or other social network members in the treatment, several factors should be assessed. First, clients must want the involvement of significant others. When clients are unwilling to involve other persons, pushing for such involvement may alienate clients and rupture the therapeutic process. Second, a client's "investment" in the other person must be determined. Research suggests that when clients are highly invested in particular social networks, there is a strong positive association between the amount of support they receive and positive therapeutic outcomes. When investment is low, social network members have relatively little impact on therapeutic outcomes (Longabaugh, Beattie, Wirtz, Noel, & Stout, 1995). Third, the significant others' attitudes toward substance use and treatment must be clarified. Ideally, only those significant others who are supportive of treatment and recovery should be involved in the treatment process. Fourth, the willingness and ability of the others to get involved in the treatment process must be determined. For example, the involvement of spouses who are contemplating divorce or siblings who have been badly "burned" by, and are bitter about, a person's addictive behaviors should be minimized until a clinician can rule out the possibility of any adverse consequences.

To maximize the benefits and to minimize disruptive aspects of involving significant others, it is essential to specify their precise roles in the treatment process (Burke, Vassilev, Kantchelov, & Zweben, 2002; Zweben & Barrett, 1993). Significant others can take on two primary roles—as witnesses or as active participants. In the witness role, they are asked only to share and receive information about the addiction and its consequences. This role is useful when clients are highly invested in these individuals but do not view their active involvement as important to recovery, or when those significant others have little desire to invest actively in the treatment process. Family members or friends who assume the role of active participant, in contrast, become directly involved in treatment planning and in strengthening the client's commitment to change. This role is appropriate when there is a higher level of interpersonal investment between the participants. The client still maintains primary responsibility, however, in determining the limits of these individuals' involvement.

When spouses and others have experienced a great deal of distress with the substance abuser, their involvement in treatment should be minimized or discouraged. In fact, it may be necessary to encourage them to disengage from the client, focus on their own concerns, and eliminate any enabling patterns in which they are involved.

CONCLUSION

This chapter has reviewed the concept of motivation in addiction treatment, and it has suggested that clinicians should take an active role in assessing clients' motivational readiness to change and in enhancing their motivational levels. Motivational interviewing is an empirically supported, client-centered clinical approach that provides a viable alternative to the more aggressive confrontational tactics that have been prominent in the addictions field for many years (Project MATCH, 1997, 1998). Through collaborative interaction that communicates empathy and understanding and encourages reasoned decision making, clients' motivation and commitment to changing addictive lifestyles can be strengthened.

Motivational interviewing seems to be especially well suited to primary care settings as well as any locations where clinicians encounter persons who are abusing alcohol or other drugs, but who are not seeking assistance for such problems, and who may be unaware of the impact of alcohol and other drugs on their lives. This interviewing format is also useful in child welfare (Hohman, 1998) and geriatric settings (Barry, Oslin, & Blow, 2001; Hanson & Gutheil, in press). It can be applied alone or used with other therapeutic strategies such as skill-building treatments, self-help approaches, and contingency management strategies.

Clinical practice is being shaped increasingly by managed care and other cost-containment efforts. Clinicians and clinical researchers must explore further the applicability of motivational enhancement strategies and other brief methods to ensure that clients receive quality treatment that will help them to live fulfilled lives. In particular, for whom brief motivational strategies are most useful must be determined as well as how these strategies can be adapted to make them responsive to the needs of a wide range of clients.

REFERENCES

Alcoholics Anonymous. (1957). *Alcoholics Anonymous comes of age: A brief history of AA*. New York: Alcoholics Anonymous World Services.

Applebaum, A. (1972). A critical re-examination of the concept of "motivation for change" in psychoanalytic treatment. *International Journal of Psychoanalysis, 53*, 51–59.

Bandura, A. (1997). *Self-efficacy: The exercise of control*. New York: Freeman.

Barber, J. G. (1994). *Social work with addictions*. New York: New York University Press.

Barber, J. G. (1995). Working with resistant drug abusers. *Social Work, 40*, 17–23.

Barry, K. L., Oslin, D. W., & Blow, F. C. (2001). *Alcohol problems in older adults: Prevention and management*. New York: Springer.

Bien, T. H., Miller, W. R., & Tonigan, J. S. (1993). Brief interventions for alcohol problems: A review. *Addiction, 88*, 315–336.

Breton, M. (1994). On the meaning of empowerment and empowerment-oriented social work practice. *Social Work with Groups, 17*(3), 23–37.

Burke, B. L., Vassilev, G., Kantchelov, A., & Zweben, A. (2002). Motivational interviewing with couples. In W. R. Miller & S. Rollnick, *Motivational interviewing: Preparing people for change* (2nd ed., pp. 347–361). New York: Guilford Press.

Chafetz, M. E. (1967). Motivation for recovery in alcoholism. In R. Fox (Ed.), *Alcoholism: behavioral research, therapeutic approaches* (pp. 110–117). New York: Springer.

Connors, G. J., Donovan, D. M., & DiClemente, C. C. (2001). *Substance abuse treatment and the stages of change: Selecting and planning interventions*. New York: Guilford Press.

Cox, W. M., Klinger, E., & Blount, J. P. (1991). Alcohol use and goal hierarchies: Systematic motivational counseling for alcoholics. In W. R. Miller & S. Rollnick, *Motivational interviewing: Preparing people to change addictive behavior* (pp. 260–271). New York: Guilford Press.

DiCicco, L., Unterberger, H., & Mack, J. E. (1978). Confronting denial: An alcoholism intervention strategy. *Psychiatric Annals, 8,* 596–606.

DiClemente, C. C., Fairhurst, S. K., & Piotrowski, N. A. (1995). The role of self-efficacy in addictive behaviors. In J. Maddux (Ed.), *Self-efficacy adaptation, and adjustment: Theory, research, and application* (pp. 109–142). New York: Plenum Press.

Gold, N. (1990). Motivation: The crucial but unexplored component of social work practice. *Social Work, 35,* 49–56.

Goldstein, E. G. (1995). *Ego psychology and social work practice* (2nd ed.). New York: Free Press.

Hanson, M., & Gutheil, I. A. (in press). Motivational strategies for alcohol-involved older adults: Implications for social work practice. *Social Work*.

Hester, R. K., & Bien, T. H. (1995). Brief treatment. In A. M. Washton (Ed.), *Psychotherapy and substance abuse: A practitioner's handbook* (pp. 204–222). New York: Guilford Press.

Higgins, S. T., & Silverman, K. (Eds.). (1999). *Motivating behavior change among illicit drug users: Research on contingency management interventions*. Washington, DC: American Psychological Association.

Hohman, M. M. (1998). Motivational interviewing: An intervention tool for child welfare case workers working with substance-abusing parents. *Child Welfare, 77,* 275–289.

Janis, J. L., & Mann, L. (1977). *Decision-making*. New York: Free Press.

Johnson, V. (1986). *Intervention: How to help someone who doesn't want help*. Minneapolis, MN: Johnson Institute Books.

Keller, M., McCormick, M., & Efron, V. (1982). *A dictionary of words on alcohol* (2nd ed.). New Brunswick, NJ: Rutgers Center of Alcohol Studies.

Kurtz, E. (1991). *Not God: A history of Alcoholics Anonymous*. Center City, MN: Hazelden Foundations.

Levin, J. D. (1991). *Recovery from alcoholism*. Northvale, NJ: Aronson.

Longabaugh, R., Beattie, M. C., Wirtz, P. W., Noel, N., & Stout, R. (1995). Matching treatment focus to patient social investment and support: 18–month follow-up results. *Journal of Consulting and Clinical Psychology, 63,* 296–307.

Marlatt, G. A. (1994). Addiction, mindfulness, and acceptance. In S. C. Hayes, N. S. Jacobson, V. M. Follette, & M. J. Dougher (Eds.), *Acceptance and change: Content and context in psychotherapy* (pp. 175–197). Reno, NV: Context Press.

Marlatt, G. A., Baer, J. S., & Quigley, L. A. (1995). Self-efficacy and addictive behavior. In A. Bandura (Ed.), *Self-efficacy in changing societies* (pp. 289–315). New York: Cambridge University Press.

Matza, D. (1969). *Becoming deviant*. Englewood Cliffs, NJ: Prentice-Hall.

Milam, J. R., & Ketcham, K. (1981). *Under the influence: A guide to the myths and realities of alcoholism.* Seattle, WA: Madrona.

Miller, G. A. (1999). *Learning the language of addiction counseling.* Boston: Allyn & Bacon.

Miller, S. D., Duncan, B. L., & Hubble, M. A. (1997). *Escape from Babel: Toward a unifying language for psychotherapy practice.* New York: Norton.

Miller, W. R. (1983). Motivational interviewing with problem drinkers. *Behavioural Psychotherapy, 11,* 147–172.

Miller, W. R. (1985). Motivation for treatment: A review with special emphasis on alcoholism. *Psychological Bulletin, 98,* 84–107.

Miller, W. R. (1995). Increasing motivation for change. In R. K. Hester & W. R. Miller (Eds.), *Handbook of alcoholism treatment approaches: Effective alternatives* (2nd ed., pp. 89–104). Boston: Allyn & Bacon.

Miller, W. R. (1996). Motivational interviewing: Research, practice, and puzzles. *Addictive Behaviors, 21,* 835–842.

Miller, W. R. (1998a). Enhancing motivation for change. In W. R. Miller & N. Heather (Eds.), *Treating addictive behaviors* (2nd ed., pp. 121–132). New York: Plenum Press.

Miller, W. R. (1998b). Why do people change addictive behavior? The 1996 H. David Archibald lecture. *Addiction, 93,* 163–172.

Miller, W. R., Andrews, N. R., Wilbourne, P., & Bennett, M. E. (1998). A wealth of alternatives: Effective treatments for alcohol problems. In W. R. Miller & N. Heather (Eds.), *Treating addictive behaviors* (2nd ed., pp. 203–216). New York: Plenum Press.

Miller, W. R., & Baca, L. M. (1983). Two-year follow-up of bibliotherapy and therapist-directed controlled drinking training for problem drinkers. *Behavior Therapy, 14,* 441–448.

Miller, W. R., Benefield, R. G., & Tonigan, J. S. (1993). Enhancing motivation to change in problem drinking: A controlled comparison of two therapist styles. *Journal of Consulting and Clinical Psychology, 61,* 455–461.

Miller, W. R., & Rollnick, S. (2002). *Motivational interviewing: Preparing people for change* (2nd ed.). New York: Guilford Press.

Miller, W. R., Taylor, C. A., & West, J. C. (1980). Focused versus broad spectrum behavior therapy for problem drinkers. *Journal of Consulting and Clinical Psychology, 48,* 590–601.

Miller, W. R., Zweben, A., DiClemente, C. C., & Rychtarik, R. G. (1992). *Motivational enhancement therapy manual* (Project MATCH Monograph Series, Vol. 2). Rockville, MD: National Institute on Alcohol Abuse and Alcoholism.

Najavits, L. M., & Weiss, R. D. (1994). Variations in therapist effectiveness in the treatment of patients with substance use disorders: An empirical review. *Addiction, 89,* 679–688.

Nelsen, J. (1980). Support: A necessary condition for change. *Social Work, 61,* 388–392.

O'Farrell, T. J. (1993). *Treating alcohol problems: Marital and family interventions.* New York: Guilford Press.

Oxley, G. B. (1966). The caseworker's expectations and client motivation. *Social Casework, 47,* 432–437.

Patterson, G. A., & Forgatch, M. S. (1985). Therapist behavior as a determinant for client noncompliance: A paradox for the behavior modifier. *Journal of Consulting and Clinical Psychology, 53,* 846–851.

Perlman, H. H. (1979). *Relationship.* Chicago: University of Chicago Press.

Prochaska, J. O., & DiClemente, C. C. (1982). Transtheoretical therapy: Toward a more integrative model of change. *Psychotherapy: Theory, Research, and Practice, 19,* 276–288.

Prochaska, J. O., DiClemente, C. C., & Norcross, J. C. (1992). In search of how people change: Applications to addictive behaviors. *American Psychologist, 47,* 1102–1114.

Project MATCH Research Group. (1997). Matching alcoholism treatments to client heterogeneity: Project MATCH posttreatment drinking outcomes. *Journal of Studies on Alcohol, 58,* 7–29.

Project MATCH Research Group. (1998). Matching alcoholism treatments to client heterogeneity: Project MATCH three-year drinking outcomes. *Alcoholism: Clinical and Experimental Research, 22,* 1300–1311.

Riedel, M., & Hanson, M. (1998, May). *Motivational interviewing: Differential responses by women and men.* Workshop presented at 30th Annual Alcoholism Institute, National Association of Social Workers, New York City Chapter, New York.

Ripple, L., Alexander, E., & Polemis, B. (1964). *Motivation, capacity and opportunity.* Social Science Monographs. Chicago: University of Chicago Press.

Rollnick, S., & Miller, W. R. (1995). What is motivational interviewing? *Behavioural and Cognitive Psychotherapy, 23,* 325–334.

Rollnick, S., & Morgan, M. (1995). Motivational interviewing: Increasing readiness for change. In A. M. Washton (Ed.), *Psychotherapy and substance abuse* (pp. 179–191). New York: Guilford Press.

Roman, P. M. (1981). From employee alcoholism to employee assistance: Deemphasis on prevention and alcohol problems in work-based programs. *Journal of Studies on Alcohol, 42,* 244–272.

Schilling, R. F., El-Bassel, N., Finch, J. B., Roman, R. J., & Hanson, M. (2002). Motivational interviewing to encourage self-help participation following alcohol detoxification. *Research on Social Work Practice, 12,* 711–730.

Scott, M. (1989). *A cognitive-behavioural approach to clients' problems.* London: Tavistock/Routledge.

Shea, S. C. (1998). *Psychiatric interviewing: The art of understanding* (2nd ed.). Philadelphia: Saunders.

Sterne, M. W., & Pittman, D. J. (1965). The concept of motivation: A source of institutional and professional blockage in the treatment of alcoholics. *Quarterly Journal of Studies on Alcohol, 26,* 41–57.

Thomas, E. J., Polansky, N. A., & Kounin, J. (1967). The expected behavior of a potentially helpful person. In E. J. Thomas (Ed.), *Behavioral science for social workers* (pp. 313–321). New York: Free Press.

Tiebout, H. M. (1957). The ego factor in surrendering to alcoholism. *Quarterly Journal of Studies on Alcohol, 15,* 610–621.

Velasquez, M. M., Maurer, G. G., Crouch, C., & DiClemente, C. C. (2001). *Group treatment for substance abuse: A stages-of-change therapy manual.* New York: Guilford Press.

White, R. K., & Wright, D. G. (1998). *Addiction intervention: Strategies to motivate treatment-seeking behavior.* New York: Haworth Press.

White, R. W. (1959). Motivation reconsidered: The concept of competence. *Psychological Review, 66,* 297–333.

Whitfield, C. L. (1984). Stress management and spirituality during recovery: A transpersonal approach. *Alcoholism Treatment Quarterly, 1*(4), 1–54.

Wright, J. H., & Davis, D. (1994). The therapeutic relationship in cognitive-behavioral therapy: Patient perceptions and therapist responses. *Cognitive and Behavioral Practice, 1,* 25–45.

Yablonsky, L. (1967). *Synanon: The tunnel back.* Baltimore: Penguin Books.

Zweben, A., & Barrett, D. (1993). Brief couples treatment for alcohol problems. In T. J. O'Farrell (Ed.), *Treating alcohol problems: Marital and family interventions* (pp. 353–380). New York: Guilford Press.

CHAPTER 3

The Clinical Practice of Harm Reduction

Belinda Housenbold Seiger

Harm reduction is a public health model that has been utilized successfully throughout the world to reduce the harm associated with chemical dependence. This model allows for broad-based treatment outcomes that do not insist upon abstinence as the sole measure of success. This form of intervention initially gained visibility in the United States as a result of the need to curtail the spread of HIV/AIDS and other blood-borne illnesses associated with intravenous drug use. Harm reduction has been successfully expanded and applied as a clinical intervention for individuals with a variety of substance use problems.

Some manifestations of harm reduction may initially seem novel or even surprising to social work clinicians accustomed to the predominant disease model of assessment and intervention. However, the principles of harm reduction share the same client-centered values as those espoused by the social work profession. The underlying concepts and clinical skills are congruent with biopsychosocial and psychodynamic principles, and integrate easily with cognitive, ego, and relational psychology, making it a valuable resource for social work clinicians. This chapter introduces the theoretical underpinnings and principles of harm reduction and provides a case example illustrating clinical interventions conducted within this perspective.

DEFINITION AND PRINCIPLES
OF HARM REDUCTION

Harm reduction has been referred to as a paradigm shift, an emergent philosophy, a new treatment approach, and a novel perspective (Erickson, 1995; Marlatt, 1998; Single, 1995b). Whichever label best describes it, harm reduction is theoretically grounded in a model of public health that subscribes to a set of assumptions over a century old. These assumptions include the acceptance of drug use, including alcohol and illicit substances, in our culture as a reality. Although not condoning usage, the public health perspective seeks to reduce or ameliorate the health risks associated with the use of alcohol and other drugs on the individual and the community at large. The public health model provides the foundation for emphasis on improving communal and individual health in relation to substance abuse (Erickson, 1995). The specific emphasis of harm reduction is on reducing the negative consequences of substance abuse by employing practical, achievable goals aimed at the safer use of drugs and the minimization of the harmful effects associated with continued drug use. Although this approach may lead to, or include the possibility of, abstinence, it does not require it. The issue of abstinence in relation to harm reduction can be somewhat confusing. Some clinicians view the values underlying harm reduction and those of abstinence as being on opposite ends of the continuum of care. Others, however, view abstinence (i.e., the total cessation of use) as one of several means of minimizing the problems associated with drug use and therefore encompassed under the umbrella of "harm reduction."

The harm reduction model expands the definition of success to include the many smaller steps that may precede or replace abstinence. The essence of harm reduction was encapsulated in a 1988 presentation by Newcombe and Parry, who described it as a "user-friendly" attempt to attract drug users to a variety of services while simultaneously empowering and possibly motivating them to change their substance-using behavior. Priority is placed on encouraging substance abusers' access to and utilization of social, health, and other community services. Harm reduction is also characterized by the belief that it is possible to encourage drug users to modify their behavior and the conditions in which they use substances in order to reduce some of the serious risks that drugs pose to individual and public health and safety (MacCoun, 1997; Zinberg, 1984).

G. Alan Marlatt (1998), a pioneer in the field of clinically applied harm reduction, provides a concise articulation of the primary values guiding this paradigm. In the spirit of public health, he views harm reduction as a viable alternative to the moral/criminal and disease models of drug use and addiction. According to Marlatt, harm reduction recognizes the benefits of abstinence as an ideal outcome but accepts that there may be incremental steps to reducing the harm associated with continued use. He emphasizes the advantages of involving substance users in the planning and advocacy of programs on their own behalf. This successful "bottom-up" approach contrasts with "top-down" judicial approaches in which administrators and policymakers prescribe what is best for the entire population of substance users. Harm reduction promotes low-threshold access to services as an alternative to traditional approaches that frequently make it difficult for active users by requiring abstinence or other lifestyle changes. Finally, according to Marlatt and others, harm reduction is based on "compassionate pragmatism," not moralistic idealism (Marlatt, 1998).

Some of the guiding concepts of harm reduction have been outlined by the Harm Reduction Coalition (www.harmreduction.org) as the following:

- accepts, for better and for worse, that licit and illicit drug use are part of our world and chooses to work to minimize the harmful effects rather than simply ignore or condemn them
- ensures that drug users and those with a history of drug use routinely have a real voice in the creation of programs and policies designed to serve them, and both affirms and seeks to strengthen the capacity of people who use drugs to reduce the various harms associated with their drug use
- understands drug use as a complex, multi-faceted phenomenon that encompasses a continuum of behaviors from severe abuse to total abstinence, and acknowledges that some ways of using drugs are clearly safer than others.
- establishes that the quality of communal and individual life can be improved not only by the cessation of use, but by a variety of intermediate changes in use
- calls for the non-judgmental, non-coercive provision of services and resources to people who use drugs and to the communities in which they live in order to assist them in reducing attendant harms
- recognizes that the realities of poverty, class, racism, social isolation, past trauma, sex-based discrimination and other social inequalities affect both people's vulnerability to and capacity for effectively dealing with drug-related harms
- does not attempt to minimize or ignore the many real and tragic harms and dangers associated with licit and illicit drug use.

THE EMERGENCE OF HARM REDUCTION

The predominant treatment model for substance abuse/dependence in the United States since the 1930s has been the abstinence-based disease approach derived from the 12 steps of Alcoholics Anonymous (Musto, 1997). Nonetheless, harm reduction has existed since the 1960s and was the underlying premise for the establishment of methadone maintenance treatment programs in the United States (Musto, 1997; Nadlemann, 1998b). In addition to methadone maintenance, the other most commonly recognized example of the harm reduction strategy is syringe exchange. Despite ongoing controversy, increasing attention has been paid to harm reduction during the past decade, given the association between HIV/AIDS and drug use, particularly injected drug use, and the increasing need for risk reduction among this cohort (Roche, Evans, & Stanton, 1997; Single, 1995a; Springer, 1991).

The HIV/AIDS epidemic had an impact on all health care providers by highlighting the risks associated with substance use. As a result of grassroots organization and advocacy, primarily accomplished by at-risk individuals, health care providers were forced to reevaluate the abstinence-only approach to the provision of services to high-risk and HIV-positive, substance-using clients who were unable or unwilling to become abstinent but were in need of services nevertheless. Harm reduction, a public health model already in place throughout Europe, Australia, and Canada, was seen as offering effective strategies for reducing the harm associated with substance use (DesJarlais, Friedman, Peyser, & Newman, 1995).

Harm reduction has since been adapted as an intervention for binge drinking and other forms of alcohol abuse, crack and cocaine dependence, as well as polysubstance usage in a myriad of settings, including private psychotherapy practice (Hill, 1998; Marlatt, Larimer, Baer, & Quigley, 1993; Tatarsky, 1998). Empirical studies point to the effectiveness of its strategies in reducing substance abuse, associated medical harmful effects, such as HIV and hepatitis, and drug-related crimes (DesJarlais et al., 1996; Marlatt et al., 1993).

COMPATIBLE VALUES: HARM REDUCTION AND SOCIAL WORK

Social workers, like most other health care providers, were introduced to the harm reduction model in the context of AIDS prevention and risk reduction strategies. Although often viewed as conflicting with the traditional drug-free missions of most substance abuse treatment agencies in which social workers are employed, harm reduction actually shares fundamental values with those guiding social work practice. Both emphasize client self-determination, empowerment, and a sense of agency associated with clients' active involvement in their own treatment planning.

Social workers are traditionally taught that the point of entry into the client system begins "where the client is"; often, stepping in on this level may entail the provision of concrete services to clients in order to allow time for engagement and the establishment of rapport between the clinician and client. Respect for the individual's freedom and his or her right to choose the intervention goals are values that underlie both the social work and the harm reduction perspectives. Harm reduction recognizes that some chemically abusing/dependent individuals are unable or unwilling to become abstinent from some, or all, drug use at present. Nevertheless, such persons may require health care services, concrete assistance, or other social work intervention. Coinciding with the edict to begin where the client is at, harm reduction seeks to identify clients' objectives and to engage them at their current level of motivation. Consequently, harm reduction programs offer interventions that enhance clients' motivation to reduce the harms of their drug-taking behavior even while they are still using substances. Harm reduction thus "lowers the threshold" (Denning, 2000, p. xii; Marlatt, 1998) for obtaining services by not requiring abstinence as a criterion for receiving assistance.

Such efforts to minimize obstacles to accessing necessary services are also a long-standing value of the social work profession. At times, the disease model has negatively impacted this premise by prohibiting or limiting access to services for individuals who are active substance users. As pointed out by a social worker who is also a pioneer in the field of harm reduction,

> there is a belief in the (traditional) drug treatment world... that active users cannot benefit from any other intervention except treatment leading to abstinence . . . you can provide education, assistance with strategy development, risk-reduction interventions and support . . . and drug users can certainly benefit from the provision of concrete services. (Springer, 1991, pp. 142–144)

The harm reduction model challenges the stigmatizing view of substance abusers and encourages a differential view of each individual and his or her unique circumstances, rather than a one-size-fits-all treatment approach. It includes the concepts of mutuality and reciprocity and the involvement of users/clients in the development of programs and treatment planning on their own behalf. This transactional aspect of the relationship between helpers and clients is one that social work has always considered relevant.

APPLICATION OF THE PUBLIC HEALTH MODEL

The public health approach to substance use and chemical dependency incorporates an interdisciplinary perspective that draws on epidemiology, pharmacology, toxicology, and social and medical sciences to conceptualize alcohol and other drug (AOD) problems. It provides an alternative approach to the war on drugs by designing user-friendly approaches to AOD problems.

The popularity of public health concepts applied to substance abuse emerged in response to the HIV/AIDS epidemic. In support of the grassroots organization and self-advocacy of drug users, public health advocates stepped to the forefront of the movement that instigated the syringe exchange programs (SEPs). This was the first time in the United States that injecting drug users became vocal advocates for services on their own behalf. The harm reduction perspective reflected a change in thinking about drug problems from one of individual psychological or moral inadequacies to one that focused on the external factors that contribute to drug use and the resultant threats to public health (Erickson, 1990). Models of the public health approach of harm reduction in action can be seen in condom distribution programs in high schools and the step-down approach to smoking cessation.

THEORETICAL UNDERPINNINGS OF THE HARM REDUCTION MODEL

Since harm reduction is not a unified paradigm in itself, it is impossible to identify a single theoretical influence that has shaped this perspective as it exists today. Rather, there have been, and continue to be, numerous influences that contribute to this emerging framework. An author who recently coined the term "harm reduction psychotherapy" considers harm reduction to be a "holistic perspective which incorporates psychodynamic as well as cognitive influences" (Denning, 2000, p. xiii).

Harm reduction remains close to its grass-roots origins in its humanistic, client-centered philosophy. It relies on seminal ideas from the client-centered psychology of Carl Rogers (1951), from the motivational interviewing techniques of Miller and Rollnick (1991), and from the transtheoretical stages-of-change process described by Prochaska and DiClemente (1982). The latter two approaches have assisted in operationalizing harm reduction principles into practical strategies and interventions.

Prochaska and DiClemente (1982) and Miller and Rollnick (1991) provide two models for the assessment of, and intervention with, substance users who may not be motivated to change their drug-taking behavior, or who may be at an early stage in the process of change. These models emphasize the clinical task of matching interventions to the motivational level of the client. An integrated model of harm reduction allows for the incorporation of motivational and abstinence-based strategies as one aspect of a larger plan guided by client-centered values.

As more and more mental health providers become aware of the clinical usefulness of harm reduction, they contribute their own theoretical interpretations and methodology, thereby enhancing the theory and practice in this area. For example, the underlying values of harm reduction have gained some recognition among contemporary relational psychoanalysts who recognize that its primary concepts are congruent with object relations and self psychology models of change. Cognitive-behavioral psychologists are also potential partners, given their emphasis on the complex processes of human motivation and behavioral change.

Interventions based on harm reduction are user friendly and designed to increase the opportunity for substance abusers to come into contact with services that are provided within a trusting milieu. For example, harm reduction programs for adolescents may be integrated into an after-school program that also provides meals or transportation home; or programs for sex workers are offered in a mobile van on the streets where they work and may include showers and basic health care amenities. A harm reduction program for single mothers may offer a drop-in child-care center and family style meals along with counseling for substance abuse.

Motivational interviewing questions a common assumption made in the chemical dependency field that "resistance is the result of pernicious personality traits (e.g., 'denial'), and that clients are inherently unmotivated to change" (Miller & Rollnick, 1991, p. 14). Rather, research evidence points to nonspecific factors that serve as determinants of change. The therapist's style is one of the main nonspecific factors impacting motivation and therapeutic outcomes. From this perspective, motivation, rather than being a fixed personality trait, is viewed as a "state of readiness or eagerness to change which may fluctuate from one time or situation to another. This state is one that can be influenced" (Miller & Rollnick, 1991, p. 14). Influencing and encouraging motivational levels within a client-centered relational context contributes to the clinical process of harm reduction strategies. Although the actual means of achieving harm reduction are borrowed from motivational interviewing, the stages of change model, public health strategies, and behavioral psychology, the approach is not limited to these methods. There is room within harm reduction to incorporate abstinence- and sobriety-enhancing approaches such as trigger recognition and relapse prevention. In this light, harm reduction can be viewed as a transtheoretical model or an integrative approach to intervening with individuals who have substance use problems.

Prochaska and DiClemente (1982) conceptualized a circular model of how change occurs, whether with or without therapeutic assistance. They understand that change takes place in identifiable stages common to all behavioral patterns about which individuals are ambivalent. The six stages—precontemplation, contemplation, determination, action, maintenance (or permanent exit), and relapse—are conceptualized as a wheel of change to convey the cyclical nature of this process. From this perspective, it is considered normal for individuals to go around in the circle of stages several times before a commitment to change is established and the new behavior is maintained. Slips and relapse are understood as normal phases in the process of change. Each slip or relapse is viewed as bringing the individual closer to the next stage of change, not as a failure. In this model, the therapist helps clients remain hopeful about their progress and ability to change rather than feel discouraged and demoralized about slipping.

INCLUSION OF PSYCHODYNAMIC PERSPECTIVES

Although many harm reduction pioneers had no understanding of object relations, psychodynamics, self psychology, or intersubjectivity, they did recognize that the drugs served many functions for individuals who abused them. From a therapeutic perspective, it is useful to understand psychodynamic theory, which, like harm reduction, allows for the exploration of the presenting symptom of substance abuse without making abstinence a requirement for receiving treatment services.

The works of Wurmser (1978) and Khantzian (1995, 1997), in addition to the self psychology theory of Kohut (1971), provide a conceptual framework for understanding how substance abuse/dependence may serve a compensatory role in the maintenance of self-esteem and affect regulation. According to Khantzian (1997), substance abusers suffer not only from the fragmentation of the self but also from the defenses they employ to cover these deficits. He views the drug of choice for each individual as pertinent to an understanding of the flaws in the self structure and the associated affects against which the individual defends. Khantzian perceives the ongoing addiction not as an attempt at self-destruction but rather as a desperate attempt to *care for* the self. The first priority of treatment for substance-abusing individuals is to assure their "comfort, safety and control." He advocates for a combination of "therapeutic elements (clinical and self-help) in meeting such patients' needs . . . [and recommends that] clinicians play multiple roles and be flexible to assure that patient needs are met" (Khantzian, 1997, pp. 97–98). Khantzian's view that most substance-abusing individuals are able to benefit from a psychoanalytically oriented approach stems from his belief that substance abusers possess a range of psychological capacities, which, in his view, has often been underestimated. This concept of substance abuse/dependency treatment allows for the empathic acceptance of individuals' drug use or alcohol as their attempt at self-regulation, while also leaving room for reducing the harm associated with the substance use and forging a potential therapeutic rapport. Thus this perspective parallels the underlying principles of harm reduction and offers theoretical legitimacy for the harm reduction approach as a valuable psychodynamic tool.

Wurmser's (1978) views also may be seen as consistent with those of harm reduction, because he did not believe that a disease called *alcoholism* existed, nor did he subscribe to the concept of the addictive personality or the one-treatment-fits-all approach (Sashin, 1995). Other psychodynamic theorists recognize the necessity to understand substance-abusing individuals' lives and the role of the substance to them as a precursor to embarking on behavior change. In this view, failure to acknowledge the value of the substance *to the individual* can—and does—thwart their recovery (Dodes, 1995).

CASE ILLUSTRATION

Jan is a 29-year-old single woman who self-referred to treatment because of her increasing difficulty managing the stress she experienced in her job. Her symptoms included frequent headaches, difficulty sleeping, and a general feeling of malaise and lethargy.

Jan works as a financial analyst in a large corporation and has a great deal of responsibility in her position. Her family immigrated to the United States from South America when Jan was about 2 years old. She was the older of two children.

Jan lives in a large city where she has many friends. She described an active lifestyle with many activities outside of work, yet she regularly experiences a sense of isolation and disconnection from other people. Most, if not all, of Jan's social activities involve drinking and sometimes cocaine usage.

Exploration revealed that Jan had had at least two periods of clinical depression in the past. The most recent occurred when she was a graduate student 6 years ago. At that time she sought counseling through the university health center and was prescribed an antidepressant, which she took for about 3 months. She stated that she was drinking quite frequently at the time as well as experimenting with other drugs and that she had felt concern about mixing the antidepressants and the recreational drugs, so she discontinued the medication. Jan clearly articulated her understanding that she had used many of these substances as an attempt to escape from feelings of depression. She was concerned that she might be returning to this pattern because she had been feeling stressed and slightly depressed again

Jan was highly motivated to reveal the details of her current substance use, and she readily verbalized concern about her behavior. She described herself as a recreational cocaine user who also drank to mitigate the effects of too much coke. She also drank when she had not used cocaine in an attempt to get to sleep. At times Jan would use cocaine at work when she knew that she would be working very late. She observed that many of her colleagues also relied on cocaine or other drugs to get them through the demanding work hours. Most of Jan's drinking was done socially, and she commented that "everyone" seemed to drink as much as she did. She was somewhat confused about whether she was actually drinking too much or not, even though she had described becoming so drunk on several occasions that she was uncertain as to how she had gotten home.

The initial assessment included obtaining information about types and amount of substances used and usage patterns. Jan seemed concerned about her cocaine use because she was using it more regularly then she would have liked and she associated her use to work stress and underlying depression. Jan also articulated some concern about her alcohol use but was admittedly less concerned about that habit. She felt that her substance use had not affected her productivity at work, and she was free to work at home and often worked irregular hours.

While conducting the assessment, the therapist explored Jan's ambivalence about the consequences of her substance use in contrast to the pleasures associated with it. Jan viewed the negative consequences of her substance use as an increasing feeling of dependence on the cocaine to stay up very late and maintain a high level of focus, and the cycle of depression that followed the high. Regarding her alcohol use, Jan regretted having had several unsafe sexual encounters while drunk or high and was concerned about contracting a sexually transmitted disease, particularly AIDS.

As emphasized by the harm reduction model, the clinician attempted to elicit Jan's concerns rather than prematurely expressing judgment about her behavior or issuing edicts about her need to become abstinent from all usage. The assessment also included identifying Jan's location on the wheel of change, or the stages of change, set forth by Prochaska and DiClemente (1982). Jan's views about where she was on the wheel of change were considered along with the clinician's.

Determining whether Jan was in the precontemplation, contemplation, preparation, or action stage allowed the clinician to ask questions about her motivational level rather than make treatment decisions and suggestions that she might have rejected. After several sessions, it was clear that Jan was in the contemplation stage, which is characterized by the "yes-but" feeling. During this phase, the therapist assesses the benefits and disadvantages of the client's substance use and encourages the client to express any concerns and ambivalence about such use (Denning, 2000). The goal is to amplify the client's ambivalence and subjective discomfort about substance use without prematurely confronting him or her and eliciting the reaction that is then labeled as "resistance." Such assessment and exploration was the initial focus of the first 4–6 months of the clinical work with Jan.

Over several months, Jan became more certain that she wanted to make a change in her drug-taking behavior; however, she was uncertain as to what change would be. Initially, she decided to cut down on her drinking but was not sure how she would change her life to support that decision. This uncertainty characterized Jan's preparation stage of change. She indicated the desire to change, was imagining what the change would look like, and actually experimented with cutting down. However, Jan's behavior had really not changed in any conclusive way. The clinician then asked Jan to imagine what her life would be like if she did make the changes she mentioned. Eliciting both positive and negative aspects of the proposed change and assisting the client in creating a decisional balance that highlighted her ambivalence allowed both clinician and client to identify the obstacles to change.

For several weeks Jan experimented with moderating her alcohol intake, but it became obvious to her that her difficulty sleeping and her increasing cocaine usage were even bigger problems then she had initially realized. To change her behavior, she realized that she needed to acknowledge her depression and the interpersonal issues troubling her in parallel with looking at her substance use. During weekly or biweekly sessions during the preparation stage of change, underlying psychodynamic issues of depression, perfectionistic work standards, and Jan's feelings of disappointment in her achievements were addressed. Some sessions focused specifically on her substance use and her own growing perception of her lack of control over both the cocaine and the alcohol use. Stress management methods, relaxation techniques, and cognitive reframing were also introduced.

Jan's motivation to change her drug-use patterns gradually increased. She experimented with cutting down her alcohol consumption or not using cocaine during the workday. Psychiatric evaluation was recommended to address her depression. However, Jan was quite ambivalent about taking that step because she viewed the need for antidepressant medication as a sign of weakness. Each session contained a period in which Jan discussed her substance use during the prior week and described her depressive symptoms. Her ability to identify and manage overwhelming feelings, particularly those associated with her job and interpersonal relations, improved throughout this period. Harm reduction principles were utilized to reduce the risks associated with Jan's drinking and cocaine use, even while she continued to use these substances. Initially, Jan decided to limit the number of drinks that she would allow herself, and she was able to stick to that commitment. She also decided not to purchase any more cocaine but to use up the amount that she had already bought. Safer-sex practices were discussed and options for carrying them out were explored. Jan also agreed to see a psychiatrist for a consultation to discuss her depressive symptoms. The clinician also proposed inpatient detoxification as an option, should that become necessary.

At one point, about 5 months into treatment, Jan had several very difficult weeks in which she lost control over her use of cocaine. This bingeing was followed by her decision to stop using cocaine completely. She was also successful in cutting down on her alcohol use for about 3 weeks. Jan then began drinking more alcohol than she had planned, and she was disappointed in herself. Rather than focusing solely on Jan's self-directed disappointment, however, the clinician assisted Jan in exploring the changes she had already made and those she hoped to make.

The treatment with Jan had progressed for approximately 1 year before she reached the action stage of change characterized by a commitment to altering her behavior. At this point she decided that an inpatient detoxification process would be helpful to her, and she entered an inpatient unit at a hospital for that purpose. It was during that period that Jan was able to come to terms with her need for antidepressants and increased support for making the changes she identified as necessary for herself. These changes included abstinence from all substances and involvement in a cognitive-behavioral support group addressing coping skills and relapse triggers. Jan also decided to attend Alcoholics Anonymous meetings as part of her treatment plan.

Jan's commitment to utilize various treatment options to maintain her progress points to the maintenance stage on the wheel of change. Throughout the treatment process, the stance of the clinician remained one of partnership, interest, and respect for the client's varying levels of motivation to change.

This case illustrates how harm reduction principles may inform the selection of treatment options and allow for an integration of therapeutic elements that are useful to a particular client. In this particular case, attention was given to reducing the harm associated with Jan's substance use even while she continued to use alcohol and cocaine. Simultaneously, the balance between her level of ambivalence and motivation for change was constantly aligned with her self-determined goals. Of course, not all clients end up concluding that abstinence is the best way for them to reduce the risks associated with their drug use; however, in this case, that is what Jan chose for herself.

It is a challenge for each clinician to work within the individual client's process and to devise treatment goals in accordance with that client's motivational level and readiness for change. By providing a smorgasbord of treatment options that may include moderation, stress management and relaxation techniques, cognitive-behavioral intervention, 12-step programs, harm reduction support groups, psychopharmacology, or any combination of these approaches, clients may feel empowered to choose what works for them rather than feeling forced to fit into only one perspective that may not be an ideal match for them. It is worth noting that according to Denning (2000), between 50 and 80% of clients actually choose abstinence on their own, even when other options are made available to them.

TRANSFERENCE ISSUES IN CLINICAL HARM REDUCTION SETTINGS

For most clinicians who are trained in the disease model and abstinence-only approach, utilizing harm reduction methods can be somewhat anxiety provoking, especially if they do not have collegial support for this perspective. Even experienced clinicians cannot help feeling somewhat ambivalent about the process, because it does not take a predictable route or have a prescribed set of steps to follow. For example, the clinician's countertransference reactions throughout the process of working with Jan included fears of enabling her to continue using substances, concerns about her well-being, shared excitement at her insights, and occasional impatience and frustration with the fluctuations that punctuated her process of change.

CONCLUSION

Working with clients who continue to use drugs can elicit powerful feelings on the part of most clinicians. Challenging the status quo to the abstinence-based model of working with substance-abusing clients requires a commitment to a larger vision of success. The harm reduction approach provides an opportunity for social workers to explore empirically proven public health methods for reducing the harm when clients continue to use or abuse substances. This method allows for the achievement of incremental steps toward improved client self-care, which may eventually include abstinence from alcohol and other drugs. Clients are viewed as consumers who are an integral part of the intervention process and therefore included, from the beginning of treatment, in the tasks of choosing the goals and methods of interaction. Coercion is avoided, although specific recommendations (such as attending a support group) may be offered (Peele, Bufe, & Brodsky, 2000).

Certainly harm reduction is controversial and has been criticized for its lack of structure, although this is changing thanks to the recent publication of several excellent resource books. To some degree, some of these criticisms may be valid. However, in light of the fact that an abstinence-only approach does not work for many clients, the use of harm reduction in clinical practice with substance-abusing clients offers an additional approach that can be incorporated into our proverbial toolboxes. Questions about how to define treatment goals, concerns regarding what supervisors or colleagues might think about working with clients who are still using drugs, and a lack of institutional support remain stressful for clinicians attempting to incorporate the harm reduction model into their own practices. Collegial and supervisory support is essential in managing these feelings and in providing a forum for learning new applications of harm reduction methodology.

REFERENCES

Bayer, R., & Oppenheim, G. (1993). *Confronting drug policy.* New York: Cambridge University Press.

Brehm, N., & Khantzian, E. (1997). Psychodynamics. In J. Lowinson, P. Ruiz, R. Millman, & J. Langrod (Eds.), *Substance abuse: A comprehensive textbook* (3rd ed., pp. 90–99). Baltimore: Williams & Wilkins.

Burke, A., & Clapp, J. (1997a). Ideology and social work practice in substance abuse settings. *Social Work, 42*(6), 552–562.

Burke, A., & Clapp, J. (1997b). Supervisor ideology and organizational response: HIV/AIDS prevention in outpatient substance abuse treatment units. *Administration in Social Work, 21*(1), 49–64.

Carey, K. (1996). Substance use reduction in the context of outpatient psychiatric treatment: A collaborative, motivational, harm reduction approach. *Community Mental Health Journal, 32*(3), 291–306.

Davies, D. L. (1962). Normal drinking in recovered alcohol addicts. *Quarterly Journal of Studies on Alcohol, 23*, 94–104.

Denning, P. (2000). *Practicing harm reduction psychotherapy: An alternative approach to addictions.* New York: Guilford Press.

DesJarlais, D. (1993). Systems issues. In R. Robertson (Ed.), *Management of drug users in the community* (pp. 39–53). London: Arnold Press.

DesJarlais, D., Benny, J., Marmor, M., Paone, D., Titus, S., Shi, Q., Perlis, T., & Friedman, S. (1996). HIV incidence among injecting drug users in New York City syringe-exchange programmes. *Lancet, 348,* 987–991.

DesJarlais, D., & Friedman, S. R. (1993). AIDS, injecting drug use and harm reduction. In N. Heather, A. Wodak, E. Nadelmann, & P. O'Hare (Eds.), *Psychoactive drugs and harm reduction: From faith to science* (pp. 297–309). London: Whurr.

DesJarlais, D., Hagan, H., & Friedman, S. (1997). Epidemiology and Emerging Public Health Perspectives. In J. Lowinson, P. Ruiz, R. Millman, & J. Langrod (Eds.), *Substance abuse: A comprehensive textbook* (pp. 591–596). Baltimore: Williams & Wilkins.

DesJarlais, D., Marmor, M., Paone, D., Titus, S., Shi, Q., Perlis, T., et al. (1996). HIV incidence among injecting drug users in New York City syringe exchange programs. *The Lancet, 348,* 987–991.

DesJarlais, D., Paone D., Friedman, S., Peyser, N., & Newman, R. (1995). Regulating controversial programs for unpopular people: Methadone maintenance and syringe exchange programs. *American Journal of Public Health, 85,* 1577–1584.

Diwan, S. (1990). Alcoholism and ideology: Approaches to treatment. *Journal of Applied Social Sciences, 14*(2), 221–246.

Dodes, L. (1995). Psychic helplessness and the psychology of addiction. In S. Dowling (Ed.), *The psychology and treatment of addictive behavior* (American Psychoanalytic Association Monograph 8, pp. 133–145). Madison, WI: International Universities Press.

Drake, R. (1996). Substance abuse reduction among patients with severe mental illness. *Community Mental Health Journal, 32*(3), 311–314.

Drucker, E., & Hantman, J. (1995a). Harm reduction drug policies and practice: International developments and domestic initiatives. *Bulletin of the New York Academy of Medicine, 72*(2), 335–338.

Drucker, E., & Hantman, J. (1995b). Harm reduction: A public health strategy. *Current Issues in Public Health, 1,* 64–70.

Duncan, D., Nicholson, T., Clifford, P., Hawkins, W., & Petosa, R. (1994). Harm reduction: An emerging new paradigm for drug education. *Journal of Drug Education, 24*(4), 281–290.

Dupont, R. (1990). A public health approach to demand reduction. *Journal of Drug Issues, 20*(4), 563–575.

Dupont, R. (1995). Harm reduction: What it is and is not. *Drug and Alcohol Review, 14*, 283–285.

Dupont, R. (1996). Harm Reduction and decriminalization in the United States: A personal perspective. *Substance Use and Misuse, 31*(4), 1929–1945.

Erickson, P. (1990). A public health approach to demand reduction. *Journal of Drug Abuse Issues, 20*(4), 563–575.

Erickson, P. (1995). Harm reduction: What it is and is not. *Drug and Alcohol Review, 14*, 283–285.

Fingarette, H. (1988). *Heavy drinking: The myth of alcoholism as a disease.* Berkeley: University of California Press.

Freeman, E. M. (1992). *The addiction process: Effective social work approaches.* New York: Longman.

Hart, P. (1994). *Americans see the drug problem as bad and getting worse.* Unpublished paper. Washington, DC: Peter D. Hart Research Associates.

Hawks, D., & Simon, L. (1995). Harm reduction in Australia: Has it worked? A review. *Drug and Alcohol Review, 14*, 291–304.

Heaney, C., & Burke, A. (1995). Ideologies of care in community residential services: What do caregivers believe? *Community Mental Health Journal, 31*(5), 449–462

Heather, N. (1995). Groundwork for a research program on harm reduction in alcohol and drug treatment. *Drug and Alcohol Review, 14*, 331–336.

Hill, A. (1998). Applying harm reduction to services for substance-using women in violent relationships. *Issues of Substance, 3*(3), 1–13.

Hubbard, R. L. (1989). *Drug abuse treatment: A national study of effectiveness.* Chapel Hill: University of North Carolina Press.

Imhof, E. M. (1960). *The disease concept of alcoholism.* New Haven, CT: Hillhouse Press.

Jonas, S. (1997). Public health approaches. In P. Lowinson, P. Ruiz, R. Millman, & J. Langrod (Eds.), *Substance abuse: A comprehensive textbook* (pp. 775–785). Baltimore: Williams & Wilkins.

Khantzian, E. (1995). Self-regulation vulnerabilities in substance abusers: Treatment implications. In S. Dowling (Ed.), *The psychology and treatment of addictive behavior* (American Psychoanalytic Association, Monograph 8, pp. 17–41). Madison, WI: International Universities Press.

Khantzian, E. (1997). The self medication hypotheses of substance use disorders: A reconsideration and recent applications. *Harvard Review of Psychiatry, 4*, 231–244.

Klingman, H. (1991). The motivation for change from problem alcohol and heroin use. *British Journal of Addiction, 86*, 727–744.

Klingman, H. (1997). Drug treatment in Switzerland: Harm reduction, decentralization and community response. *Addiction, 91*(5), 723–736.

Kochems, L., Paone, D., DesJarlais, D., Ness, I., Clark, J., & Friedman, S. (1996). The transition from underground to legal syringe exchange: The New York City experience. *AIDS Education and Prevention, 8*, 471–489.

Kohut, H. (1971). *The analysis of the self.* New York: International Universities Press.

Krystal, H. (1995). Disorders of emotional development in addictive behavior. In S. Dowling (Ed.), *The psychology and treatment of addictive behavior* (American Psychoanalytic Association, Monograph 8, pp. 65–100). Madison, WI: International Universities Press.

MacCoun, R. (1997). The psychology of harm reduction: Comparing alternative strategies for modifying high-risk behaviors. The 1996 Wellness Lectures. *Drug Policy Research Center*, 4–27. Santa Monica, CA: RAND.

Marlatt, G. A. (Ed.). (1998). *Harm reduction: Pragmatic strategies for managing high-risk behaviors.* New York: Guilford Press.

Marlatt, G. A., & Gordon, J. R. (1985). *Relapse prevention: Maintenance strategies in the treatment of addictive behaviors.* New York: Guilford Press.

Marlatt, G. A., Larimer, M., Baer, J., & Quigley, L. (1993). Harm reduction for alcohol problems: Moving beyond the controlled drinking controversy. *Behavior Therapy, 24,* 461–504.

Miller, N., & Gold, M. (1990). The disease and adaptive models of addiction: A reevaluation. *Journal of Drug Issues, 20*(1), 29–35.

Miller, W. R., & Page, A. (1991). Harm turkey: Other routes to abstinence. *Journal of Substance Abuse Treatment, 8,* 227–232.

Miller, W. R., & Rollnick, S. (1991). *Motivational interviewing: Preparing people to change addictive behavior.* New York: Guilford Press.

Musto, D. (1997). Historical Perspectives. In J. Lowinson, P. Ruiz, R. Millman, & J. Langrod (Eds.), *Substance abuse: A comprehensive textbook* (pp. 1–10). Baltimore: Williams & Wilkins.

Nadelmann, E. (1998a). Commonsense drug policy [Online]. *Foreign Affairs, 77*(1). Available at www.foreignaffairs.org

Nadelmann, E. (1998b). Experimenting with drugs [Online]. *Foreign Affairs, 77*(1). Available at www.foreignaffairs.org

Nadelmann, E., McNeely, J., & Drucker, E. (1997). International perspectives. In J. Lowinson, P. Ruiz, R. Millman, & J. Langrod (Eds.), *Substance abuse: A comprehensive textbook* (pp. 22–39). Baltimore: Williams & Wilkins.

Newcombe, R., & Parry, A. (1988). *The Mersey Harm-Reduction Model: A strategy for dealing with drug users.* Presentation at the International Conference on Drug Policy Reform, Bethesda, MD.

Paone, D., Caloir, S., Clark, J., & Jose, B. (1995). Operational issues in syringe exchanges: The New York City tagging alternative study. *Journal of Community Health, 20* 111–123.

Paone, D., Des Jarlais, D., Gangloff, R., Milliken, J., & Friedman, S. (1995). Syringe exchange: HIV prevention, key findings, and future directions. *International Journal of Addictions, 30,* 1647–1683.

Peele, S., & Brodsky, A. (1991). *The truth about addiction and recovery.* New York: Simon & Schuster.

Peele, S., Bufe, C., & Brodsky, A. (2000). *Resisting 12-step coercion: How to fight forced participation in AA, NA, or 12-step treatment.* Tucson, AZ: Sharp Press.

Prochaska, J. O., & DiClemente, C. (1982). Transtheoretical therapy: Toward a more integrative model of change. *Psychotherapy: Theory, Research, and Practice, 19,* 276–278.

Roche, A., Evans, E., & Stanton, W. (1997). Harm reduction: Roads less traveled to the Holy Grail. Section III: Health service issues in addiction. *Addiction, 92*(9), 1207–1212.

Rogers, C. (1951). *Client centered therapy: Its current practice, implications, and theory.* Boston: Houghton Mifflin.

Rosenberg, H. (1993). Prediction of controlled drinking by alcoholics and problem drinkers. *Psychological Bulletin, 113.* 129–139.

Salmon, R., & Salmon, R. (1983). The role of coercion in rehabilitation of drug abusers. *International Journal of the Addictions, 18* 9–21.

Sashin, E. (1995). Psychoanalytic studies of addictive behavior: A review. In S. Dowling (Ed.), *The psychology and treatment of addictive behavior* (American Psychoanalytic Association Monograph 8, pp. 3–15). Madison, WI: International Universities Press.

Single, E. (1994, October). *Harm reduction and alcohol problem prevention.* Paper presented at the Conference on Harm Reduction: An Emerging Public Health Perspective, Honolulu.

Single, E. (1995a). Defining harm reduction. *Drug and Alcohol Review, 14,* 287–290.

Single, E. (1995b, May). *Harm reduction, drugs and alcohol: Future directions.* Paper presented at the Annual Conference of the Ontario Federation of Community Mental Health and Addiction Programs, Toronto.

Single, E. (1997). The concept of harm reduction and its application to alcohol: The 6th Dorothy Black Lecture. *Drugs: Education, Prevention and Policy 4*(1).

Springer, E. (1991). Effective AIDS Prevention with Active Drug Users: The Harm Reduction Model. In M. Shernoff (Ed.), *Counseling chemically dependent people with HIV illness* (pp. 141–157). New York: Haworth Press.

Springer, E. (1996). The spectrum of harm reduction. *Harm Reduction Communication, 3,* 20–21.

Tatarsky, A. (1998). An integrative approach to harm reduction psychotherapy: A case of problem drinking secondary to depression. *Session: Psychotherapy in Practice, 4,* 9–24.

Westermeyer, R. (1997a). *Inducing harm: A very good idea.* Available at www.fullspectrumrecovery.com

Westermeyer, R. (1997b). *Harm reduction and moderation as an alternative to heavy drinking.* Available at www.fullspectrumrecovery.com

Williams, G., & Williams, S. (1990). American drug policy: Who are the addicts? *Iowa Law Review, 75* 1119–1133.

Wodak, A. (1999, February 4). How needle exchange protects us all. *Sydney Morning Herald,* p. 13.

Wurmser, L. (1978). *The hidden dimension: Psychodynamics in compulsive drug use.* New York: Jason Aronson.

Wurmser, L. (1995). Compulsiveness and conflict: The distinction between description and explanation in the treatment of addictive behavior. In S. Dowling (Ed.), *The psychology and treatment of addictive behavior* (American Psychoanalytic Association Monograph 8, pp. 43–64). Madison, WI: International Universities Press.

Yalisove, D. (1998). The Origins and Evolution of The Disease Concept of Treatment. *Journal of Studies on Alcohol, 59,* 469–476.

Zinberg, N. (1984). *Drug, set and setting.* New Haven, CT: Yale University Press.

CHAPTER 4

Working with Mandated Substance Abusers

The Language of Solutions

Insoo Kim Berg
Kathryn C. Shafer

The past decade has seen an increasing number of clients mandated into substance abuse treatment by various sources. The criminal justice system increasingly views diversion to substance abuse treatment as a viable alternative to incarceration because of the possibility of rehabilitation, especially for first-time offenders, and as a less costly alternative to imprisonment (Massaro & Pepper, 2000; Vigdal, 1995). The changing public assistance requirements also have led to a growing number of substance-abusing individuals who are mandated into treatment in order for them to receive benefits. Many other individuals are brought to the attention of substance abuse treatment centers through child welfare agencies. Since 1976 child welfare departments across the country have seen an increase of more than 330% in child abuse and neglect reports, and it is estimated that at least two-thirds of the families known to child welfare agencies have substance abuse problems (Howard, 2000). Clients are also mandated into substance abuse treatment by employers concerned about poor work performances, and many are forced into treatment by their family members. Therefore, there is a clear need for a practice model that not only elicits the cooperation of clients but also empowers them to take responsibility for finding and enacting their own solutions.

This chapter introduces clinicians to solution-focused therapy (SFT) and the language and practice skills that are useful when working with clients who are mandated for substance abuse treatment by external authorities. First, we define and clarify the language and practice methods used in the traditional, problem-focused approaches and then offer an alternative view from the solution-building perspective (DeJong & Berg, 1998). Next, we provide useful practice techniques for building client-centered and empowering therapeutic relationships with mandated individuals. Case examples are used to illustrate how to negotiate workable goals, enhance motivation for change, and build solutions that are acceptable and more readily implemented by mandated clients.

CURRENT PERSPECTIVES ON MANDATED CLIENTS

The language used by clients mandated to substance abuse treatment often mirrors the language of the criminal justice system. Mandated clients often describe the treatment as a matter of "doing time." They focus on the "release date" and are more concerned with meeting the requirements recommended by the judge, probation officer, child welfare department, public assistance system, the employer, the family, or some other monitoring authority than with the successful completion of clinical goals established by the treatment center. The flip side of this lexicon is the language used by treatment providers to describe the mandated client. Words such as *mandated, involuntary,* or *criminal justice* elicit certain preconceived notions in clinicians, such as difficult, resistant, oppositional, or defiant, as well the other commonly used description of clients as "in denial" or as "minimizing the seriousness of the problems." It is not a big leap to then interact with the client in a manner that conveys the perceived truth of these descriptions. Before long, the client indeed displays many of the signs of being "noncompliant" and having a "bad attitude."

Frustrated clinicians often wonder, "How can I make this client admit that he is in denial?" "What can I do to make her think about her kids first, before she goes for the drugs again?" "How can I help him see that following a schedule and maintaining abstinence will help him keep a job [or stay out of jail]?" Even though, on a cognitive level, most experienced practitioners know that no one can change another person, when faced with "resistant" clients who are literally killing themselves with alcohol or other drugs, or harming their children or other people, it is extremely difficult to admit that one is helpless to change others. However, only the clients can change themselves; the job of the clinician is to attempt to help clients identify and move toward a type of change that is congruent with their own idea of what is "better" for them.

CLINICIANS' VIEWS OF THE MANDATED CLIENT

Because most current treatment models are based on clinical work with voluntary clients, existing literature is generally not helpful in providing guidelines on how to work with mandated or involuntary clients (Ivanoff, Blythe, & Tripodi, 1994). What is indicated in the literature is the need to engage clients through active and empathic listening; only when trust and cooperation are established is the clinician encouraged to move on to problem-solving efforts. Although this approach may be appropriate for many clients, it does not necessarily work for those who are forced into treatment by others. Such clients often feel that they have been unjustly and unfairly treated by the system, and they may not stay around long enough to develop a trusting relationship with a helping professional. They are often not convinced that the suggested changes would be helpful or useful to them; what is more, at times they view them as harmful.

Working with involuntary clients is also difficult for the staff. Many complaints of "burnout" stem from practitioners' frustration at knowing their own limitations in making a difference and feeling as if they were fighting a losing battle. When the clinician or the treatment program has an agenda for the treatment outcome of the client, "resistance" by all parties involved seems to grow, and "successful outcome" becomes more elusive. Discouraged by the continued breaking of promises, involvement in criminal activity, and relapses, family members, employers, treatment providers, and clients themselves give up, believing that they must indeed "hit bottom" in order to become motivated to change (Fishman, 1995).

A growing literature is emerging, however, that advocates the need for a better fit between client motivation and provided services (Prochaska, DiClemente, & Norcross, 1992). Trotter (1999), for example, suggests that practitioners pay attention to the positive or prosocial comments or behaviors that clients show and openly praise them. He also emphasizes the advisability of challenging or confronting antisocial comments or behaviors—but of doing so cautiously. Rooney (1992) advocates a four-stage process: (1) emphasizing client choice whenever possible, (2) informing clients about what to expect during treatment and their part in it, (3) contracting with clients around goals and treatment procedures, and (4) fostering client participation throughout treatment. These strategies offer a greater degree of choice and control to clients, orient them to the treatment process, and give them a sense of responsibility for success or failure in achieving the treatment goals that they themselves have established.

DeJong and Berg (2001) support the work of Rooney (1992) and believe that giving clients a sense of choice and control is essential when working with those who are mandated into treatment. Moreover, they contend that SFT casts a different light on client goals and introduces new perspectives on thinking, motivational interviewing for change, and interviewing the mandated client, as can be seen in the following sections.

THE SOLUTION-BUILDING PROCESS

The traditional problem-solving paradigm, also described as the scientific or medical model, begins with a detailed assessment or identification of the problems. It is based on the belief that an understanding of the problem will aid in the next step of selecting the matching solution(s). This second stage is the task of the expert. It is generally thought that the finer and more detailed the biopsychosocial assessment or diagnosis, the better fit we will find between the problems and the solution. In the third step, the clinician prescribes or recommends a solution to the client, who then must agree to implement the procedures of the solution in a given time frame. The fourth and final step involves an evaluation of progress, making finer adjustments as new information emerges, and if necessary, changing the course of treatment (DeJong & Berg, 2001). This methodology is reasonable when the client is voluntary or is desperate for guidance and has some investment in changing. However, most mandated clients do not want to stay in treatment long enough to see the results, nor do they see the benefit of following suggested remedies they see as useless, inconvenient, or even harmful. Thus there is a fundamental disconnection between what the expert clinician believes is helpful to clients, and what clients believe is helpful to them. When this disjuncture occurs, it is usually the client who is labeled *noncompliant, resistant,* or *oppositional and defiant.*

In contrast, SFT begins with finding out what the *client* wants. The therapist asks clients to describe their view of their own future. How do they want their lives to be different? How confident are they that they can make these changes happen? These questions set the direction and tone for the treatment endeavor. SFT is a therapeutic model, developed inductively and qualitatively, based on what clinicians observed to be effective in clinical settings (Berg & Miller, 1994; Berg & Reuss, 1998; DeJong & Berg, 2001; De Shazer, 1985, 1988, 1994; Miller & Berg, 1995). It is easy to see why this solution-building process is described as collaborative, since clients play an important role in setting the direction and making necessary changes according to their idea of how they want to shape their life. Research studies (Gingerich & Eisengart, 2000; Lee, Sebold, & Uken, 2002; Lindforss & Magnusson, 1997; Uken & Sebold, 1996) have found that the SFT approach (1) has similar and/or better treatment outcomes with fewer number of sessions than traditional approaches, and (2) that it reduces recidivism rates among incarcerated men and domestic violence offenders, resulting in substantial savings in criminal justice expenses and social cost.

Because the client's goals play a significant role in the treatment process, the SFT approach pays a great deal of attention to the process and outcome of the client's goal-attainment efforts. This first step opens the client to think about all the possibilities and choices that life has to offer ("miracle questions") and what he or she wants out of life. The second step is to find out what capacities the client can exert toward achieving these goals. This step is accomplished by learning about past and current successes ("exceptions to problems") and finding out the details of what actions, however small, the client has taken toward achieving his or her goal. The third step is to keep the client on the success track by helping him or her monitor any progress toward the goal ("scaling questions"). Because clients set their own goals according to their own dreams and aspirations, and determine the pace of how to achieve them based on their own understanding of personal and situational limitations, resistance is greatly diminished or nonexistent.

Most of us are usually much more invested in implementing our own ideas than those imposed by someone else. Furthermore, the more respected we feel, the more confident we are in carrying out even a difficult task (Shafer & Greenfield, 2000). This notion is consistent with the social work philosophy of beginning where the client is at and respecting the client's right to a self-determination. It is clearly more productive for the practitioner to begin by cooperating with the client and not making "the resistance" an issue in treatment.

Language, beliefs, and imagination are tools that people can use to negotiate and transform the meaning that events or incidences hold for them (Shafer & Greenfield, 2000). Thus paying close attention to the exact words, beliefs, and images clients use to describe themselves and their lives makes it possible for clinicians to gain access to clients' inner world. Designing steps for solutions that fit the client's frame of reference requires a careful and creative use of language. Helping clients see themselves living in a new way helps pave the way for them to *actualize* this new perception.

In the traditional problem-solving approach (DeJong & Berg, 1998, 2001), therapists unwittingly encourage clients to emphasize undesirable parts of their lives by focusing on the details of the problems that brought them to treatment, thereby highlighting their deficiencies rather than whatever competencies they may have. Although this traditional view maintains that talking about problems "dis-solves" them, we have found that such problem-focused conversation often highlights and amplifies the client's failures. Through talking, we selectively build or ignore certain aspects of the story, thus creating a sense of reality and conveying a belief in the existence of certain problems or solutions. Each repetition of the same story, whether positive and negative in slant, makes the story more real and reinforces the sense of failure or success. It is easy to see how detrimental it can be to focus only on the problems when working with substance-abusing clients who are mandated into treatment, since they already have experienced numerous failures and disappointments. Therefore, instead of focusing on clients' past failures or deficits, we focus on even a small "success," such as a time when they achieved a week, or even a day, of sobriety, which becomes a step that can be built upon further (Berg & Reuss, 1997).

THE SOLUTION-FOCUSED TREATMENT APPROACH

To effectively "begin where the client is at" when working with mandated clients, the following treatment steps are suggested: (1) Assess the person, not the problem; (2) take the "not-knowing" posture; and (3) find ways to cooperate with the client.

Assessing the Person, Not the Problem

The traditional social work concept of looking at the person in the environment has made a tremendous contribution to our awareness of the importance of assessing the person first, and not the problem. We need to pay attention to the clients' "expertise" regarding the circumstances that led them to being mandated to treatment, thus respecting their way of understanding and making sense of their world. We also need to listen to clients' understanding of what led to their present life situation and find ways to utilize this understanding, without correcting or educating clients on their "wrong" or "inadequate" perception of the seriousness of their problems. Lastly, we need to find out what is important to clients, what *they* value, what beliefs *they* hold about themselves, and what *they* want in life.

The following questions are useful in helping clients "see" how they are thinking about their problem:

- "Tell me about your family and how you spend your time at home. What are your best traits? Who in your family is most supportive of you?"
- "What kind of previous treatment experience has been most helpful for you?"
- "Would you please describe, in your own words, what led you to come and see me today?"
- "Whose idea was it that you should come and talk to me? What is _____ [the judge, your spouse, your job, child welfare, etc.] expecting to come out of your meeting with me that would be useful to you?"
- "What are you hoping will come out of your talking to me?"
- "How would _____ [the judge, probation officer, etc.] tell that your talking to me is helpful to you?"

When asked the above questions, clients frequently show a considerable degree of understanding and respond in a positive and cooperative manner that indicates an ability to differentiate what is confrontational and what is not. In the process of talking about solutions, clients voluntarily offer information about the way they see the problem. Some clients may respond in a manner the practitioner may not approve of, such as using evasion, minimizing the problem, or blaming others for their difficulty. Rather than taking offense at such answers or immediately labeling the client as unmotivated or lacking insight, it is more helpful to explore further how the client sees his or her situation from his or her perspective.

The following dialogue exemplifies how a worker's questions can shape the client's answers:

RUTH: I don't know what you can do for me. I don't even think I belong here. Nothing against you personally, but, you know, I really am not an alcoholic, like most people think I am. I am a good mother, you know. I just lost my head and got carried away and got a little rowdy. Don't get me wrong. I'm a good mother and I try my best, but somebody got this idea that I'm a bad person.

WORKER: I can see that it is very important to you that you are a good mother. I can also see that you are the kind of person who knows what you are and what you are not. It's important to know the difference. So I'm impressed with how you decided to come here even though you realize that you may not belong here. What made you to decide to come here today?

RUTH: I was told by that judge that I have to come here if I want my children back with me. The judge don't know nothing about me. He never saw me before, so how can he decide I'm not a good mother? But he says I have to come here. So I came, and I don't want to lose my kids, because they are everything to me.

Even if the client says "I don't belong in a place like this," the worker can stay neutral and continue to negotiate the client's goal while remaining supportive.

WORKER: I'm really impressed that you decided to follow through on this judge's order, even though you disagree with him. I guess you are one of these people who really want to do what's right and what's good for yourself and your children.

By framing the client's protest as reasonable and sensible, the worker makes it easy to return to the negotiation of what the client wants in more detail. Certainly getting the credit for keeping the appointment is likely *not* what the client expected to hear. Such statements frame the clinical interaction in a positive light.

From this brief exchange, it is clear that Ruth values her role as a mother and that it is very important to her to keep her children. With this knowledge about Ruth, the worker can continue the conversation about what Ruth values, what she might be motivated to work toward, and where she learned to be such a "committed mother." Once Ruth establishes her identity as a committed mother, she is more likely to want to work making it a reality. By staying with what is important to Ruth, the worker can then explore her understanding of what she is supposed to do in the treatment program and how her children will benefit from whatever she decides to do as a result of this conversation.

TAKING THE "NOT-KNOWING" POSTURE

The "not-knowing" (Anderson & Goolishan, 1992) posture assumed by the clinician conveys the message that clients have certain knowledge and expertise about their own life circumstances and that they basically know what to do in order to achieve their goals without needing to be told. By utilizing the client's knowledge, the clinician can help a woman such as Ruth to build her own future in the way that she believes is good for herself and her children. In doing so, the worker learns about Ruth's frame of reference, how she thinks, what she believes in, and what aspirations, hopes, and dreams she might harbor. Getting to know and connect with Ruth, for example, also means accepting her perceptions of, and disagreements with, the mandating authority without the clinician having to defend or take sides. This approach allows the client to be the expert of his or her life (Shafer & Greenfield, 2000).

- "Which part of what you were told to do by coming to this agency do you agree with, and which part do you disagree with?" *Comment*: By separating the list of mandates the client is required to do, the practitioner helps Ruth sort out what she might be willing to tackle first.
- "What are you hoping I can do to help so that you will get your children back? Can you tell me exactly what I can do to be helpful to you?" *Comment*: By eliciting more details of what Ruth wants from the encounter, the worker clarifies further what she is motivated to do first. It is important not to assume that professionals know what is best for the client.
- "Suppose you get your children back, what would they say they like best about living with you?" *Comment*: By bringing in the children's perspective of what they might want from their mother, the worker is inviting the mother to look at a wider view of who else is invested in her success.

Rather than making demands that the client change, the worker addresses the mother's relationship with her children by asking her to think about her children's views of what would improve their lives. This indirect approach reduces the need to confront the mother, without letting her "off the hook." It also addresses the important issue that was already established by the mother. This sort of questioning assumes that the client may or may not agree with the mandate for treatment, and that the practitioner is willing to listen to both sides of the story. Such a neutral position reduces clients' need to defend their position or attack the mandating authority.

- "So, now that you are here, what do you suppose needs to come out of this meeting between you and me, so that this is useful to you? Suppose your children were here and I were to ask them, 'What do you want your mom to do today that would be most helpful for you?' What would they tell me? What would your children tell me they like the best about the things you do with them?" *Comment*: By asking about the client's desires and hopes for the session, the clinician immediately frames the meeting as potentially "useful" to the client, not something that simply must be tolerated. The clinician is interested in learning about what and who the client values as important. Bringing other people's perception into the conversation makes the focus much more relevant to the client, even though those people cannot be present physically. Since the worker has previously learned that Ruth's children are important to her, the focus is kept on that relationship. Such an approach reduces the likelihood that the client will resist or engage in combative or uncooperative behavior.

Finding Ways to Cooperate with the Client

Cooperating with clients means learning how to stand side by side with them, not facing against them, as if in a competition. It is our professional obligation to honor and cooperate with the client first, thus "leading from one-step behind" (Cantwell & Holmes, 1994). Doing so requires that we see things from clients' perspectives and eliminate the "professional posture" of judging them. Clients do not need one more failure or one more label as "incompetent" or "difficult." The most important contribution a practitioner can make during the initial contact is to shape clients' experience in a way that is different from any other negative professional experiences they may have encountered in the past. Clients need the opportunity and the latitude to make choices instead of feeling coerced to comply; to feel understood instead of being labeled. This side-by-side approach supports clients' choices as well as their acceptance of responsibility for the consequences of these choices (Shafer & Greenfield, 2000). By viewing the world from clients' perspectives, while maintaining their own, clinicians are able to help clients build a bridge from their world of failure and loneliness to one of belonging, in which they feel that they can, as one client phrased it, "walk tall, with my head up straight."

ASSESSING FOR SUSTAINABLE SOLUTIONS

All clients have some ideas for solutions to their difficulties: Some may be reasonable and realistic; others, outlandish. Of course, when the client's ideas for solutions are reasonable and realistic, it is easy to be supportive and encouraging. Maintaining a respectful stance toward the client means, however, that the practitioner must withhold his or her judgment when the client's solutions seem outlandish or unrealistic, and to continue to ask many open-ended questions to elicit the client's ideas more fully.

The following case suggests some useful questions to ask when the client seems unrealistic in his or her assessment of what is doable:

> André and Melinda, a young couple with two small children, live in a semirural area that has no public transportation. Melinda worked in a nursing home, a job that she found extremely stressful. As her feelings of being trapped and stressed increased, so did her drinking, especially on her way home from work. One day on her way home, she was stopped by the police because of her erratic driving and arrested for drunk driving. Melinda lost her driver's license and was told that she must attend mandatory driving under the influence (DUI) classes in order to regain it. In addition, she had to pay a hefty fine and fees for the classes.
>
> In reaction to the financial pressure, she began to drink more. During a loud shouting match with André about his lack of support and their lack of money, the police were called by a neighbor who heard her threatening to harm the children, herself, and to "end it all." The police called Social Services and the children were tempo rarily placed with their maternal grandparents, who live nearby.
>
> Shamed and remorseful, Melinda found herself in deeper despair and in greater financial trouble. She promised to do everything the mandating agents demanded from her: attend the DUI class for 10 weeks, visit the children daily at the grandparents' house 5 miles away, and keep her job (which was about 15 miles away)—all without any means of transportation. André needed to use his truck in his long hours of work in construction and was unable to drive her to and from work. Melinda agreed to go to couple counseling with André, where she was told that she needs to work on her drinking problem and her anger at the world. After her session with the counselor, Melinda attempted to end her troubles by overdosing on medications she had stolen from the nursing home. She was rushed to a hospital emergency room, where she was successfully treated. She was discharged the following morning, with a recommendation to follow up with outpatient treatment. Melinda readily agreed.

Is it realistic to expect Melinda to accomplish all these goals? Of course not! It is not only unrealistic, it sets up the client to fail one more time. It is easy to imagine how Melinda would be tempted to drive without her driver's license, thus compounding her problems even more. A sensible clinician would question the client's willingness to comply, out of desperation with all the suggestions and requirements, however insurmountable. In situations such as this one, a realistic assessment of what is manageable is needed. Taking a not-knowing posture and having clients explain the situation can help them assess how realistic is it is for them to agree to all the recommended services. The following comments and questions helped Melinda get grounded in the reality of what she could, and could not, reasonably accomplish:

- "I wonder, what do you know about yourself that tells you that you can do all these tasks? It seems like an awful lot for anybody to do."
- "Can you explain to me how you are planning to get to these places without a car?"
- "I can see that you cannot quit your job because you are concerned that, even if you find another job closer to your home, you may not earn the same wage you are earning now. With this in mind, can you tell me in more detail how you plan to accomplish all this?"
- "Knowing you as well as he does, what would André say about how likely it is that you are going to be able to do all this?"
- "If I were to ask your best friend—you say her name is *Laurie*—how confident would she be that you could do all this?"
- "Of all the things you need to do, what small thing can you can do right away that will make the greatest difference in your life?"
- "What will tell you that you are making progress?"

EXCEPTIONS TO PROBLEMS

The basic assumption of SFT is that all problematic situations, even chronic problems such as substance abuse and mental illness, contain periods when these problems either do not happen or are less severe. It is the clinician's task to uncover these circumstances during the initial conversation, thereby helping clients recognize that they have had times when they could have gotten drunk, taken a pill, or lashed out at someone, but somehow managed not to do so. Such an *exception* is a significant indication that the client can repeat this small success, and even expand on it. The important step is for the clinician to ask about the details surrounding the exceptions, the "forgotten successes," which allowed for the successful mastery of a problematic behavior or urge. A detailed discussion of how the client was able to have a day of sobriety, for example, reminds the client of all the steps he or she had taken to be successful, even for a brief time period. Such detailed recounting of a successful experience helps the client re-peat these steps, as the following dialogue illustrates.

WORKER: I can see that you are very concerned about your tendency to promise yourself that you are not going to drink and then you end up drunk. This certainly can be pretty discouraging, I'm sure. So, tell me about the most recent times when you made this promise to yourself and you *were able* to keep your word to yourself?

TODD: I don't know . . . it seems like I've been doing a lot of drinking lately.

WORKER: So, when would you say was the most recent time when you could have gotten drunk but somehow you decided against that?

TODD: I guess last week, Friday night. Of course I showed up at the bar as usual, but you know, I decided that I wanted to know what I was do-ing and not make a fool of myself, as usual, when I get drunk. I sat there and drank soda instead of my usual booze. I was sure other guys were going to razz me about drinking soda, but you know what, no-body said anything. I was surprised. I got to thinking about this and I guess they all know how much I drink and what happens to me when I do. I guess it's not a pretty picture.

WORKER: Wow, sounds like you learned a lot from this little experiment Friday night. You could have easily fallen into your usual Friday-night habit. What made you decide that you wanted to drink soda instead?

TODD: I just wanted to find out if I could do it or not. You know, you won-der about that sometimes, you know what I mean?

WORKER: Yeah, many people tell me the same thing that you are telling me now. So, what did you learn from this little experiment?

TODD: What I learned from this is that I must look pretty stupid when I get drunk, and nobody told me that before. Actually, my family has been telling me that, but I usually don't listen to them. I sat there and watched everybody, and some of my old drinking buddies looked pretty stupid, all slobbering and wobbling when they walked.

WORKER: So, say that again, what did you learn about yourself from this experiment?

TODD: I'm sure I looked just as dumb as all these people at the bar, and I decided, *that's not me*, I don't want to be that stupid anymore. That's why I'm here.

WORKER: I see you already have a pretty good sense of what you want to be and what you don't want to be. I would say you have a very good start. So, what kind of person do you want to be instead?

TODD: I'll tell you that I don't want to spend my life being a drunk. I messed up my life already, but maybe I can turn things around yet—I'm still young and maybe there is a hope for me.

Once an exception to the problem has been identified, as with Todd's decision not to "make a fool of myself" and somehow having had enough control to stay away from "drinking as usual," the important task is to discuss how to repeat that one exception on a regular basis and how such an ability may change other aspects of the client's life. Exceptions point to potential solutions that clients do not even realize that they are capable of achieving. When clients recognize these forgotten successes, they become more confident of their abilities, which reinforces their resolve to repeat the successes. At times, just recognizing small successes is enough to instill in clients a sense of hope about their future and their own capacities to achieve change.

SCALING QUESTIONS

It is a common human impulse to measure, score, and compare ourselves with others. By taking advantage of this human tendency to measure and compare, *scaling questions* (Berg, 1994; Berg & de Shazer, 1993; Berg & Reuss, 1998; DeJong & Berg, 1998) invite clients to step back and assess their own situation in various areas: their level of motivation to change, how much progress they have made toward their goals, how hopeful or optimistic they are in their abilities to achieve their desired goals, the seriousness of the problem, feelings of confidence or level of depression over time, and a host of other issues that surface in treatment. Examples of scaling questions that might have been used with Melinda and Ruth follow:

- "I am going to ask you a different kind of question this time. Let's just say that *10* stands for how you want your life to be; that is, get your children back from the foster home, have a place of your own, and feel and act like the good mother that you want to be. That's *10*. Now *1* stands for how terrible you thought your life was when you were in the middle of drug use and your life fell apart. Those days stand for *1*. In terms of a scale between 1 and 10, where would you say you are now?"
- "What tells you that you are at 4 now? What else have you done to go all the way up to 4?"
- "What would it take for you to move up to 4.5? When you move up to 4.5, what would be different with your life?"
- "Suppose I were to ask your best friend where she thinks you are on this scale of 1–10. What would she say?"

- "This time, *10* stands for how much you are willing to work to get your children back to live with you, and *1* stands for not lifting a finger to make it happen. Where would you put yourself?"
- "Suppose I ask your probation officer how motivated she believes you are. Were would she put you on this scale? What would she do differently if she believed that you had moved up 1 point higher on the scale?"

The variation and flexibility of scaling questions are limitless. Scaling questions can been used in a variety of therapeutic modalities, including individual, family, and group settings. Many creative clinicians have adapted the scaling questions when working with young children or with clients who are described as developmentally challenged.

RELATIONSHIP QUESTIONS

Substance abusers affect other people around them; they are also affected by other people, especially their family members or best friends. Therefore, it is important to bring the views of these important people into the conversation with a client, because they can either undermine or support and reinforce the changes the client makes while in treatment. In addition, these significant persons are potential resources for treatment because they are generally knowledgeable about the client's strengths as well as shortcomings. Furthermore, any clinical suggestion for change must fit into the client's natural social context. The following questions show how the SFT approach includes the client's perception of his or her impact on others and helps the practitioner obtain a richer view of the client's social network:

- "What do you suppose your children would say about how close you've come to having them come home? What about your mother? Your best friend? What about the judge [probation officer]?"
- "What would your daughter say that she likes best about you being sober when she visits with you?"
- "Wow, you managed not to drink for a whole month!? How did you do this? You must worked very hard to achieve this. What would your mother [spouse, best friend] say about how you are different now that you've been sober for a whole month?"
- "How confident would your mother say she is that you will stay clean this time, on a scale of 1 to 10, with 10 being that she is as confident as can be, and 1 the opposite?"
- "What would your mother say about how you are different now that you are stable, working again, and spending more time with

your children and family? How is she different with you when she sees these positive changes your are making?"

COPING QUESTIONS

At times, practitioners may lose hope about a client and convey this feeling to him or her; or a client may already have reached a point where life seems hopeless. In such situations, *coping questions* are useful tools for eliciting clients' strengths and internal resources. When asked with compassion, curiosity, and admiration for the client's ability to "hang in there" despite what appears to be monumental odds against him or her, such questions can make the client more aware of the internal and external supports that are sustaining him or her and awaken hope. For example:

- "Most people would have a tough time getting out of bed when faced with such problems. How did you manage to get out of the bed this morning?"
- "Wow, you have lived through some tough situations! How do you keep going?"
- "What keeps you going, day in and day out, in the middle of so many problems?"
- "Most people in similar situations would have given up long time ago. How do you cope with such impossible circumstances, day in and day out?"
- "How come you are doing as well as you are doing, considering all the difficulties you have to cope with?"
- "Where did you learn to be so strong, to keep going, to keep your family together?"

For many mandated clients, being asked how they have coped with so many demands of the mandating systems or how they have found the stamina and will to follow through on the many non-negotiable conditions forced on them generates a much-needed sense of pride and a recognition of their own successes. Such an approach enhances clients motivation—their tenacious will to succeed—and strengthens their fortitude and determination not to give in to despair. It also points out their hidden resources that perhaps no one has recognized or given them credit for having.

THE MIRACLE QUESTIONS

The *miracle question* is used to assist clients in generating a vision of life that is free of their current problems. It helps clients consider possibilities they may have never thought of before, thereby shifting their whole belief system. Exploring the miracle question can provide a vision of a life that they have not dared to dream. The resulting new insight or belief often seems to transform the person.

The miracle question works best when asked in the following manner, in a slow, soft voice:

> "I am going to ask you a rather strange question. (*Pause.*) Let's say that after we talk here today, you will do whatever you normally do for the rest of today. (*Pause.*) Then tonight you go to bed and fall asleep. While you are sleeping, a miracle happens. And the miracle is that all the problems you have been telling me about that brought you here have been solved, just like that. (*Snap your finger; long pause.*) But because you are sleeping, you have no idea that a miracle has occurred. (*Pause.*) So, when you are slowly coming out of your sleep, what will be the first, small sign that will let you know that the problem is all solved?"

Even when using this carefully phrased sentencing, which is based on years of experimenting with different wording, the client is likely to say, "I don't know." However, if the clinician waits patiently, the client slowly begins to formulate a reply, such as "Well . . . I suppose I would feel like I'm not hung over . . . I would want to get up and face the day, and not pull the cover over my head . . . Then I would go get some coffee . . . and not look for the bottle behind the couch." The clinician can then ask: "What would you do instead?" One client answered: "I would walk straight to the kitchen and get a glass of milk and a cup of coffee and sit down with a bowl of cereal." Another client, a mother of two who has been using cocaine for several years, answered, "I would get up in the morning and comb my daughter's hair." Since the significance of such an ordinary act as "comb[ing] my daughter's hair" was lost on the clinician, the client was asked to clarify the significance of this miracle. The mother responded that this meant that she would not have used drugs the night before, because when she does, she is unable to get up in the morning with the children to send them off to school. This vision becomes the first small step toward building an alternative solution to an existing problem.

DEALING WITH RELAPSES

Relapse during the recovery process is a common phenomenon among substance abusers (Fisher & Harrison, 2000). When there is only a single criterion for success—such as total abstinence—the chances of failure increase, regardless of the problem one is trying to solve. Instead of viewing relapse as a failure, it is more helpful to think in terms of success, because there can be no relapse without *any* success. It is also important to help the client see recovery as a process, so that each relapse episode does not compound a client's already discouraged and demoralized state of mind, leading to even lower morale. Because the client already feels ashamed, embarrassed, and guilty, it is not useful to reprimand him or her about another failure and get into the details of this failure. Instead, practitioners can use the following five steps to quickly help the client get back on the path to recovery:

Step 1

Approach the client who has recently relapsed with a positive mindset and a genuine belief that tomorrow can be the beginning of a new future. As discussed earlier, most substance abusers have experienced exceptions to their current problems, and it is those exceptions that need to be focused on now. Ask the client how long it has been since the last relapse. Then ask how the client managed to stay substance free for so long (for some, staying free of substance use for a day can be a huge success) and find out the details of what has worked in the past. Many clients are surprised to find that they have forgotten about these small successes. The following questions are very useful to expand on exceptions:

- "How do you explain to yourself that you stayed clean for so many days?"
- "What do you suppose your family would say you did that was most helpful for you to stay clean, even for a day?"
- "What would it take for you to be able to repeat this success?"
- "How confident are you that you can do this again?" If the client says, for example, that attending AA meetings was helpful in staying sober, ask what it would take for him or her to return to those meetings. This reminder of a successful period following a prior relapse can be very encouraging to a client.

Step 2

Whenever you hear a report of a relapse from the client, ask the details of how he or she *stopped* the drinking or drug taking when he or she did, instead of having the client recount how he or she started drinking or drug taking again. Nothing can be gained by recounting the failure. What is important in building solutions is finding out what the client did successfully, even in the midst of failure, such as making sure that the children were under the supervision of a babysitter and that they had enough food in the house. Also find out about specific cues the client picked up, either internally or from the environment, that made him or her stop at 12 beers instead of continuing to drink the 13th one. The idea behind this approach is that if the client knows exactly what he or she did to stop at the 12th beer, then he or she can recognize that it is possible to stop at the 10th, 8th, or 5th drink, and so on. This perspective shows clients that they have some control, however small, which can become a building block for the future.

Step 3

Clients rarely seek help in the midst of an active relapse unless they are forcibly brought to a treatment center by police, family, or other health care workers. The majority of those who have relapsed usually show up at the treatment facility after they have stopped using the substance once again. It is helpful to find out what the person has done since he or she stopped drinking or doing drugs: for example, taking a shower, going back to work, apologizing to family or friends, returning to care for the children, and so on. These are all solutions, generated by clients, that need to be brought to their awareness so that they can repeat these useful strategies earlier next time. It is also important to elicit the perceptions of significant others by asking relationship questions, such as, "What would your family say they liked the most about what you did first after you stopped drinking?" This line of questioning shifts the focus from the client to the family or other important people with whom the client may be interested in having a better relationship—or in getting them "off my back."

Step 4

Find out what and how this current relapse is different from the last one. Although the word "relapse" may imply that all relapses are the same, each relapse is different from the one before; this time, for example, the client may have stopped sooner, used a little more or less alcohol or drug, or done something different such as calling a sponsor sooner, asking for help from friends or family, or behaving less nastily toward her child. These small details can make a big difference during the next relapse, because by emphasizing them clients start to realize that they have the power to make a difference, and that what happens is not an accident over which they have no control.

Step 5

During this final step, it is helpful to discuss what lessons clients may have learned from this relapse episode, and what concrete, detailed, behavioral, and measurable changes they will implement immediately in their daily life. What has she learned about her drinking? What new information has he gained this time and what difference will this knowledge make in his life? How will others respond to her when her sobriety continues for a longer stretch of time? How will he take advantage of the next period of sobriety? What kind of lifestyle changes will she implement from now on? How exactly will she do this? What difference does he expect this lesson will make in his life when this change continues for a while?

Again, we find that when the practitioner remains calm and hopeful about the client's future, always looking for a grain of success in the midst of problems, the client can maintain hope for him- or herself. Instilling such hope in clients is the greatest gift practitioners can offer.

CULTURAL COMPETENCE

SFT, with its not-knowing posture and deep respect and appreciation of the client's unique perspectives and ways of doing things, is highly congruent with our desire to honor and work within the client's cultural frame of reference. Whether it is a religious, cultural, or ethnically driven remedy, if it is valuable to clients and works for them, we must have the humility to honor it. This perspective means that our concept of normative behaviors is much broader, whereas the concept of pathology is rarely discussed. The guiding framework of SFT is based on the following three main principles:

1. If it works, don't fix it.
2. If it worked once, do it again.
3. If it doesn't work, don't do it again. Do something different.

CONCLUSION

The guiding assumption of SFT has been greatly influenced by social constructionism and its view that what is real—what is viewed as acceptable behaviors and a host of other rules of conduct—are all socially constructed. That is, the definitions of psychopathology or mental health, of how much substance use is acceptable or not, under what condition, by whom, and so on, are all socially negotiated. It is further understood that these negotiations take place within the context of language, since our primary tool is talking.

It is easy to see how all clinical interventions are selective in their choice of what they ask about and what they ignore, and that they are shaped by the underlying assumptions about what is useful and helpful for clients. SFT practitioners believe that through talking, we can trigger change, alter and rewrite our history, and create a different reality that is useful to clients as they navigate in the world around them. How we look at an event influences what we see and what we believe, and this, in turn, influences what we do, and so on, in a domino-like manner.

Guiding clients to participate in treatment by finding their own solutions—that is, finding what works for them—is not only respectful of their uniqueness but also empowers them to view themselves as agents of change who can shape their own lives. Helping clients take responsibility for and focus on "what works," or what is "different," or how they are changing contributes to their construction of different perspectives and beliefs about themselves. This chapter has presented the guiding assumptions of SFT and offered some practical ways to help clinicians provide more effective client-centered ways of working with individuals who are mandated into treatment.

REFERENCES

Anderson H., & Goolishan, H. (1992). The client is the expert: A not-knowing approach to therapy. In S. McNamee & K. J. Gergen (Eds.), *Therapy as social construction* (pp. 25–39). London: Sage.

Berg, I. K. (1994). *Family based services: A solution-focused approach.* New York: Norton.

Berg, I. K., & de Shazer, S. (1993). Making numbers talk: Language is in therapy. In S. Friedman (Ed.), *The new language of change: Constructive collaboration in psychotherapy* (pp. 5–24). New York: Guilford Press.

Berg, I. K., & Miller, S. (1992). *Working with the problem drinker.* New York: Norton.

Berg, I. K., & Reuss, N. H. (1998). *Solutions step by step: A substance abuse treatment manual.* New York: Norton.

DeJong, P., & Berg, I. K. (1998). *Interviewing for solutions.* Pacific Grove, CA: Brooks/Cole.

DeJong, P., & Berg, I. K. (2001). *Interviewing for solutions* (2nd ed.). Pacific Grove, CA: Brooks/Cole

de Shazer, S. (1985). *Keys to solution in brief therapy.* New York: Norton.

de Shazer, S. (1988). *Clues: Investigating solutions in brief therapy.* New York: Norton.

de Shazer, S. (1994). *Words were originally magic.* New York: Norton.

Fisher, G. L., & Harrison, T. C. (2000). *Substance abuse: Information for school counselors, social workers, therapists, and counselors.* Boston: Allyn & Bacon.

Fishman, C. H. (1995). The resistant substance abuser: Court mandated cases pose special problems. In M. R. Winchester-Vega (Ed.), *Substance abuse: Considerations for social workers* (pp. 75–78). Boston: Allyn & Bacon.

Gingerich, W., & Eisengart, S. (2000). Solution-focused brief therapy: A review of the outcome research. *Family Process, 39*(4), 477–498.

Howard, J. (2000). *Substance abuse treatment for persons with child abuse and neglect issues.* Treatment Improvement Protocol (TIP) series, No. 36. Rockville, MD: Center for Substance Abuse Treatment, Substance Abuse and Mental Health Services Administration.

Ivanoff, A., Blythe, B. J., & Tripodi, T. (1994). *Involuntary clients in social work practice: A research-based approach.* New York: Aldine de Gruyer.

Lee, M. Y., Sebold, J., & Uken, A. (2002) *Accountability for solutions: Domestic violence offender treatment.* London: Oxford University Press.

Lindforss, L., & Magnusson, D. (1997). Solution-focused therapy in prison. *Contemporary Family Therapy, 19*(1), 89–103.

Massaro, J., & Pepper, B. (2000). The relationship of addiction to crime, health, and other social problems. In J. Massaro & B. Pepper (Eds.), *Treatment for alcohol and other drug abuse: Opportunities for coordination* (pp. 11–23). Rockville, MD: U.S. Department of Health and Human Services, SAMHSA Technical Assistance Publication Series, No. 11.

Miller, S., & Berg, I. K. (1995). *Miracle method.* New York: Norton.

Prochaska, J., DiClemente, C., & Norcross, J. (1992). In search of how people change: Application to addictive behaviors. *American Psychologist, 47*(9), 1102–1114.

Rooney, R. H. (1992). *Strategies for work with involuntary clients.* New York: Columbia University Press.

Shafer, K., & Greenfield, F. (2000). *Asthma free in 21 days: The breakthrough mind–body healing program.* San Francisco: HarperCollins.

Trotter, C. (1999). *Working with involuntary clients: A guide to practice.* London: Sage.

Uken A., & Sebold, J. (1996). The Plumas Project: A solution-focused goal-directed domestic violence diversion program. *Journal of Collaborative Therapies, 4*(2).

Vigdal, G. (1995). *Planning for alcohol and other drug abuse treatment for adults in the criminal justice system.* Treatment Improvement Protocol (TIP) series No. 17. Rockville, MD: U.S. Department of Health and Human Services Administration, Center for Substance Abuse Treatment.

CHAPTER 5

Assessment and Intervention with Clients Who Have Coexisting Psychiatric and Substance-Related Disorders

Lois Orlin
Margaret O'Neill
Jenna Davis

The coexistence of substance abuse and severe and persistent mental illness has been well documented over the years. Hall (1979) found that 58% of 57 consecutive patients admitted to a psychiatric unit reported a history of drug abuse. Similarly, a study of young patients with chronic mental illness found that 37% abused alcohol and another 37% abused drugs (Pepper, Kirshner, & Ryglewicz, 1981). McKelvy, Kane, and Kellison (1987), in a study of patients in a state psychiatric hospital, learned that the 10–15% estimate of patients with a dual diagnosis on their arrival was vastly underestimated, and that, in fact, 60% of those admitted met the criteria. More recent studies of prevalence indicate that the coexistence of psychiatric and substance-related disorders ranges from 30 to 60% in the psychiatric population (Koegel, Sullivan, Burnam, Morton, & Wenzel, 1999; Menezes et al., 1996) and from 37 to 84% in the substance-abusing population (Regier, Farmer, & Rae, 1990; Ries, 1994). Studies of patients diagnosed with schizophrenia found that 47% also have a substance-related disorder (Ries, 1994). In a nationally representative study, Kessler and colleagues (1997) determined the co-occurring lifetime prevalence rate of alcohol dependence and psychiatric diagnoses using DSM-III-R. They found that 78.3% of the male respondents who met criteria for alcohol dependence also met criteria for at least one other psychiatric diagnosis, and 86% of the women met the criteria for alcohol dependence and at least one other psychiatric diagnosis. It is important to note that of those who met the criteria for alcohol dependence, 40.6% of the men and 47.1% of the women also met criteria for drug abuse or dependence. Hence, both psychiatric and addiction services face the challenge of treating individuals with coexisting disorders.

Given the decrease in available state hospital beds and the limited number of supervised psychiatric residential facilities and single-room occupancy dwellings (SROs) staffed with mental health teams, more individuals with severe and persistent mental illness find themselves homeless and vulnerable to alcohol and other drug use. Many of the same people may be seen on separate occasions in alcohol and drug detoxification or psychiatric units within the same hospital. How a patient presents him- or herself in the emergency room frequently determines the treatment disposition. Some patients become acquainted with the distinct admission criteria of each unit and spare the staff diagnostic uncertainty by delineating the symptoms that would most likely gain them admission to the unit of their choice. Their success with this strategy results in inadequate treatment (i.e., for only one disorder) and discharge planning.

Patients with coexisting psychiatric and substance-related disorders are often perceived as difficult because of their diagnostic complexities and high rates of recidivism and rehospitalization (Haywood et al., 1995), poor compliance with medication, violent and criminal behavior, and poor response to traditional substance abuse and/or mental health treatment (Osher & Kofoed, 1989). The comorbidity of substance-related and psychiatric disorders has been consistently associated with poor treatment outcomes. Often, these patients are not engaged successfully in traditional treatment systems due to a lack of clarity regarding diagnostic classification, the paucity of specialized services, and poor communication between personnel from substance abuse services and those from mental health services (Drake, Mercer McFadden, et al., 1998).

The purpose of this chapter is to discuss assessment and treatment issues for patients with a dual diagnosis and to describe how existing psychiatric and substance abuse treatment models can be utilized to work effectively with this population. A dual diagnosis treatment model provides quality care to those suffering with two diseases; in this era of capitation and managed care, the cost-effectiveness of such treatment makes the use of separate and parallel treatments obsolete.

DEFINITION OF DUAL DIAGNOSIS

Any person suffering from two diseases can be considered dually diagnosed. For the purpose of this chapter, the patient with a dual diagnosis is defined as an individual who has both a major (Axis I) psychiatric disorder, such as schizophrenia, and a psychoactive substance-related disorder (Axis I; Singer, Kennedy, & Kola, 1998).

Mental health providers frequently experience diagnostic dilemmas when a potential patient presents with a myriad of symptoms: mania, depression, anxiety, paranoia, hallucinations, and incoherence. Even if the patient is able and willing to document current and past chemical use, there is still a question as to which triggered which: Did the painful symptoms lead to drug use, or did the drug use precipitate the symptoms? It is even more difficult for emergency room staff and intake workers to make a primary diagnosis, since the symptoms of crack/cocaine use and schizophrenia are similar. Given the pressures of time, patients can easily be misdiagnosed and given improper treatment. Too often, persons with major psychiatric illnesses may be dismissed from treatment facilities with the suggestion that they seek help for their abuse of alcohol or other drugs, and substance abusers may be mislabeled as psychiatric patients, medicated and discharged. In neither case will the patients be accepted at most treatment facilities for substance abusers once they display or relate their psychiatric symptoms. As a result, these patients consistently receive one basic treatment—that of "referral therapy."

DIFFERENTIAL ASSESSMENT

Many patients enter psychiatric settings with suspected or documented substance abuse. To assess and treat all patients as one diagnostic category is to miss the important distinction that there are *two types* of clients with dual diagnosis: the primary psychiatric patient and the primary chemical abuser.

The primary psychiatric patient, also referred to as MICA (i.e., mentally ill chemical abuser), uses drugs and/or alcohol in response to the discomfort of mental illness. Such patients self-medicate to relieve the nagging voices in their heads, to feel less frightened of the imagined forces tormenting them, and to experience a high and a sense of control that prescribed antipsychotic medications do not provide. Many patients report that the only time they feel safe on the street, free from symptoms of paranoia, is when they are high or stoned. Furthermore, drug use has a secondary advantage for those with mental illness: In addition to numbing the disease symptoms, it gives them an opportunity to interact with individuals and groups outside the mental health system—to be "in the mainstream." The purchase of the drugs, the communal use, "makes me feel like a big shot," reported Ray, a previously shy and isolated schizophrenic. Thus the primary psychiatric patient who has suffered the pain, stigma, and social limitations conferred by the disease is extraordinarily vulnerable to the seeming benefits of drug and/or alcohol abuse. Unfortunately, the pleasures are short-lived and lead to decompensation and rehospitalization. Then, if the patient is not treated for both disorders, the cycle of abuse, decompensation, and rehospitalization is repeated.

The second category of dual diagnosis applies to the primary substance abuser. Such clients may have long histories of depression, anxiety, and poor psychosocial adjustment, but it can be documented that when they experience more florid symptoms, such as hallucinations, delusions, or thought disorder, these symptoms are secondary to substance abuse.

Ideally, when a psychiatric patient presents in an acute phase of illness, a urine toxicology is ordered immediately, whether or not there is clear evidence or history of substance use. Furthermore, little or no antipsychotic medication is instituted until staff have the opportunity to observe the patient in a drug-free state. Symptoms of psychosis will persist if unmedicated; symptoms due to chemical use will abate with abstinence (Wanck, 1987). The following case illustrates this point.

Marsha, a 25-year-old single white female was brought to a psychiatric emergency room by her parents. She was delusional, disoriented, and paranoid. According to her parents, Mr. and Mrs. A., she had a 9-year history of treatment in a variety of psychiatric outpatient settings. Most recently, she had stopped treatment when she moved away from home to live with a man whom Mr. and Mrs. A. suspected of being a drug abuser. When asked by the emergency room psychiatrist if Marsha used drugs, her parents assured him, "that is not her problem." They continued to document a pattern in which Marsha's condition would improve for a brief period and then deteriorate again. They were disheartened to be seeking help once again and were greatly relieved when admission to the hospital's psychiatric inpatient unit was offered.

Marsha's mental status on admission and the history given by her parents supported a diagnosis of schizophrenia, and she was promptly treated with antipsychotic medication. Her rapid improvement in the first 2 days of hospitalization seemed to confirm this diagnosis. Marsha avoided lengthy sessions with her therapist, but she was oriented and willing to participate in ward activities. On the third day of hospitalization, she developed a dystonic reaction (i.e., painful stiffening of her neck, eyes rolling back) to medication, and it was necessary to discontinue it. The staff were concerned that her symptoms might not be manageable without medication, but Marsha continued to improve. At this point, her therapist was able to get a more extensive psychiatric history. He learned that she had drunk alcohol and smoked marijuana throughout high school, and at age 18, prior to her first "breakdown," had begun to broaden her use to include LSD, Quaaludes, and cocaine. She knew that her family would disapprove, and since they paid for her treatment, she did not confide her substance use disorder to any of her therapists. It never occurred to her that her substance abuse and psychiatric disorder might be related. Marsha was discharged with a diagnosis of polysubstance dependence and a referral to a drug treatment program.

Had Marsha not developed the dystonic reaction to the prescribed medication, she would have left the hospital without the help she needed. Marsha is an example of a patient with a dual diagnosis whose primary diagnosis is a substance-related disorder. Once drug use is initiated, she presents with symptoms resembling a psychiatric disorder.

ASSESSMENT TOOLS

Although time is the most reliable assessment tool, taking a history that reflects the course of both diseases and their possible interaction is essential for accurate diagnosis and very helpful to both clinician and patient. One tool for obtaining such a history is the Dual Diagnosis Assessment Form that we have developed. Filling out this form (see Figure 5.1) (1) chronicles the diseases, treatment, and periods of remission, (2) identifies triggers for both, and (3) provides an understanding of how the patient experiences any positive or negative consequences of the illnesses. The form is equally useful in helping to identify the patient's perception of the two disorders and in determining whether any connections between the two can be made. Figure 5.1 shows the use of the Dual Diagnosis Assessment Form in the following case.

Orlando, a 24-year-old Hispanic male, was referred to an outpatient psychiatric clinic on the day of his discharge from the hospital's inpatient psychiatry unit. The referral stated that he had schizophrenia, had had three acute hospitalizations in 14 months, and had shown very poor follow-up with outpatient treatment recommendations.

The intake social worker discovered how frustrated Orlando was by his frequent hospitalizations and how hopeless he was feeling. This state of distress prompted her to examine the triggers of his relapses. He acknowledged that he did not think he needed medication, so he never took it for very long: "I feel better on my own." He was asked,

FIGURE 5.1. Dual Diagnosis Assessment Form.

Patient: Orlando V.

HISTORY	PSYCHIATRIC	SUBSTANCE USE/ABUSE
1. *Age of onset and circumstances*	At age 18, paranoid symptoms; delusional about family members. Hospitalized for 1 month.	At age 17, used cocaine and alcohol with friends.
2. *Treatment history* a. Hospitalizations/ detoxifications	Total of five hospitalizations (ages 18 and 20; three in the last 14 months).	No drug/alcohol treatment.
b. Outpatient treatment involvement (include rehabilitation and residential programs)	Attended clinic sporadically for past 2 years.	
c. Medications prescribed (include compliance, length of time) Helpful/not helpful to patient	c. Thorazine, Klonopin; poor compliance. Does not like effects; feels "lifeless." Has not found any treatment helpful in the past.	
3. *Periods of remission* Length of time and circumstances	Never symptom free outside of the hospital.	Other than hospitalizations, 2 months when in summer work program at age 21.
4. *Triggers for return of symptoms/use of substances*	With help can identify drinking and stopping medication.	Boredom, frustration, loneliness.
5. *Positive consequences of illness(es) for patient*	Cannot identify.	Takes away pain.
6. *Negative consequences of illness(es) for patient*	a. Fights with mother. b. Loss of faith. c. "Being locked up."	Same.
7. *Patient's understanding of illness(es). Does he/she see connections?*	Patient believes, "I have schizophrenia, but God may cure me someday."	Just beginning to see that alcohol may stimulate psychiatric symptoms.
8. *Family history of illness(es)*	Maternal grandmother "depressed" and had many hospitalizations.	Father—alcoholism Brother— heroin addiction
9. *Family responses to patient's illness(es)*	"Mother worries and wants me to go to clinic."	Drinking minimized and not seen as a disorder by any family members.

"How do you handle any problems? He replied, "I have a few drinks and I feel good." As the worker explored further, it became evident that Orlando's alcohol consumption had increased rapidly and that this increase had heightened his paranoia and isolation. Given this information, the worker charted each relapse with him—the triggers and the consequences—utilizing the Dual Diagnosis Assessment Form. Orlando was able to see, for the first time, that there might be some connection between his psychiatric symptoms and his drinking.

The Drug Diary, in which a patient records the circumstances of substance use, is another tool that can be helpful, in either individual or group treatment, in assessing the extent of addiction and psychiatric disorder. The diary helps clients understand the connection between their two disorders and the notion that substance use is triggered by circumstances and feelings of discomfort. For clients who find it helpful, the diary can also provide concrete evidence of progress.

Figure 5.2 shows how the Drug Diary was used in the following case:

Andy, a 32-year-old white male, was referred by his psychiatric day treatment program, which described his escalating drug and alcohol use as making him "impossible to treat" in their setting. Andy was pleasant and cooperative in his first appointment, but he had difficulty staying on a subject and appeared to be responding to a voice other than that of the interviewer's.

Andy was able to inform the interviewer that during the past 10 years, he had never been drug- or alcohol free for more than 5–7 days, but he had managed to avoid hospitalization for as long as 3 years. Because he was totally unaware of what triggered his substance use and could not describe or name his psychiatric symptoms, the intake worker sent him home with copies of the Drug Diary. He was directed to abstain from all chemicals, but if he was unsuccessful in doing so, he was to record his use in the diary. When Andy returned with his completed diary (see Figure 5.2), it was clear to the intake worker that he was having psychiatric-related symptoms. She explored what it meant to have his "head on fire" and learned, "That's my sister's voice telling me I'm a bad person." Getting high was his attempt to medicate the symptoms. Andy's response to question 5 about how he felt afterward illustrated his ambivalence about wanting and not wanting treatment. In reviewing the diary with him, the intake worker was able to help him express his mixed feelings. Andy realized that the relief obtained from crack was temporary, and he expressed a willingness to see the program psychiatrist to get better stabilized on his medication. Andy has continued to use the Drug Diary in his individual appointments. He is very pleased to bring it in with notations of "clean, clean, clean."

FIGURE 5.2. Drug Diary.

Patient: <u>Andy P.</u>

1. DRUGS USED   AMOUNT   TIME

   a. *Crack*   a. *$25*   a. *2–3 P.M.*

   b.   b.   b.

   c.   c.   c.

   None: _____

   Because: _____

   _____

2. I knew I would use drugs today because

   I got my allowance today and had nothing to do.

3. Before I used, I felt

   I have a pain in my back and my stomach. I want to lighten my head. My head's on fire.

4. When I was using drugs, I felt

   Not high. Nothing. Is this really power?

5. Afterward I felt

   I don't know if I want these drug programs to help. Maybe I'm crazy. I want you to arrest me.

ASSESSMENT OF MOTIVATION FOR TREATMENT

In both mental health and substance abuse facilities, a prospective client's motivation for treatment is part of the assessment. Whether one is motivated or unmotivated may determine acceptance or rejection into a treatment program. In actuality, neither disorder promotes motivation for treatment. The high incidence of patients leaving both detoxification units and psychiatric wards "against medical advice" demonstrates this fact. Treatment, whether for singly or dually diagnosed disorders, is associated with powerlessness and stigma; self-medication or taking no medication at all gives the patient options and some sense of control.

If treatment slots are limited, it is more realistic to assess whether treatment leverage exists for a potential client with a dual diagnosis. Is there a compelling reason for this individual to enter treatment? What will the client lose or gain? A job, housing, financial benefits, family support, and custody of one's children are all excellent points of leverage that providers can use to engage patients in treatment. It is important that clinicians appreciate that *leverage* is a far better indicator than motivation for treatment engagement and that they employ this knowledge in their work. Two cases, those of Belinda and George, illustrate the issue of treatment leverage:

Belinda, a 24-year-old single African American mother, was admitted to the hospital for an acute psychotic episode. Her mother reported that Belinda had had three similar admissions in the past 2 years but, when discharged, always refused to continue in treatment. As Belinda became less psychotic and more trusting of staff, it was learned that she had been using crack to treat her paranoia, anxiety, and mood swings. She had never taken medication outside the hospital because she was convinced it would harm her and hamper her ability to care for her 4-year-old son. She had temporarily lost custody of her son, and she was willing to do anything to get him back.

Staff worked to educate Belinda about the nature of her two disorders and the benefit of treatment. It was made clear that only through participation in treatment could she hope to regain custody of her son. This realization helped Belinda to follow up by joining the hospital's dual diagnosis treatment program upon discharge.

George, a 54-year-old single Irish American male with a documented history of bipolar disorder and alcohol dependence, was referred from the inpatient unit to the dual diagnosis program at the same time as Belinda. George, like Belinda, met the dual diagnosis criteria for admission: that is, diagnosis of a major psychiatric disorder and a substance use disorder. Program staff worked to engage him, making home visits when he did not attend. Unfortunately, they could find no point of leverage. His housing and benefits were intact. He had no family or friends who were affected by his disorders. His health was good despite his years of drinking. When he did attend groups, he was unresponsive to the concerns of his fellow members. Within 3 months, he dropped out of treatment.

Programs treating persons with dual diagnoses have had some success in using harm reduction, as opposed to abstinence, as an initial treatment goal. For persons who have little or no social and vocational life but do have disturbing psychotic symptoms, the use of drugs and alcohol is the only daily activity experienced as pleasurable—it is the one thing to look forward to experiencing. To advise such patients that treatment would involve cessation of all drug and alcohol often undermines the clinician's ability to engage new clients. However, an abstinence-oriented approach is important to consider, based on the client's circumstances and is an option clinicians may also find useful (Ries, 1994).

The harm reduction approach is certainly not without its critics, who argue that if substance abuse is life threatening, it is clearly unethical to give credence to the mere limitation of its use. However, one primary con-

cern must be the engagement of the client in treatment. Thus, if harm reduction as an early treatment goal is more likely to encourage a client to
return for appointments, take medication as prescribed, and consider reducing drug and/or alcohol intake, then it is an approach that offers
greater benefit and safety to the client. For example:

> Tom, diagnosed with schizoaffective disorder and polysubstance de-
> pendence, was hospitalized frequently over a 25-year period. His his-
> tory indicated that he never connected, beyond the first visit, with any
> of the outpatient service referrals he received upon discharge.
>
> Three years ago, Tom was hospitalized and once again referred
> for aftercare. The clinician assigned to see Tom in outpatient treat-
> ment realized that there would be no treatment if she could not engage
> him in their initial session. Rather than highlight abstinence as a goal,
> she chose to stress avoidance of rehospitalization—something Tom
> could agree to work on with her. Objectives included his keeping his
> appointments, taking prescribed medication, and discussing his sub-
> stance use and the possibility that it might undermine his goal to stay
> out of the hospital.
>
> In an early session Tom was obviously high on marijuana, and he
> was amazed and embarrassed that his therapist could detect this. The
> following week he returned and announced, "I've stopped smoking."
> Several sessions later, Tom complained of getting fat. The therapist
> used this opportunity to educate Tom regarding the connection be-
> tween his weight gain and his consumption of a six-pack of beer
> nightly. She proposed a plan in which he would slowly decrease his in-
> take of beer. After a month, he was proudly alcohol free and 7 pounds
> lighter.

ASSESSMENT OF FAMILY

Knowing how a family has responded to mental illness and substance
abuse in the past and is responding in the present is essential to assessment.
Are these disorders minimized or acknowledged? And if acknowledged, are
concern and support or frustration and helplessness expressed? It should
be highlighted that denial on the part of persons who are dually diagnosed
and their families is an important consideration in assessment. Given the
persistence and painful symptoms involved in either a psychiatric or addictive disorder, it is not surprising that people suffering from both have great
difficulty acknowledging them. To compound their own conflicts, they are
constantly confronted with the stigma that either or both disorders engen-
der in their families, the health care personnel, and the larger community.

Families who cannot or will not support the need for medication create a tremendous dilemma for the client with a dual diagnosis, and this di-

lemma must be addressed in treatment. In dual diagnosis treatment, the families need to receive the same education and support as the primary patients, because their responses have a profound influence on treatment outcome.

SIMILARITIES OF THE DISORDERS

For all who work in the helping professions, there must be a secure sense that the treatment skills used are congruent with the needs of the client population. To work effectively with people who have persistent psychiatric illness, mental health professionals learn to understand the biopsychosocial aspects of schizophrenia and affective disorders and to set realistic expectations for their patients as well as for themselves. Yet, when these same skilled clinicians are confronted with a client who has a dual diagnosis, instead of applying this body of knowledge to the second disorder, they typically feel inadequate in the face of addictive illness and unsure of what action to take. The addiction is mistakenly viewed as a negative behavior that can be extinguished if the patient is "motivated" or has "willpower." On the other hand, the skilled clinician specializing in the area of substance-related disorders understands that drug/alcohol dependence is a disease and that to engage a client in the struggle to gain sobriety or achieve a substance-free state is a tremendous undertaking, not just a matter of motivation. Yet, once mental illness is diagnosed, they, too, react with concern that their skills are not adequate to provide successful treatment. Prejudice based on lack of knowledge, pessimism, and concern regarding professional competence sustains the current gap in services. It is, therefore, important that mental health and addiction practitioners realize that they *do* share a common concern about patients as well as a common knowledge base. Therefore, before discussing the issue of treatment, it is important to identify those aspects of the two disorders that are alike and must be considered during treatment planning.

It is essential that service providers understand how similar the disorders are in order to appreciate that the skills they have and the treatment they offer can be of immense benefit to those with a dual diagnosis. Both persistent psychiatric and substance-related disorders, singly or in combination, produce the following:

1. *Impairment in many or all areas of functioning.* Family relationships, school or job performance, financial stability, health, and ability to socialize can be negatively affected by either disorder.
2. *Loss of control.* When an acute episode begins, both the use of substances and the psychiatric symptoms render the patient powerless to manage his or her life.

3. *Persistence and relapse.* Treatment brings remission, but to remain free of psychotic symptoms and substance abuse requires constant vigilance on the part of the patient, the family, and the treatment providers.
4. *Denial as a primary defense.* For the person with psychosis who is also abusing drugs or alcohol, coming to terms with either illness is painful and anxiety provoking.
5. *Social isolation.* When either disorder goes untreated, the patient is severely limited in his or her interactions with others; typically fearful and secretive, the patient's relationships are superficial, at best.
6. *Inattention to physical health.* Untreated mental illness and substance abuse prevent conscious attention to one's health. Minor and serious health problems go unattended, often in the context of increased exposure to health risks.
7. *Extremes in behavior.* For either disorder, there is no consistency in patient behavior. The disorders can produce passivity, aggression, impulsivity, and, in the extreme, suicidal and homicidal behavior.
8. *Impact on family.* Both disorders have a profound impact on family members; feelings of anger, shame, depression, and helplessness are common and can promote enabling and/or blaming behavior.

INTERVENTION WITH CLIENTS WHO HAVE COEXISTING DISORDERS

Given the similarities in the impact of the disorders on patient and family, effective treatment of dual diagnosis (or coexisting) disorders closely resembles the services offered by psychiatric facilities as well as by drug and alcohol treatment programs. This treatment includes the following components.

Psychoeducation

Becoming educated regarding every aspect of each disease is fundamental to recovery for patients with a dual diagnosis. The nonjudgmental, didactic group format that confirms that the illnesses are diseases, not moral or behavioral issues, with documented symptoms, progressions, and side effects, arms patients with information that they can use to understand and protect themselves. The learning is enhanced in the group setting, as members give examples and identify together the common threads of the diseases' impact. The therapist offers information and facilitates discussion and mutual aid.

The following is a list of psychoeducational topics of use for patients with a dual diagnosis:

1. Defining mental illness and addiction. *Purpose*: To identify characteristics of each disorder, their similarities and differences, and how they interact.
2. Theories of mental illness and addiction. *Purpose*: To explore environmental, genetic, and moral models of etiology.
3. Triggers for relapse in mental illness and addiction. *Purpose*: To identify triggers (i.e., people, places, and things) that precipitate relapse in either or both disorders and to highlight similarities.
4. Symptoms of mental illness and addiction. *Purpose*: To identify symptoms of both disorders and note their similarities and differences.
5. Tracing the progression and patterns of mental illness and addiction. *Purpose*: To understand how the disorders progress and distinguish between acute stages and remission.
6. Family role and involvement in mental illness and addiction. *Purpose*: To understand the impact on families when a member suffers from two disorders and to discuss the various responses patients can expect.
7. Good drugs and bad drugs. *Purpose*: To explore the effects of street drugs, alcohol, and psychotropic medications.
8. Social and political issues in mental illness and addiction. *Purpose*: To review sociopolitical views of the disorders and their impact on patients.
9. Treatment planning for mental illness and addiction. *Purpose*: To learn about the variety of treatments available and identify what works and what does not.

Supportive Counseling

A one-to-one relationship with a caring professional provides structure and safety, positive feedback on strengths and progress, hope, and validation that the patient can get better and has the ability to control his or her illness and life. The clinician's focus is not on personality change but on helping the patient make gradual behavioral changes. Interventions are geared toward presenting the patient with options and fostering self-esteem and empowerment. Confrontation, pointing out discrepancies between words and actions, and reality testing are all employed.

Crisis Intervention

With either disorder, patients are always at risk. Patients often handle stress poorly, abruptly stopping medications and/or returning to substance abuse. Any missed appointment is a signal to the treatment staff that the patient is having difficulties. A "slip" in substance use or the cessation of psychiatric medication can herald a downward spiral. Providing follow-up with a phone call or a home visit by staff can help the patient return to treatment before the disorder reaches an acute phase.

Relapse Prevention

Both psychiatric and drug- or alcohol-dependent patients are prone to relapse. To prevent repeated suffering and hospitalizations, patients must learn what circumstances—people, places, or things—trigger an acute episode. Individual, group, and family treatment must stimulate the patient to identify past patterns and ways in which future vulnerability can be diminished. The discovery and rapid arrest of early relapses may help to prevent later ones (Osher & Kofoed, 1989).

The following excerpt from a dual diagnosis education group illustrates the helpfulness of the psychoeducational model and the importance of relapse prevention training.

At the weekly education workshop led by a social worker, the leader announced the day's topic: Identifying Triggers. On the board she wrote headings for two lists to be made by the group: "Emotional illness" and "Addiction."

"Let's start by recalling the situations and feelings that have led to the relapse of people's illnesses." Mark answered, "Nerves," explaining that when he feels anxious, he smokes marijuana. After putting *anxiety* under the heading of "Addiction," the leader asked if anyone else had experienced anxiety as a possible trigger of their emotional illness. Mary raised her hand to say "yes." Once, when she had started a volunteer job, she became very nervous, and her voices became "noticeable, like when I was in the hospital." Offering the next trigger, Julia said, "When I forget I have a sickness." She related how she had become so involved in an art project last winter that she had stopped going to Narcotics Anonymous and the dual diagnosis program. She figured that she was "cured." After the project was completed, Julia, diagnosed with schizoaffective disorder and crack addiction, found herself celebrating her accomplishments with what she thought would be only "one or two hits" off the crack pipe. Julia described a rapid return to daily use. Her poignant tale prompted the leader to ask if members knew the term used to describe this "forgetting" or "ignoring" phenomenon. "Denial," chimed in several members. Writing *denial* under the "Addiction" heading, the leader wondered if denial of emotional illness could potentially trigger the same kind of relapse. Tracy said, "Yeah, like when I stop my meds because I've been feeling good." Tracy explained that he had discontinued his antidepressants in the past when he felt good, figuring he had his disease "licked." The members continued to construct their list of triggers, finding that most triggers belonged under both headings.

Emotional illness	*Addiction*
Anxiety	Anxiety
Denial (forgetting)	Denial (forgetting)
Depression	Depression
Family and peer pressures	Family and peer pressures
Feeling paranoid	Feeling paranoid
Loneliness	Loneliness
Anger	Anger
Holidays and anniversaries	Holidays and anniversaries
	Physical craving for substance
	Too much money

Group Treatment

Denial, isolation, lack of socialization skills, and absence of pleasurable activities can best be remedied in structured groups. Giving and receiving aid, learning to listen, to articulate thoughts and feelings, to be understood, and to have fun are some of the goals of group treatment.

Assertiveness training, psychodrama, art, music, and recreational therapy are effective in achieving these goals. The following vignette demonstrates how group treatment is effective for patients with a dual diagnosis, providing both mutual aid and an increased understanding of the diseases:

Edward complained that "recovery is boring." There is "no zing" without drugs. He reminded the group that he had now been clean for 40 days, "my longest time ever," and asked, "When will anything be fun again? Will there be any zing ever again?" He added that "it is hard to feel feelings now." Without the high of cocaine, all feelings are dulled and interactions with others are difficult and awkward. The leader normalized what Edward described as a commonly experienced stage of early recovery and wondered if others had had similar experiences and/or ideas for how Edward might cope and maintain his psychiatric stability and clean time.

Another member, Tina, agreed wholeheartedly and discussed ways in which she allows herself to use drugs occasionally, at least once or twice a month, "to have something to look forward to, to have some fun." Margie, recently recovering from a third relapse, responded that she understood, but that just this week she had surprised herself. She had gone to a neighborhood flea market and found herself spending several pleasurable hours just browsing.

Jack, 6 months substance free and psychiatrically stable, turned to Edward to say, "Oh, you'll just get used to it." "How?" queried Edward. Jack, a recovering amphetamine addict with schizophrenia, described how, after a while, he had realized that having "average days" is what everyone, even people without a dual diagnosis, have. Jack said it took time to get used to talking to people without a "high on" and, smiling, added that he had just made a comedy video with other members of his residence—an activity he would never have been able to do when he was abusing.

Carla, diagnosed with bipolar disorder and alcohol dependence, remembered how, before her last relapse, she had been missing that zing, or high-energy feeling, she gets when she goes off her lithium. Asked by the leader to name that symptom, Carla replied, "My mania." Carla then told Edward and the group how her mother tells her she "makes sense" now that she is back on her medicines and off alcohol. She added, "Edward, you make sense to me."

Assertive Case Management

People who are recovering, whether they have psychiatric or substance-related disorders or both, have a host of concrete problems directly related to the chaos precipitated by an acute phase of their illness. They need help to partialize and prioritize the issues that need attention, such as securing benefits, housing, education, or job training; following up on medical concerns; and coordinating the prescribed treatment plan (Drake, McHugo, et al., 1998).

Family Involvement

Both mental illness and substance use have a major impact on family members. All family members should be involved in treatment in order to better understand the disorders, to support the patient's progress, and to get the support they need for themselves.

Jane, a 21-year-old suffering from a schizoaffective disorder and cocaine addiction, was living with her older sister Nora and had frequent contact by phone with her parents. When she relapsed after 4 months of drug-free time, her social worker invited the family to come in and discuss what was happening and elicit their ideas on how best to help Jane.

What emerged early in the family meeting was how differently each family member perceived what would be helpful to Jane. Nora, who in earlier meetings with the social worker had had great difficulty acknowledging the psychiatric disorder, was consistent in this thinking: "All Jane needs is a job. The real problem is the drugs, and if she is working, she'll be busy and won't have time to think about them." Jane's mother, Mrs. S., believed that the most helpful thing everyone in the family could do is "detach." Mr. S. had another view: He did not think either work or detaching were good ideas; rather, "Jane just needs all the treatment she can get; from early in the morning to late at night, she should be going to groups and attending the program."

The social worker was made aware of how difficult these conflicting family views were for Jane, increasing her stress rather than alleviating it. She acknowledged the caring feelings of each family member as well as the pain Jane's two illnesses had created for them. She took this opportunity to educate them about the complexity of the two diseases.

With this information, Nora realized that her thoughts about getting a job might have felt more like a demand to Jane at this point in her illness. Her genuine concern was evident when she asked, "Can my sister ever get better?"

Mrs. S. began to understand that her daughter still needed her support and that, perhaps out of her own pain for Jane, "I have detached too much." Mrs. S. agreed that it would be helpful to Jane if she became reinvolved to support Jane in taking her medication and continuing treatment for her addiction. Mr. S. was able to understand that although treatment was essential, too much would create additional stress.

This session gave the family members an opportunity to learn more about Jane's illnesses and to plan a more consistent and realistic kind of support. It also further engaged them in working with the treatment staff to get the information and support they needed for themselves.

USE OF MEDICATIONS

Conventional antipsychotic medications treat the positive symptoms of psychosis effectively. Taking these medications, as prescribed, has decreased or even eliminated the discomfort of paranoia, delusions, and hallucinations for many. In the early 1990s, four new antipsychotic medications became available for use in the treatment of schizophrenia. Classified as "atypical" antipsychotics, these drugs are clozapine (Clozaril), risperidone (Risperidal), quetiapine (Seroquel), and olanzapine (Zyprexa). In mid 2000, a fifth atypical antipsychotic medication, ziprasidone (Zeldox), was made available. The new medications thus far have far fewer side effects. What is most relevant for persons who are dually diagnosed is that these medications target negative symptoms as well as positive ones. Negative symptoms such as depression, low energy, and anxiety are significant triggers for self-medication efforts with alcohol and other drugs. These new medications hold promise for all persons diagnosed with a psychotic disorder. Of greatest value for individuals with dual diagnoses would be the development of an atypical antipsychotic that is injectable. Such medication would be likely to enhance compliance among clients who tend to have difficulty managing their daily oral medications.

TREATMENT MODIFICATIONS

Certain modifications in expectations and treatment must be made by addiction or psychiatric clinicians to provide comprehensive dual diagnosis treatment.

Modifications for Drug and Alcohol Treatment Providers

1. *A longer timeframe to achieve abstinence.* Unlike in the case of the person with a single diagnosis of a substance-related disorder, acceptance for treatment cannot carry the expectation that the patient immediately become free of alcohol or drugs. More slips and relapses can be anticipated and should not be viewed as failure on the part of either the patient or the staff. There are two illnesses from which the patient must recover. Any period of abstinence within the first year of treatment is promising.

2. *The value of psychotropic medication.* Traditionally, the addiction treatment approach has required abstention from *all* chemicals, prescribed as well as nonprescribed. Most patients suffering from major psychiatric disorders that have significant biological components, however, must be maintained on medication to prevent relapse and to enable them to participate fully in the treatment offered. Stopping psychiatric medication is a trigger for relapse in both diseases.

3. *Modification of confrontation techniques.* Although patients with a dual diagnosis must be taught that they frequently exhibit behavior that is in direct opposition to their well-being, they will not benefit from the traditional confrontation techniques used in therapeutic drug communities. Confrontation must be gentler and directed only at behaviors, never at the patients themselves.

4. *The concept of enabling.* The concept of enabling, which is viewed as a negative enforcer of illness by addiction specialists—that is, as protecting patients from the consequences of their behavior (Levinson & Straussner, 1978)—must be considered in a different light with patients who have dual diagnoses. If a patient appears to be at risk for relapse, staff must respond promptly with appropriate interventions, such as daily appointments, accompanying the client to an appointment, or facilitating negotiations of difficult systems.

5. *Psychiatric availability.* The availability of a psychiatrist to evaluate and monitor mental status and to prescribe and follow patients taking medication is essential. Furthermore, many patients with a dual diagnosis have fewer relapses when on injectable medication.

6. *Harm reduction.* This approach offers particular promise in the early phases of treatment, especially during the engagement phase.

Modifications for Mental Health Providers

1. *Assess and monitor substance abuse.* Mental health staff have to fully assess and monitor substance abuse. Psychiatric programs treating clients with a dual diagnosis must help them understand the effects and consequences of chemical dependency and offer ongoing individual and group education and support.

2. *Urine monitoring and breathalyzers.* Such monitoring devices need to be used regularly when patients are not able to discuss their current substance use openly.

3. *Participation in 12-step program.* Patients need active encouragement to participate in 12-step self-help groups such as Alcoholics Anonymous (AA), Narcotics Anonymous (NA), Cocaine Anonymous (CA), or Double Trouble (DT), and family members should be referred to Al-Anon, Nar-Anon, or Co-Anon.

4. *Policy on attendance.* A clear policy should prohibit any patient from being seen in out-patient treatment when "appearing" to staff to be high or intoxicated. Since it is impossible for staff to convince a patient that he or she is high when the patient denies this, basing the rules on appearance rather than factual evidence eliminates arguments and helps to stress the importance of a drug-free environment for all patients participating in recovery.

TREATMENT MODEL FOR PATIENTS WITH A DUAL DIAGNOSIS

The ideal treatment progression for the patient with a dual diagnosis consists of three steps:

1. Brief psychiatric hospitalization to assess, stabilize, and, when necessary, provide supervised detoxification.
2. Rehabilitation treatment in a residential setting targeted to both disorders for 6–12 months.
3. Psychiatric outpatient services and 12-step program attendance.

Given the limited number of residential treatment facilities for clients with a dual diagnosis, a more realistic model consists of outpatient day treatment, with brief hospitalization when needed. The mental health staff should include a counselor who is recovering from an addiction; such a person brings a very special dimension to the treatment of patients by leading 12-step groups and providing a tangible example that recovery is a hope that can be fulfilled. All members of the treatment team need to utilize the following guidelines:

1. Both illnesses are acknowledged and discussed in every patient contact.
2. Abstinence is a goal of, not a precondition to, treatment.
3. Patient admissions of substance abuse are treated as a health concern, not grounds for discharge from treatment.
4. Despite the nonpunitive climate of dual diagnosis treatment, breathalyzers are used and urine testing is done; these are objective instruments that allow clinician and patient to monitor progress and to support treatment.
5. Participation in self-help groups (AA, NA, CA, DT) is strongly encouraged, as is provision of both on-site meetings and staff accompaniment of patients to outside meetings until the patients are connected.
6. Patients sign a contract that clearly prohibits treatment attendance when they appear to be intoxicated or high and indicate their agreement to be hospitalized when either disease is assessed to be acute by staff.
7. Treatment of a dual diagnosis condition is a team effort. A single practitioner cannot provide all the support essential to recovery; team members bring different subspecialty skills to the many patient crises that are inherent to both disorders.

CONCLUSION

The client who is dually diagnosed suffers from a major psychiatric disorder as well as a substance-related disorder; both are primary disorders and require specific and concomitant treatment approaches. *Treatment that targets only one disorder will not be successful.*

Given the many similarities in the two disorders and their impact on clients and their families, it is not surprising that the traditional treatment models have much in common. The difficulty in integrating psychiatric and addiction treatment approaches is rooted in philosophical differences as well as fear and prejudice due to lack of knowledge. These differences can be resolved if practitioners are willing to expand their thinking. Mental health service providers can work effectively with this population with only a few modifications in their existing treatment skills, and substance abuse providers need to understand that some patients *do* need to be maintained on medication and do need some modification in their treatment regimes.

To encourage the expansion of comprehensive dual diagnosis treatment in psychiatric facilities, it is important to highlight the similarities of the disorders, instead of the differences. Given the enormity of the needs and numbers of persons with primary psychiatric and substance-related disorders, there is no alternative.

REFERENCES

Drake, R. E., McHugo, G. J., Clark, R. E., Teague, G. B., Xie, H., Miles, K., & Ackerson, T. H. (1998). Assertive community treatment for patients with co-occuring severe mental illness and substance use disorder: A clinical trial. *American Journal of Orthopsychiatry*, 68(2), 201–215.

Drake, R. E., Mercer-McFadden, C., Mueser, K. T., McHugo, G. J., & Bond, G. R. (1998). Review of integrated mental health and substance abuse treatment for patients with dual disorders. *Schizophrenia Bulletin*, 24(4), 589–608.

Hall, R. C. (1979). Relationship of psychiatric illness to drug abuse. *Journal of Psychedelic Drugs*, 11, 337–342.

Haywood, T. W., Kravitz, H. M., Grossman, L. S., Cavanaugh, J. L., Jr., Davis, J. M., & Lewis, D. A. (1995). Predicting the "revolving door" phenomenon among patients with schizophrenia, schizoaffective and affective disorders. *American Journal of Psychiatry*, 152(6), 856–861.

Kessler, R. C, Crum, R. M., Warner, L. A., Nelson, C. B., Schulenberg, J., & Anthony, J. C. (1997). Lifetime co-occurrence of DSM-III-R alcohol abuse and dependence with other psychiatric disorders in the national comorbidity survey. *Archives of General Psychiatry*, 54, 313–321.

Koegel, P. Sullivan, G., Burnam, A., Morton, S. C., & Wenzel, S. (1999). Utilization of mental health and substance abuse services among homeless adults in Los Angeles. *Medical Care*, 37(3), 306–317.

Lehman, A. F., Meyers, C. P., & Corty, E. (1989). Assessments and classification of patients with psychiatric and substance abuse syndromes. *Hospital and Community Psychiatry*, 40(10), 1019.

Levinson, V. R., & Straussner, S. L. A. (1978). Social workers as "enablers" in the treatment of alcoholism. *Social Casework*, 59(1), 14–20.

McKelvy, M. J., Kane, J. S., & Kellison, K. (1987). Substance abuse and mental illness: Double trouble. *Journal of Psychosocial Nursing*, 25, 20–25.

Menezes, P. R., Johnson, S., Thornicroft, G., Marshall, J., Prosser, D., Bebbington, P., & Kuipers, E. (1996). Drug and alcohol problems among individuals with severe mental illness in South London. *British Journal of Psychiatry*, 168(5), 612–619.

Osher, F. C., & Kofoed, L. L. (1989). Treatment of patients with psychiatric and psychoactive substance abuse disorders. *Hospital and Community Psychiatry*, 40(10), 1025–1029.

Pepper, B., Kirshner, M. C., & Ryglewicz, H. (1981). The young adult chronic patient: Overview of a population. *Hospital and Community Psychiatry*, 32(7), 463–469.

Regier, D. A., Farmer, M. E., & Rae, D. S. (1990). Comorbidity of mental disorders with alcohol and other drug abuse. *Journal of the American Medical Association*, 264, 2511–2518.

Ries, R. (1994). *Assessment and treatment of patients with co-existing mental illness and alcohol and other drug abuse*. Rockville, MD: Center for Substance Abuse Treatment, the Substance Abuse and Mental Health Services Administration.

Safer, D. (1987). Substance abuse by young chronic patients. *Hospital and Community Psychiatry*, 38, 511–514.

Singer, M. I., Kennedy, M. J., & Kola, L. A. (1998). A conceptual model for co-occurring mental and substance related disorders. *Alcoholism Treatment Quarterly,* *16*(4), 75–89.

Wallen, M. D., & Weiner, H. (1989). Impediments to effective treatment of the dually diagnosed patient. *Journal of Psychoactive Drugs, 21,* 161–168.

Wanck, B. (1987). Addiction and mental illness: Assessing the difference. *Mediplex* *Medical Update, 3*(1), 1–4.

CHAPTER 6

12-Step Programs as a Treatment Modality

Betsy Robin Spiegel
Christine Huff Fewell

For centuries people with similar interests and concerns have banded together and formed what have more recently been termed *self-help groups*. Thus, some of our religious institutions were "self-help" groups before they became institutions. Research estimates that more than 25 million Americans have been involved in self-help groups at some point during their lives (Kessler, Mickelson, & Zhao, 1997). The most impressive and well known of the self-help groups is Alcoholics Anonymous, which has been the prototype of other groups for substance-abusing individuals, such as Cocaine Anonymous, Narcotics Anonymous, Pills Anonymous, and Methamphetamine Anonymous, as well as groups for family members, such as Al-Anon, Alateen, and Adult Children of Alcoholics. Khantzian and Mack (1994) contend that "beyond achieving abstinence and providing support, AA is effective because it is a sophisticated psychological treatment whose members have learned to manage effectively and/or transform the psychological and behavioral vulnerabilities associated with alcoholism" (p. 21). The purpose of this chapter is to illuminate the potent therapeutic potential of these groups and the 12 steps by utilizing psychodynamic theory and case examples.

CHARACTERISTICS OF 12-STEP PROGRAMS

No analysis of self-help groups can omit a discussion of the phenomenal growth of these groups during the past two decades. Twelve-step programs are commonplace in our national vernacular, on television and in print. Almost everyone knows someone who has benefited from one of them. Membership in the 12-step programs was originally focused exclusively on helping alcoholics and their families. Later additions to the 12-step family include Overeaters Anonymous, Emotions Anonymous, Parents Anonymous, Sex Addicts Anonymous, Self-Mutilators Anonymous, and Gamblers Anonymous.

The tradition of anonymity is the fulcrum of a 12-step program. It bestows an immediate freedom on the member who can feel able to share without fear of rejection or betrayal, and it aids in rapidly creating an atmosphere of trust. All 12-step programs include regularly scheduled meetings, a telephone network for immediate intervention, outreach to others, and sponsorship. Sponsorship is a mutually beneficial relationship in which a long-term member provides support and advice to the newcomer.

ALCOHOLICS ANONYMOUS

Alcoholics Anonymous (AA) officially began in May 1935 when Bill Wilson, a formerly hopeless alcoholic then trying to stay sober, met with Dr. Bob Smith, another floundering "drunkard." They found that by supporting each other and helping other individuals with alcoholism, they were able to attain and maintain sobriety. Bill Wilson had been a member of the Oxford Group, which was an international movement in the 1920s and 1930s based on the spiritual teachings of the early Christians. Some of the ideas and spiritual beliefs of AA, particularly the 12 steps, are derivatives of this movement. The Oxford Group was a nondenominational Christian movement that advocated sharing personal experiences of pursuing a life guided by the principles of honesty, purity, unselfishness, and love (Encyclopedia Britannica, 2004). Dr. Bob said of Bill W. after the first meetings, " . . . he was the first living human with whom I had ever talked, who knew what he was talking about in regard to alcoholism from actual experience" (quoted in Robertson, 1988, p. 35). Both men had social stature, were articulate and educated, and were able to spread their ideas—first to Akron, Ohio, and then throughout the country.

Newcomers at their first AA meeting today encounter many of the same procedures as did those in the days of Bill W. and Dr. Bob 65 years ago. Many AA meetings take place in church basements because churches opened their doors to AA early in its life. A beginner usually goes down a set of stairs and is greeted by the same old slogans, such as "Easy does it," "First things first," "HALT" (don't get Hungry, Angry, Lonely, or Tired), and "Keep it simple."

A beginner is encouraged to attend 90 meetings in 90 days. In other words, almost total immersion is recommended when the person first puts down the bottle and learns to replace "booze" with people and meetings.

The following vignette describes the experience of one member, Martha, at her first AA meeting.

> Martha is a 37-year-old schoolteacher who drank periodically for 7 years. She was persuaded by an old friend to call AA after a serious binge resulted in head and leg injuries that she had no recollection of sustaining. Her call was answered by Jim B., an AA volunteer, whose direct and compassionate manner eased her fear and shame. "We alcoholics have a disease," he told her. "We have a disease of loneliness." He arranged for her to be escorted to her first AA meeting by another volunteer, Ramona M., who was a longtime member of the fellowship.
>
> The meeting was held in a church in her community in a large city. As soon as Martha walked in, she saw well-dressed smiling men and women at a table with books and pamphlets. Two older women wearing blue badges labeled "Hospitality" greeted her. Martha was stunned. Where were the bag ladies? Where were the winos? A young woman approached her with a friendly, welcoming "hello" and an offer of a telephone number. Then Martha saw plastic scrolls at the front of the room. One said "Twelve Steps" and the other "Twelve Traditions." Most of the letters were a blur, but she managed to remember the first words of the first step: "We admitted we were powerless over alcohol."
>
> Martha remembers being both frightened and exhilarated. She was especially relieved to see so many attractive professional women. It was the speaker's story that finally convinced her that she was in the right place. "I never thought I was any good," he said, "I never felt I belonged until I found alcohol."
>
> Martha does not know if it was the speaker or the heads nodding in agreement, but she began to cry. She recalls feeling safe for the first time in years. She knew she was home.

The unconditional warmth and acceptance of the group members facilitated the beginning of a strong attachment, or bonding, that enabled Martha to feel safe. This topic is discussed later in more detail in the chapter.

Attendance at an AA meeting can range from two people to 200. For each meeting there is a chairperson who opens and closes the meeting; a secretary who makes announcements and asks if there are any anniversaries, visitors, or additional announcements; and a treasurer who monitors the collection and disbursements of contributions. All contributions to AA are voluntary, and each group is self-supporting. Officers are elected and change every 6 months. *Open* meetings consist of three speakers who have a minimum of 90 days sobriety and who tell the story of their addiction and recovery. These meetings are open to all who are interested. *Closed* meetings are held exclusively for those in the fellowship; the tradition of anonymity is taken very seriously. Most meetings involve a "qualification," which is a speaker's story of drinking, bottoming out, and recovery.

The speaker usually presents a topic for discussion. A *step* meeting is one in which one of the 12 steps is read. The speaker's story or qualification is usually focused on this step, as is the discussion from the floor that follows. A *beginners* meeting addresses the tools necessary in early sobriety. Many are embodied in slogans such as "It's the first drink that gets you drunk," "Easy does it," and "First things first." Beginners are encouraged to share their concerns and feelings. Through the process of identification, beginners learn that they are not alone.

The sponsorship relationship is crucial in ending isolation and ensuring recovery. A sponsor is someone of the same sex with sober experience in AA who becomes a mentor or special friend and guides the newcomer on his or her journey of sober living. According to the 1998 AA membership survey, 75% of AA members have a sponsor, and 85% belong to a home group (Alcoholics Anonymous, 1999).

The results of the AA membership survey further revealed that, as of 1998, AA as a whole was composed of 34% women and 66% men. Among members under age 30 the ratio was somewhat narrower, with 38% women and 62% men. The average length of sobriety was more than 7 years, and the average age of an AA member was 45. The membership spans a large age range, with 2% of members then under the age of 21, and 4% over the age of 70. Most members reported attending two meetings per week. Occupationally, 13% of AA members were classified as professional, 13% as retired, 11% as other, including self-employed, 10% as managerial, and 8% as labor. Six percent categorized themselves as health care professionals. Only 6% listed themselves as unemployed. The remaining 33% of respondents fell into the categories of disabled (5%), sales worker (4%), craft worker (4%), service worker (4%), clerical worker (3%), educator (3%), homemaker (3%), student (3%), and transportation (2%).

COCAINE ANONYMOUS

Alcoholics Anonymous has had an increasing number of "offspring" that offer programs to treat addictions to everything from narcotics, pills, and cocaine, to sex, self-mutilation, and procrastination. Cocaine Anonymous (CA), founded in Los Angeles, is over 20 years old. Its members tend to be younger than those in AA. The format of CA resembles that of AA. CA offers additional tips for staying clean and sober. These include, "Throw away all your drug paraphernalia, throw away all your drugs, don't deal drugs. If the connection calls, hang up." CA also cautions against using any other mind-altering drugs. In CA much of the sharing is about the sensation of using cocaine and the high of the drug use. Many users seek to escape from profound feelings of apathy or deadness.

NARCOTICS ANONYMOUS

Narcotics Anonymous (NA) was created to serve the users of drugs and follows the same format as AA and CA, with small variations. NA was founded in California in 1953 by a number of drug addicts who wanted to recover from addiction (Narcotics Anonymous World Service Office, 1983). NA is the fastest growing 12-step group. Whereas in 1978 there were fewer than 200 groups registered in three countries, in 2000, there were 28,207 NA meetings held weekly in over 104 countries. Of the 5,000 NA members responding to an informal poll taken in 1989, 64% were male and 36% were female. Eleven percent were under 20; 37% were between 20 and 30; 48% were between 30 and 45; and 4% were over 45 (Narcotics Anonymous World Services, n.d.).

NA views the addiction as the problem without naming a particular drug. The first step of NA is worded: "We admitted that we were powerless over our addiction, that our lives had become unmanageable." The slogan is "Take people, not a hit"; for anniversaries chips are given out, with two quarters taped to one side and a phone number to the other, to encourage impulsive members to turn to people and not to the "hit."

For almost 15 years an increasing number of users have contracted the AIDS virus and hepatitis C through the use of dirty needles, and the fellowship has had to deal with the death of some of their members and the illness of many others. It is a testament to the strength of this fellowship that members continued to practice the principles and utilize NA as a support service. The culture of Narcotics Anonymous is warm and enthusiastic and attendance at these meetings continues to increase.

DUAL RECOVERY ANONYMOUS

An example of the adaptability of the 12-step model can be seen in the growth of the 12-step group called Dual Recovery Anonymous. This group, which began in 1989 in Kansas, has adapted the 12 steps of Alcoholics Anonymous for the purpose of helping individuals suffering from dual disorders to maintain abstinence from alcohol and other intoxicating drugs and manage their emotional or psychiatric illness in a healthy and constructive way (Dual Recovery Anonymous, n.d.). The message is clearly given that it is necessary to accept differences, and that some members use prescription medication whereas others do not. The program also stresses that attendance at meetings is not a substitute for professional help for psychiatric or emotional illness. Meetings are not yet as evenly available across the country as those of AA, CA, and NA, and are more concentrated in California and the Midwest.

AL-ANON

Al-Anon is the biggest and oldest group for the families and friends of alcoholics. In the early days of AA most meetings were held in people's homes. The spouses were left in the kitchen to take care of the coffee and cake; it was in these kitchens, with the help of Lois W., wife of Bill Wilson, that Al-Anon was born. According to the 1999 Membership Survey of Al-Anon–Alateen World Services, there are now over 30,000 Al-Anon and Alateen groups worldwide, over 19,500 in the United States alone (Al-Anon/Alateen, 2000). Although 85% of its members is female, it is significant that 15% is male, given the group's all-female origin. The typical Al-Anon member is a married white female who has some college training or a college degree, works in a professional, managerial, or executive job, and lives in a large city (Al-Anon/Alateen, 2000). The majority of Al-Anon members (65%) are between 35 and 54 years old, with the average age being 50. Most Al-Anon members surveyed have an alcoholic spouse or partner (78%); 36% have an alcoholic parent and 26% have a child with a problem. In addition, 46% of members have other relatives with an alcohol problem, indicating the presence of alcoholism in more than one significant relationship.

The major slogan of Al-Anon is called the 3C's: "I didn't *cause* alcoholism, I can't *control* it, and I can't *cure* it." Another slogan, which also tells the essential story, is "Keep the focus on yourself." Programs such as Nar-Anon and Co-Anon, for the families of narcotic users and cocaine addicts, follow the principles of Al-Anon.

Adult Children of Alcoholics (ACOA) originated within the Al-Anon program in 1976. In the 1980s it emerged as the fastest growing 12-step program in the country, aimed at the estimated 28 million Americans who have at least one alcoholic parent (Eigen & Rowden, 1995). Alateen is the part of the Al-Anon Family groups designed for teenagers to "recover from the effects of someone else's drinking" (Al-Anon/Alateen, 2000). A recent study by Grant (2000) indicates that one in four children in the United States lives in a family with a history of alcohol abuse, and many suffer direct negative consequences as a result.

THE THERAPEUTIC VALUE
OF THE FELLOWSHIP OF 12-STEP PROGRAMS

The anonymous programs and the 12 steps offer an opportunity for internal, structural, therapeutic change. The meetings, slogans, literature, sponsorship, and the 12 steps themselves all act as therapeutic agents. The anonymous programs provide a *holding environment*, a term first used by the British object relations theorist D. W. Winnicott (1975). Winnicott believed that the therapist, the office, and all the arrangements surrounding the therapy sessions, especially consistency, create an environment that is safe and nurturing, thereby setting and holding the stage for psychological exploration and development. Similarly, AA and the other 12-step programs with their accoutrements provide this safety and consistency.

Winnicott's (1951) concepts of transitional objects and transitional phenomena also have relevance for understanding the therapeutic action of the anonymous programs. According to Winnicott, the infant's relation to transitional objects provides an important step in the process of development toward objective reality. An object such as a blanket or teddy bear comes to symbolize the mother's image so that the child can be soothed by the object in her absence. Gradually the child internalizes the capacity for self-soothing and does not need the concrete, external object. This transitional period, when internalized, lays the foundation for a range of adult abilities, such as the ability to play with ideas, to be creative, and to enjoy cultural experiences (e.g., art and music). If the process is hindered, the young child develops what Winnicott termed a "false self." The self-image is split: The part containing the child's subjective world (i.e., the true self) is kept secret, while another part adapts to the demands of the environment (i.e., the false self). This split leaves the true self feeling empty and alienated. According to McDougall (1991), this split state may predispose people to seek what she terms "transitory objects" (p. 77), such as drugs, as a way of soothing the self (although the relief is only temporary). The AA program can be viewed as a transitional space in which the recovery process can take place. The newcomer to AA is advised to rely heavily on the meetings and on AA people outside of the meetings, both of which offer unconditional acceptance and support, unlike what is normally encountered in the everyday world. Extreme reliance on the program can be seen as serving an excellent transitional role while the person gradually internalizes less destructive and more reliable self-soothing mechanisms. This is the psychodynamic fulcrum of the program.

Whatever the degree of physical deterioration and emotional regression, all newcomers to 12-step programs share some similar traits. They are usually desperate, full of pain, and have a low sense of self-esteem. The pain and desperation shatter the wall of narcissistic pride and grandiosity that prevents the self-destructive, active alcoholic from asking for help. When the defenses crumble, access is gained to an earlier, more authentic self, which facilitates the bonding with others.

The relationship of a newcomer to AA can resemble the early bonding with the mother, as described in Bowlby's (1958) attachment theory. Those who do bond often make a very productive and exhilarating connection with the program. Here we see the sense of magic and feeling of grandiosity characteristic of the young child. In the parlance of Alcoholics Anonymous, it is called the "pink cloud." If the recovering alcoholic were to apply words to this stage, it would be something like, "The program is magic, my sponsor is magical, and everything will be all right."

Attachment theory posits that young children remain in close proximity to a caretaker for the purpose of protection and security. When the caretaker is available, helpful, and appropriately responsive, the child develops attachment bonds that provide an enduring sense of security. These bonds, in turn, enable the child to explore increasingly further afield as he or she grows and passes through adolescence (Ainsworth & Bowlby, 1991). When the caretaker is rejecting or ambivalent in his or her response, the child develops insecurity about attachment and may need to seek continual reassurance that the caretaker (and later, other emotionally invested people) is available, or to act as though it did not matter.

A drug often becomes an attachment object that can be depended on for an individual who has insecure attachment. The substance-dependent person seeks to keep the drug readily available and feels anxiety when separated from it, which may be chemically or neurobiologically, as well as psychologically, induced. Other attachment figures often fade in importance and may be replaced altogether by the drug that has assumed primary importance. AA can be seen as providing an attachment object which the newcomer can rely on to be available 24 hours a day, either through meetings or personal telephone contact. AA suggests that a new member attend 90 meetings in 90 days and encourages contact with AA members 24 hours a day via telephone, if needed. This format provides a highly available attachment group, without the need to attach to any *one* person, which might prove very threatening to a substance-dependent person who may be suffering from anxiety about attachment. Intense involvement in the program can provide what Bowlby (1988) termed "a secure base."

Once having fostered attachment to the anonymous program and its "holding environment," the Steps and other components of the program can be viewed as providing guidelines for making progress along the maturational continuum of separation–individuation (Mahler, Pine, & Bergman, 1975). Straussner and Spiegel (1996) describe how the curative process of the 12 steps can contribute to increasing differentiation and the development of healthy object relations and object constancy. For example, such elements as the "holding environment" of the program, the sponsor, unconditional acceptance, slogans, and guidelines for daily living all facilitate the gradual working through of Mahler's differentiation subphase. Straussner and Spiegel liken the phenomenon of the pink cloud to the feelings of euphoria experienced by the child in Mahler's practicing subphase. Object constancy is gradually attained as the tasks outlined in the steps are undertaken, and the recovering substance abuser is ready to lessen his or her dependency on the program.

THE PROMISES

The book *Alcoholics Anonymous* (1939) describes "The Promises," which hold out hope for change to the discouraged and confused newcomer. The promises state that if an individual rigorously adheres to the AA program, he or she will find new paths of being and relating. The promises are statements such as "You will instinctively know how to handle situations that once baffled" and "Self-seeking will slip away." The words *instinctively* and *slip* indicate that the changes are part of an unconscious process. Appropriate reality testing and mature object relations are key to the attainment of these promises.

Another promise, "You will not regret the past nor wish to shut the door on it" seems impossible to the shame- and guilt-ridden person with alcoholism. This promise speaks to the acceptance of self that is so often the result of the spiritual part of the program, and to the ability to use personal experience to help others.

Thus, the program has been used as a "good enough mother" (to borrow a phrase from Winnicott), a good object, which, once internalized, acts as a change agent. The promises hold out the hope that deep changes of character are possible.

SPONSORSHIP

The use of the sponsorship relationship is an important tool in the recovery from addiction. Many people with addictions did not experience an essentially loving relationship with their same-sex parent. Such a loving relationship fosters the idealization necessary for a positive identification that, when internalized, produces a healthy sense of one's gender and identity.

The deficit in same-sex parenting is addressed in the sponsorship relationship. The sponsor can become a confidant(e), mentor, and even a "good enough" parent. Old conflicts can surface and be resolved in the holding environment of a compassionate, understanding relationship. Sponsorship is one key that turns the lock in the door to sobriety.

THE THERAPEUTIC NATURE
OF UTILIZING THE 12 STEPS

In addition to the benefits of fellowship in the 12-step program already mentioned, the person with alcoholism or a drug addiction who is practicing the 12 steps obtains an important structure and a roadmap for recovery. The 12 steps and their tasks are as follows (W., 1953):

1. "We admitted we were powerless over alcohol—that our lives had become unmanageable." This is the admission step, which provides access into the recovery process and acknowledges the pervasiveness of the illness.
2. "We came to believe that a Power greater than ourselves could restore us to sanity." This step instills hope in the recovery process that AA offers.
3. "We made a decision to turn our will and our lives over to the care of God as we understood Him." Here, a commitment is made to accept help from an outside source that is not fully comprehended. This is an extension of the previous step into faith and a surrender of personal will to a higher order.
4. "We made a searching and fearless moral inventory of ourselves." This step focuses a member upon him- or herself and requires the listing of personal assets and liabilities.
5. "We admitted to God, to ourselves, and to another human being the exact nature of our wrongs." The appraisal of the previous step is shared and examined with others.
6. "We were entirely ready to have God remove all these defects of character." Continuing the process begun in steps 4 and 5, the individual seeks a change in attitude and becomes willing to give up negative aspects of the self.
7. "We humbly asked Him to remove our shortcomings." Going beyond the previous step, the member surrenders to a deeper level of change, seeking help from an external source to do so.
8. "We made a list of all persons we had harmed, and became willing to make amends to them all." Here the person accepts responsibility for past negative actions and alters his or her attitude toward others.
9. "We made direct amends to such people whenever possible, except when to do so would injure them or others." Now active restitution is implemented for any destructive behavior identified in the previous step.
10. "We continued to take personal inventory and when we were wrong promptly admitted it." This step fosters daily self-appraisal of behavior and corrective action.
11. "We sought through prayer and meditation to improve our conscious contact with God as we understood Him, praying only for knowledge of His will for us and the power to carry that out." Now, on a daily basis, the individual makes a commitment to the spiritual aspects of the program, seeking an inner state of peace and harmony.
12. "Having had a spiritual awakening as the result of these steps, we tried to carry this message to alcoholics, and to practice these

principles in all our affairs." This culmination step integrates the ideals and values of the program and is a commitment to help other individuals with alcoholism.

If the steps are taken sequentially, an increasingly stronger and more flexible ego is developed. The ego function of reality testing serves as an example. A major function of the ego is to ensure the individual's appropriate relation to reality (Spiegel & Mulder, 1986). Reality testing involves the adjustment of personal needs and impulses to the world's ever-changing roles, expectations, and circumstances. The relationship between inner and outer worlds is best mediated by firm ego boundaries and a cohesive sense of self. Reality is confronted immediately in step 1: "We admitted we were powerless over alcohol—that our lives had become unmanageable." To pierce through the denial of active alcoholism and clearly see the turmoil and damage in its wake is a painful awakening. In step 4, when the person is asked to conduct a searching and fearless inventory of self, good reality testing is essential. This step can only be accomplished with better reality-testing skills than are needed in step 1, because the recovering member must review the drinking years and acknowledge how his or her sense of reality was distorted. Reality testing is further strengthened in step 8, which calls for reviewing past harm to others and changing one's attitude toward them. And ongoing self-appraisal of the effect of one's behavior is called for in step 10.

Defense mechanisms, like other ego functions, are also admirably handled by working the steps in sequence. Maladaptive defense mechanisms are dismantled and replaced with more adaptive ones. For example, it is the primitive defense mechanism of denial that is addressed in step 1: "We admitted we were powerless . . . " The key word here is not *powerless*, but *admitted*. Projection, another primitive defense mechanism, is addressed in steps 4 and 5, when the person writes down his or her defects and shares them with a trusted person. Whereas the defense of projection permits a person to deny his or her own feelings and displace them onto someone else, making a list of defects destroys this defense; the person can no longer avoid responsibility for his or her own actions. By utilizing the steps, the person recovering from alcoholism moves toward using the higher level defense mechanism of sublimation in place of the more distorting defense mechanisms of denial and projection. In step 12 the person is asked to sublimate his or her grandiosity and aggressive power strivings into providing help to another person with alcoholism.

Yet another benefit: The internal working model of self, described by Bowlby (1988), can be altered by utilizing the 12 steps. This aspect of attachment theory posits that the interaction pattern of the caretaker's relationship with the child becomes internalized as a mental representation of how consistently available or rejecting attachment figures are, and how supportive they are of exploration. The mental representation also contains a complementary view of how acceptable or unacceptable and how worthy of care and support the individual is in the eyes of others (Marvin & Britner, 1999).

Working steps 1, 2, and 3 provides the opportunity to alter an existing internal working model. Step 1 sets the stage when the individual acknowledges that he or she is powerless to manage the current situation. In children, it is the recognition of powerlessness that promotes the formation of attachment bonds. Admitting powerlessness opens the possibility of revising the original internal working model. Step 2 requires a belief that someone else can be relied on for help. Step 3 further requires that a commitment be made to trust in this possibility. Inherent in accepting steps 2 and 3 is the assumption that the person is worthy of receiving such help. Accepting this assumption begins the development of an internal working model of the self as a person who is worthy and capable of receiving nurturing and care.

Spiegel and Mulder (1986) describe how working the steps also aids in relaxing a harsh and punitive superego. A person with alcoholism is usually his or her own most severe critic. However, a softening of the superego is essential to sobriety. This softening can be inaugurated by focusing on assets as well as liabilities (step 4). A harsh superego can interfere with accurate reality testing just as much as a grandiose and infantile ego.

The ego function of object relations is also developed through the 12 steps. Early object relations are characterized by striving for self-gratification and preoccupation with one's own survival. Later, as object relations become more cohesive, good and bad aspects of others and the self can be integrated. Eventually, the pervasive fear of abandonment subsides. It is significant that the pronoun used in all of the 12 steps is *we*; the person with active alcoholism likely has not thought in terms other than *I* in a long time. The first relationship a newcomer is asked to form is with a "Power greater than ourselves." As seen in step 3, members are asked to turn their life and their will over to "God as we understand Him." This surrendering entails a transfer of personal grandiosity from the injured self to an external force, the Higher Power, which sets the stage for the breakdown in grandiosity and the reconstruction of relationships to self and others. Step 8, which suggests making a list of those people one has harmed, cannot be done without the capacity for empathic feeling for others. Certainly it cannot be done by the newcomer who still objects to the *we* in step 1. Empathic feelings lead to compassionate activity. Thus, in step 12, the last step, the member is asked to help other people with alcoholism and carry the message of AA to all who still suffer. Successful and genuine 12-step work produces mature feelings, healthy boundaries, and solid reality-testing abilities.

What happens in meditation and prayer is best explained by looking at what happens to the ego during the state of creative inspiration. Ernest Kris (1952) states that "impulses, wishes and fantasies derived from the unconscious are attributed to a supernatural being and the process of their becoming conscious is experienced as an action of this being upon the person" (p. 302). In meditation, unconscious and preconscious aspects of the self are split off, attributed to God or a Higher Power, and then reintegrated by the ego. Meditation and prayer provide the ego with a means of relating to parts of the self that have been outside of ordinary awareness. This may explain the expansive feeling that accompanies the working of step 11.

Perhaps the most sophisticated ego function is that of synthesis and integration (Goldstein, 1995), which makes a cohesive whole out of fragments of self (i.e., information and/or feelings). The last words of step 12 are "and to practice these principles in all our affairs." In order to do this, the AA member must have integrated and internalized all the principles of the program and developed an entirely new character structure—and, indeed, a new life.

AL-ANON AS A TREATMENT
MODALITY FOR CODEPENDENCY

The term *codependency* emerged in the chemical dependency field in the 1970s as a way to describe the mutual involvement of the non-substance-abusing partner in the interactive process of maintaining the addiction. Many authors have written about the growing dependence and preoccupation of the codependent person with the needs of others, to the detriment of self-care and self-esteem. Although a spouse who is codependent may appear to be highly competent, defensive functioning that complements that of the actively addicted spouse frequently serves to maintain the status quo. This behavior, elicited by the systemic pull of addiction, combines with the intrapsychic needs of the individual to create the state of codependency.

Recent attachment theory research provides a conceptual model for understanding the interaction in relationships where addiction and codependency are present. In the past decade, attachment researchers (Bartholomew, 1990) have developed a new model of adult romantic relationship that describes four styles of attachment: (1) The *secure* adult is comfortable with intimacy and autonomy; (2) the *dismissing* individual manifests denial of attachment and acts in a counterdependent manner; (3) the *preoccupied* individual is overly dependent and hypervigilant about the attachment or rejecting behavior of others; and (4) the individual who is *fearful* of attachment is socially avoidant (Feeney, 1999). Research has shown that relationships involving a preoccupied female and a dismissing male are more common than other pairings, and that they tend to be relatively stable (i.e., they endure; Collins & Read, 1990). Clinical description of the type of codependent relationships seen in substance abuse treatment agencies dovetails with the description of a dismissing–preoccupied couple. As relational theory points out, the problem of a codependent woman paired with a substance-abusing man could be viewed as manifesting a difficulty in connection rather than a failure to separate (Zelvin, 1999). Such a shift in understanding could have an enormous impact on the field's ability to help codependent women disentangle themselves from the destructive elements of their relationship.

The recovery process for codependent people in Al-Anon is similar to that of alcoholic individuals in AA. Both programs utilize the same structure: meetings, sharing, sponsorship, literature, and slogans. In many ways the plight of the codependent person is equally serious. His or her life is filled with catastrophe that must be kept a secret. It is this deception that ultimately destroys the individual, as he or she hides behind a rapidly crumbling wall of artifice. Both the identification with others in meetings and the relationship with a sponsor who has suffered similarly decrease the poisonous isolation with its accompanying need for deceit. The stability and acceptance of the group afford the member the opportunity to begin to experience an alteration of internal working models of attachment (Bowlby, 1988). In place of the anxious uncertainly about whether dependency needs will be met, the group member is able to begin to internalize newly consistent models of the self as worthy of care and concern, and others as able to provide both. The sponsorship relationship also can be regenerative, as it meets the underlying dependency needs of the codependent. It is not unusual for a husband and wife to undergo parallel recoveries in two separate 12-step programs. Often each partner evidences similar resistance and progress. It is also likely that the person's attachment to Al-Anon will be similar, initially, to that of the early caretaker in his or her life, as illustrated in the following example.

> Mary Ellen was a young woman in her early 30s who worked as a secretary in a brokerage firm. She dressed neatly, was highly invested in her work, and was well respected in her company. Her main concern in coming for treatment was her husband Jerry, a lineman with the telephone company—and a person with alcoholism. He went on frequent drinking binges and would fail to appear for days at the house. One morning she found him asleep on the front steps. He was already in trouble at work and had been sent to rehab twice. His job was now on the line.
>
> Mary Ellen was urged by her therapist to go to Al-Anon, but she never was able to attend for one reason or another. When her therapist asked why it was so difficult for her to attend, she answered, "To

get to the meeting, I would have to take the car out of the garage."
Her resistance was so obvious that the therapist prompted her to explore what lay beneath. In anticipating what it would be like to attend
a group primarily composed of women, Mary Ellen remembered her
feelings of being excluded and hurt by her cousins who lived upstairs
when she was growing up. Unconsciously she feared this experience
would be repeated again. After this first level of resistance was addressed, she was able to begin attending Al-Anon. Mary Ellen's new
friendships in Al-Anon became the means by which she established
more satisfying experiences with others and increased her self-esteem.

An examination of the slogans in Al-Anon illustrates the psychodynamic aspects of the 12-step program. "Keep the focus on yourself" is an
Al-Anon theme that addresses the anxious need to experience life through
another person. "Let go, let God" speaks to the concomitant need for control, coupled with constant fear. It addresses members' difficulty in trusting
that their needs for soothing and contact with others will be met. "You
didn't cause it, you can't control it, and you can't cure it" speaks to poor
ego boundaries and the tendency to merge (with the alcoholic person) that
arises from the fear of being abandoned.
    Al-Anon adapts the 12 steps of AA. For the Al-Anon member the first
step of AA—"We admitted we were powerless over alcohol—that our lives
had become unmanageable"—becomes "We admitted were powerless over
the alcoholic . . . " It teaches its members that sobriety is not an end but a
beginning to a new life, just as it is for the person with alcoholism.

CRITICISMS OF 12-STEP PROGRAMS

Critics of 12-step programs claim that they are not appropriate for everyone. The most common complaint is the central focus on God or a Higher
Power. One response might be, "Think of God as Good Orderly Direction" or even "Group of Drunks." It should be remembered that in 12-step
programs, the steps are presented as "suggestions" rather than "rules."
The use of "suggestions" does not alienate people with alcoholism, who
are often oppositional in personality and spirit.
    Another criticism is that 12-step programs create the same kind of de-
pendence among the members that the members once had on the substance. This is initially true. As discussed earlier, these programs serve a
reparenting function. Whereas most people mature out of the early symbi-
osis with the program, there are those who remain highly dependent on it.
This dependence, however, is rarely life threatening or permanent, as addiction to alcohol and other drugs often proves to be. Wallace (1985)

speaks of the therapeutic value of using the "preferred defense structure" of the recovering person as a beginning step in treatment. Among other things, the individual's obsession with alcohol can be beneficially transformed into a preoccupation with sobriety and the AA program. If the individual is using the elements available in the program, such as sponsorship and working on "making a searching and fearless moral inventory," as suggested by the fourth step, he or she is more likely to develop some introspection. The increased anxiety brought about by this process often leads people to seek therapy at this juncture.

A growing concern is that the focus of 12-step programs such as AA and NA on abstinence as the only viable goal is not suitable for all individuals. Reducing the quantity of use and the negative consequences of drinking or using drugs are two goals of harm reduction efforts (Lawson, Lawson, & Rivers, 2001). It has been recognized that for some individuals the timetable for achieving abstinence must be slower or more flexible—for example, in the case of individuals dually diagnosed with a psychiatric disorder and substance dependence (Orlin & Davis, 1993), or those with a physical disability such as a hearing impairment (Heinemann, 1997). Both AA and NA promote abstinence as the goal because of the belief that any use of mood-altering substances will trigger the person's loss of control. However, the programs do encourage members who are actively using to return to meetings, although they are requested not to participate if they are under the influence. The programs state that "The only requirement for membership is a *desire* to stop drinking" or "taking drugs."

The 12-step programs have been remarkably flexible in accommodating people who have felt the need to identify with others who share common characteristics. There are special groups for women, gay men, lesbian women, police officers, lawyers, plumbers, pilots, social workers, nurses, and doctors, among others. Many Spanish-speaking formats also are available. Meetings in additional languages, such as Russian and Chinese, continue to appear as members recognize the need. As indicated previously, people who are dually diagnosed with a psychiatric disorder in addition to substance dependence also have found that they sometimes benefit by separate meetings, such as those offered by the Dual Recovery and Double Trouble groups, where their use of psychotropic medications is more fully understood and accepted.

WOMEN AND THE 12-STEP PROCESS

AA and other 12-step groups emerged mainly from the experiences of men. Therefore, some of the written and informal suggestions given in these programs need to be adjusted to meet the needs of women. As Coker (1997) states, "Despite the increase in female membership, women have had little influence over long-standing traditions and attitudes" (p. 266).

Carol Gilligan (1982) describes the psychological development of young girls as one in which they must ultimately identify with the same person (the mother) who nurtures them. Thus the issue of separation and connection is central for women. Whereas men often enter a 12-step program because of a failure to master a task, or mastery, women may bottom out because their web of attachments has fallen apart or someone important has left them (Straussner, 1997).

Because women often define themselves in terms of their relationships, the program's suggestion to avoid new relationships during the first year of sobriety may present a hardship for them. Another common 12-step suggestion for early recovery is to avoid situations wherein anger is likely to be provoked. This can also present conflict for women. Whereas for men, anger can be dangerously overstimulating, many substance-abusing women find that directly manifesting their anger can be a positive breakthrough from their lifelong pattern of passive–aggressive behavior.

Covington (1997) points out that due to the high correlation of physical, sexual, and emotional abuse and addiction in women, it is essential that both issues are addressed. Women need to address the shame they feel about the physical, sexual, or emotional abuse they have experienced, as well as the internalized self-reproach that usually accompanies substance abuse. This goal is often accomplished in special early recovery women's groups where a female counselor is able to provide a safe environment as well as a healthy role model.

Taking the first step of admitting powerlessness over alcohol or drugs may be interpreted differently by women and men. Men often struggle with the concept of powerlessness, seeing it as giving up rather than letting go. For men who crave power, it is generally power over others, both in the family and in the workplace. Therefore, men need to be encouraged to experience powerlessness as a positive aspect of letting go, so that a new way of relating can begin.

Women, on the other hand, are far more likely to experience powerlessness as a familiar condition, because they often feel that they have little control over their own lives. It is still common for women to defer to their partners, and conform to a society intolerant of vulnerability. For a woman, admitting powerlessness may be experienced as yet another failure and increase her feelings of shame about her seeming lack of control. Substance-abusing women need to be helped to deal with these feelings so that they can embrace the concept of powerlessness and begin the journey to recovery. Again, because of these gender differences, it is often fruitful for women in 12-step programs and treatment facilities to participate their own groups. This separation facilitates an authenticity not always present in co-ed groups.

SOCIAL WORK INTERVENTION
AND THE ANONYMOUS PROGRAMS

Social workers addressing the needs of people with addiction or co-dependent behavior patterns greatly increase their effectiveness when they understand the value of the 12-step process. The Alcoholics Anonymous 1998 Membership Survey (Alcoholics Anonymous, 1999) found that 60% of members had received counseling in the past, and 75% said it played an important part in directing them to AA. Moreover, after coming to AA, 62% of members continued to receive some type of counseling, and 83% believed it was important to their recovery. Thirty four percent of members were referred for counseling through substance abuse treatment programs or facilities, 17% were referred by health or mental health providers, and 11% by court order. This fortuitous overlap is due to increased knowledge about the recovery process and the value of 12-step programs among social workers and other mental health professionals. It also reflects efforts by AA to reach out to, and educate, the professional community about how they can work together to assist substance abusers.

Many members of Al-Anon and Alateen are also involved in treatment and counseling. The 1999 Al-Anon/Alateen Membership Survey (Al-Anon/ Alateen Membership Survey, 2000) indicates that more than half of Al-Anon members reported that psychological counseling was the single most helpful treatment received before coming to Al-Anon. Almost two-thirds (61%) of the members indicated that the treatment they received played an important role in their deciding to join Al-Anon.

In the early phase of recovery, when the need for support and the potential for relapse are both massive, the anonymous program may indeed be the primary "therapist." Some people, however, may need help in using these programs. While it is important for social workers to have knowledge about how to facilitate their clients' entry into 12-step programs, social work training in understanding individual psychodynamics is equally valuable in understanding a client's resistance to using the program, as illustrated in the following example.

John, a rather depressed young man, could not "connect" with AA. He was being seen in an outpatient clinic by a social worker who encouraged him to go to a meeting and to share his experience. John finally said that he feared losing his thoughts and feelings to the people in the room if he shared. Understanding his disturbance and boundary difficulties, the social worker replied that he was right. He was in an early phase of his sobriety—a time to take, not give. The social worker wisely suggested that he attend meetings but not speak until he felt ready to do so. This interpretation enabled John to attend AA meetings *and* to maintain his fragile sense of self.

This example illustrates how a social worker can utilize both psychodynamic knowledge and knowledge of 12-step programs in the same intervention.

CONCLUSION

Social workers can make an enormous contribution in assisting family members of all ages to understand the impact of alcohol or other drug abuse on their lives and to help them examine what they can do, realistically, to alter the situation (Straussner & Fewell, 1996). In this process, it is important that they understand and facilitate the use of such 12-step programs for families as Al-Anon, Alateen, Adult Children of Alcoholics, Nar-Anon, and Co-Anon.

Clearly, the 12 steps and the community and spirituality of the anonymous programs appeal to millions as a solution to the agony of addiction. The honest sharing, opportunity for identification, and tradition of anonymity provide an alternative to the isolation and loneliness experienced by so many in today's rootless society.

Social workers are on the front line in hospitals, mental health facilities, child and family service agencies, schools, and prisons. The social work profession emphasizes understanding of the environment and working with the community. For those in recovery, the 12-step program may indeed become their community. Understanding the value and function of this community is crucial in helping clients.

In AA there is a saying that "It's a simple program for complicated people." It is indeed simple—as well as prophetic and profound.

REFERENCES

Ainsworth, M. D. S., & Bowlby, J. (1991). An ethological approach to personality development. *American Psychologist, 46*(4), 333–341.

Al-Anon/Alateen 1999 Membership Survey. (2000, March). Virginia Beach, VA: Al-Anon Family Group Headquarters.

Alcoholics Anonymous. (1939). New York: Alcoholics Anonymous World Services.

Alcoholics Anonymous. (1999). *1998 Membership Survey* New York: Alcoholics Anonymous World Services.

Bartholomew, K. (1990). Avoidance of intimacy: An attachment perspective. *Journal of Social and Personal Relationships, 7,* 147–178.

Bowlby, J. (1958). The nature of the child's ties to his mother. *International Journal of Psychoanalysis, 39,* 350–373.

Bowlby, J. (1988). Developmental psychiatry comes of age. *The American Journal of Psychiatry, 145*(1), 1–10.

Coker, M. (1997). Overcoming sexism in AA: How women cope. In S. L. A.

Straussner and E. Zelvin (Eds.), *Gender and addictions: Men and women in treatment* (pp. 265–281). Northvale, NJ: Aronson.

Collins, N. L., & Read, S. J. (1990). Adult attachment, working models, and relationship quality in dating couples. *Journal of Personality and Social Psychology, 58,* 644–663.

Covington, S. (1997). Women, addiction, and sexuality. In S. L. A. Straussner & E. Zelvin (Eds.), *Gender and addictions: Men and women in treatment* (pp. 73–95). Northvale, NJ: Aronson.

Dual Recovery Anonymous. Retrieved April 1, 2004, from www.draonline.org

Eigen, L. D., & Rowden, D. (1995). A methodology and current estimate of the number of children of alcoholics in the United States. In S. Abbott (Ed.), *Children of alcoholics: Selected readings* (pp. 77–79). Rockville, MD: National Association for Children of Alcoholics.

Feeney, J. A. (1999). Adult romantic attachment and couple relationships. In J. Cassidy and P. R. Shaver (Eds.), *Handbook of attachment: Theory, research, and clinical applications* (pp. 355–377). New York: Guilford Press.

Gilligan, C. (1982). *In a different voice.* Cambridge, MA: Harvard University Press.

Goldstein, E. G. (1995). *Ego psychology and social work practice.* New York: Free Press.

Grant, B. (2000). Estimates of U. S. children exposed to alcohol abuse and dependence in the family. *American Journal of Public Health, 90*(1), 112–115.

Heinemann, A. W. (1997). In J. H. Lowinson, P. Ruiz, R. B. Millman, & J. G. Langrod (Eds.), *Substance abuse: A comprehensive textbook* (3rd ed., pp. 716–725). Baltimore: Williams & Wilkins.

Kessler, R. C., Mickelson, K. D., & Zhao, S. (1997). Patterns and correlates of self-help group membership in the United States. *Social Policy, 27,* 27–46.

Khantzian, E. J., & Mack, J. E. (1994). Alcoholics anonymous and contemporary psychodynamic theory. In J. D. Levin & R. H. Weiss (Eds.), *The dynamics and treatment of alcoholism: Essential papers* (pp. 347–369). Northvale, NJ: Aronson.

Kris, E. (1952). *Psychoanalytic exploration in art.* New York: International Universities Press.

Lawson, G. W., Lawson, A. W., & Rivers, P. C. (Eds.). (2001). *Essentials of chemical dependency counseling* (3rd ed.). Gaithersburg, MD: Aspen.

McDougall, J. (1991). *Theaters of the mind.* New York: Brunner/Mazel.

Mahler, M., Pine, F., & Bergman, A. (1975). *The psychological birth of the human infant.* New York: Basic Books.

Marvin, R. S., & Britner, P. A. (1999). Normative development: The ontogeny of attachment. In J. Cassidy & P. R. Shaver (Eds.), *Handbook of attachment: Theory, research, and clinical applications* (pp. 44–67). New York: Guilford Press.

Moral re-armament. Encyclopedia Britannica. Retrieved April 4, 2004, from Encyclopedia Britannica Online: www.search.eb.com/eb/article?eu=55001

Orlin, L., & Davis, J. (1993). Assessment and intervention with drug and alcohol abusers in psychiatric settings. In S. L. A. Straussner (Ed.), *Clinical work with substance-abusing clients* (pp. 50–68). New York: Guilford Press.

Narcotics Anonymous World Service Office. (1983). *Narcotics Anonymous: The basic text of recovery.* Van Nuys, CA: Author.

Narcotics Anonymous World Services. (n.d.). *Information about NA* [Brochure]. Van Nuys, CA: Author.

Robertson, N. (1988). *Getting better inside Alcoholics Anonymous.* New York: Morrow.

Spiegel, E., & Mulder, E. (1986). The Anonymous program and ego functioning. *Issues in Ego Psychology, 9*(1), 34–42.

Straussner, S. L. A. (1997). Gender and substance abuse. In S. L. A. Straussner & E. Zelvin (Eds.), *Gender and addictions: Men and women in treatment* (pp. 5–27). Northvale, NJ: Aronson.

Straussner, S. L. A., & Fewell, C., (1996). Social work perspectives on alcohol and substance abuse problems. In J. Kinney (Ed.), *Clinical manual of substance abuse* (2nd ed., pp. 140–146). St. Louis, MO: Mosby-Year Book.

Straussner, S. L. A., & Spiegel, B. R. (1996). An analysis of 12–step programs for substance abusers from a developmental perspective. *Clinical Social Work, 24*(3), 299–309.

W., B. (1953). *Twelve steps and twelve traditions.* New York: New York Alcoholics Anonymous Publishing.

Wallace, J. (1985). Working with the preferred defense structure of the recovering alcoholic. In S. Zimberg, J. Wallach, S. B. Blume, & J. Wallace (Eds.), *Practical approaches to alcoholism psychotherapy* (pp. 23–36). New York: Plenum Press.

Winnicott, D. W. (1951). Transitional objects and transitional phenomena. In *Collected papers* (pp. 229–242). New York: Basic Books.

Winnicott, D. W. (1975). *Through paediatrics to psychoanalysis.* London: Hogarth Press.

Zelvin, E. (1999). Applying relational theory to the treatment of women's addictions. *Affilia, 14*(1), 9–23.

CHAPTER 7

Relapse Prevention

Muriel Gray
Sandy Gibson

During the past 10 years there has been a proliferation of clinical interventions in the treatment of people with substance use disorders. These clinical interventions have been very effective in helping substance abusers initiate change toward a life of abstinence and a state of recovery, but they have been far less effective in helping these individuals maintain this change over time, for long-term recovery (Humphreys, Moos, & Cohen, 1997). Studies of lifelong patterns of recovery and relapse indicate that not all patients relapse. However, relapse continues to be a treatment challenge. For instance, whereas approximately one-third of patients achieve permanent abstinence from their first serious attempt at recovery, long-term (i.e., longer than 1 year) recovery rates among others are estimated to be about 35% (Dolan & Olander, 1990; U.S. Department of Health and Human Services, 1999). The likelihood of relapse is increased if a managed care delivery system provides only minimum treatment exposure (Gray, 1995). All in all, the probability of a return to substance use after an apparent period of abstinence remains a major deficit in substance abuse treatment (U.S. Department of Health and Human Services, 1996).

This chapter focuses on the use of clinical approaches and treatment interventions to prevent relapse. We present a conceptual framework, define the major components and clinical interventions in relapse prevention counseling and therapy, describe a service delivery model, provide an annotated list of instruments, and discuss the role of social workers in the treatment of people with substance use disorders, in general, and in relapse prevention treatment, in particular.

DEFINITION OF RELAPSE PREVENTION

The relationship among treatment, recovery, and relapse has been debated among substance abuse treatment professionals for years (Bellenir, 1996; Daley & Raskin, 1991; Marlatt & George, 1984). This debate focuses specifically on the role of relapse, or the interruption of an apparent state of abstinence or recovery, in the overall recovery process (or lack of recovery). Because of the prevalence of relapse, some treatment professionals accept it as a part of substance use disorders and see it as an anticipated interruption in the recovery process. Others, however, noting that some patients proceed smoothly to a state of uninterrupted recovery or experience very few relapse episodes, tend to view relapse as an indication of treatment failure (Margolis & Zweben, 1998).

Most practitioners agree that a patient cannot be in recovery and relapse at the same time. *Recovery* assumes a behavioral and emotional change toward healthful and growthful functioning; relapse assumes a reversion to a previous state of dysfunction (Annis & Davis, 1989; Gorski, 1986). Thus, relapse prevention is, by definition, a strategic set of clinical interventions and responses designed to help patients maintain a state of recovery and continued movement toward health and growth. It is an essential component of treating people with substance use disorders (Dimeff & Marlatt, 1998; Schmitz et al., 1997).

CONCEPTUAL FRAMEWORK: CONTINUUM OF CARE

The prevention of relapse is inextricably linked to the treatment process, and since there is no known cure for substance use disorders, both treatment and relapse prevention are ongoing processes. Thus defining treatment as a singular event (e.g., detoxification) or relapse as a singular event (e.g., resuming alcohol or drug use) increases the likelihood that the patient will not enter a state of recovery. Clinicians and their patients need to view treatment, recovery, and relapse as ongoing processes, and they need to be knowledgeable about the phases of each (Committee on Alcoholism and Addictions, 1998).

Treatment

The treatment of substance use disorders is delivered in many different settings (Substance Abuse and Mental Health Services Administration, 2002) and occurs in phases along a treatment continuum, with the focus of treatment changing at each phase. These phases typically are conceptualized as pretreatment, stabilization, rehabilitation, and continuing care (Washton, 1989).

Pretreatment, the first phase of treatment, actually begins before the patient enters treatment specifically for a substance use disorder. This phase is commonly seen in treatment settings when the patient presents with another problem. During this phase the clinician needs to help the client (1) identify substance abuse as a problem, (2) become motivated to change, and (3) become involved in a structured treatment regime. The focus during this phase is on getting the client involved in intensive substance abuse treatment. Brief motivational techniques have been found to be effective during this stage (Margolis & Zweben, 1998).

The *stabilization* phase focuses on detoxifying the body of drugs (including alcohol) and monitoring the physiological and/or psychological effects of drug withdrawal, stabilizing daily functioning, resolving any immediate crises, and formulating an ongoing treatment plan to help the patient respond better to the next phase of treatment. Treatment at this phase typically occurs in an inpatient medical setting, though it can occur on an outpatient basis with medical management.

The *rehabilitation* phase is an intensive, structured period during which the physical, emotional, social, and spiritual effects of the disorder are addressed. This treatment may be delivered in a short- or long-term residential setting, but is more likely to be delivered in an intensive outpatient program. Education about substance use disorders, the recovery process, the use of self-help groups, and ongoing personal care is the focus, with the goal of helping the patient abstain from substance use and feel comfortable living without substances. Although this phase of treatment does address the concept of relapse by developing an ongoing treatment plan aimed at relapse prevention and by teaching techniques to handle the stresses and strains of early recovery, relapse prevention, per se, is not the primary focus.

Relapse prevention is the focus of the *continuing care* phase of treatment, during which the patient makes the transition from the structured environment (either inpatient or outpatient) to a routinely unstructured outpatient environment. Helping the patient maintain the positive biopsychosocial changes made in the previous phase by applying the knowledge and techniques learned during rehabilitation is the focus. The patient is educated about the relapse process, its warning signs and how to assess risk factors, as well as how to continue to treat the disorder in order to prevent and/or minimize the possibility of relapse. A part of this education includes an identification and appropriate use of supportive resources, including medication, to manage cravings. Preventing relapse is so critical to the treatment of people with substance use disorders that it is viewed as a therapy in itself. Relapse prevention therapy utilizes various cognitive–behavioral strategies that facilitate abstinence and help those who experience relapse (National Institute on Drug Abuse [NIDA], 1999). This treatment typically occurs in an outpatient setting and varies in length from 6 weeks to 6 months, depending on the modality used.

The Process of Recovery

Recovery from a substance use disorder is a process of abstinence and change (Marion & Coleman, 1995). It occurs along a continuum, with different foci at each phase (Gorski, 1986; van Wormer, 1995). The phases of the recovery continuum are typically conceptualized as early, middle, advanced, and maintained recovery (Prochaska, DiClemente, & Norcross, 1992; Washton, 1989). Even though the phases are presented here as if they occurred at specified times, the timeframe is merely a rough guide to a typical patient's progress along the recovery continuum; each patient will have a unique recovery style, as he or she addresses the quality of life, lifestyle, and successful management of the various aspects of his or her life.

Early recovery (also referred to as the abstinence stage) usually refers to the first 3 months of compliance with the recovery plan. Because this is the most vulnerable time for relapse (Siegal, Rapp, Li, Saha, & Kirk, 1997), this phase focuses on (1) maintaining abstinence and monitoring patients' reactions to postacute withdrawal (PAW) and other physiological and medical conditions; (2) developing strategies for handling PAW discomfort (which may be accompanied by depression); (3) identifying and appropriately addressing predisposing factors, such as legal, family, school, or dual diagnosis problems; and (4) identifying and appropriately addressing precipitating factors, such as high-risk situations, psychological and physiological triggers, or overconfidence. Introduction to self-help groups also begins during the stabilization phase; however, involvement continues throughout the recovery process. Anecdotal retrospective analyses of patients' relapse patterns show that some patients may have a high potential for relapse during this phase because they feel "too good"; as a result they tend to see no need to comply with the recovery plan (Gorski, 1980; Ludwig, 1988).

Middle recovery begins about 3 to 12 months into the recovery process. The focus in this phase is on continuing to help patients (1) make positive, lasting lifestyle changes; (2) learn how to identify and handle emotions; (3) learn how to have fun without alcohol or other drugs; (4) learn how to effectively deal with problems, adjustments, and setbacks; (5) identify and appropriately use internal strengths; (6) identify and appropriately use external support systems; (7) increase involvement in self-help groups; and (8) heighten spiritual awareness.

Advanced recovery begins 1 to 2 years into sobriety. It is a somewhat open-ended period of time, and the issues addressed during this phase are unique to individual patients and their situations. The focus is on helping patients (1) address issues of arrested maturity, (2) solidify adaptive coping and problem-solving skills, (3) address emotional and personality issues that affect self-esteem, and (4) identify and address areas of needed growth for both patients and their families.

Maintained recovery is also an open-ended phase. Patients in this phase focus on normal life-cycle issues, supporting all their positive gains, staying motivated to avoid "old behaviors," confronting their own backsliding, and maintaining and sharing their recovery with others (Bellenir, 1996) through continued involvement in self-help groups and continued attention to the recovery plan. It also means that patients should assume a more helping role in the self-help groups by making themselves more available to others.

THE RELAPSE PROCESS

Although it may appear that relapse is a singular, discrete event characterized by resumption of alcohol or other drug use, practitioners have noted a constellation of signs and symptoms that appear to precede the relapse behavior (Dimeff & Marlatt, 1998; el-Guebaly & Hodgins, 1998; Ramanathan & Reischl, 1999). Moreover, it has also been observed (Allsop, Saunders, & Phillips, 2000; Moore & Budney, 2003; Price, Risk, & Spitznagel, 2001) that the patterns of resumed use are often incremental and have differing consequences. Individuals may "build up" to a resumption of use. Once they do resume the use of substances, the pattern may involve a temporary "slip" (lapse) characterized by a brief episode of controlled use, or a full-blown relapse characterized by an extended episode of uncontrolled use or bingeing.

The consequences of a relapse vary with each patient; some patterns are more deleterious than others. A relapse that is interrupted before resumption of substance use occurs is usually not recognized as a relapse by patients and therefore may not be viewed as deleterious. For example: Upon discharge from the intensive phase of primary treatment, Bob, a recovering cocaine addict who also abused alcohol, had a very positive attitude and a commitment to continued recovery. He agreed to a recovery plan that included weekly attendance at a minimum of four Narcotics Anonymous (NA) or Alcoholics Anonymous (AA) meetings, weekly attendance at an aftercare group, daily exercise (either a 2-mile walk or 4-mile bike ride), daily inspirational reading, no more than 10 hours of overtime work a week, regular consumption of nutritious meals, and weekly telephone or face-to-face contact with his NA sponsor. During follow-up interviews in the month after discharge, it was found that Bob was increasingly discontinuing the activities specified by his recovery plan. It was also noted that Bob's attitude had changed: He no longer believed he had a "serious drug problem" and had begun to question his need for the recovery plan. He became angry at the suggestion that he attend NA meetings and questioned his need for the support of the follow-up counselor. A urinalysis and self-report indicated that Bob was abstinent.

This example shows a constellation of signs and symptoms that indicated Bob was moving toward potential relapse. In cases where a brief episode of controlled alcohol or other drug use does occur, the consequences are more psychological than physical, often manifested as anger, guilt, and shame. In other cases, an extended period of uncontrolled drug or alcohol use often results in serious physiological and social consequences, as well as an array of psychological reactions.

The process of relapse can be interrupted at any point; clinicians can intervene after any incident, whether it is one that did not include the resumption of substance use, one that involved a brief, controlled episode of substance use, or one that extended into a binge of uncontrolled use.

Relapse can be prevented if the clinician is attuned to the symptoms that forewarn an impending episode. Among the constellation of symptoms that have been identified as leading to relapse are the following (Dimeff & Marlatt, 1998; el-Guebaly & Hodgins, 1998; Ramanathan & Reischl, 1999):

- Anger
- Poor self/health care
- Defensiveness
- Impulsivity
- Dishonesty
- Impatience
- Self-pity
- Cockiness
- Loneliness
- Unreasonable resentments
- Depression
- Irregular attendance at a self-help program

It is important to remember that patients who have not resumed substance use may find it difficult to acknowledge that they exhibit signs of relapse and are not in a state of recovery. It may be even more difficult for them to understand that unless something changes, it may only be a matter of time before they resume alcohol or other drug use. In such cases, practitioners will want to assess patients' compliance with the recovery plan or modify the recovery plan in an attempt to interrupt the relapse process.

COMPONENTS OF RELAPSE PREVENTION

Relapse prevention begins with a treatment plan, which also may be referred to as a recovery plan. It is a prescription that specifies a daily regime for healthful living and is designed to treat the dynamics of the disorder in the context of the patient's individual circumstances. It reinforces the treatment components of the rehabilitation phase while recognizing and attending to the issues appropriate for each recovery phase.

Throughout each recovery phase, the plan approaches recovery from a holistic perspective and stresses the fact that treatment of a substance use disorder is an ongoing process. The components of relapse prevention include clinical interventions to facilitate physical, emotional, social, and spiritual well-being (Alcoholics Anonymous, 1975; Dimeff & Marlatt, 1998; Gray, 1989; McLellan, Arndt, Metzer, Woody, & O'Brien, 1993) as well as the monitoring of substances use through urinalysis and breath analysis.

Physical Well-Being

Substance use disorders often have deleterious physical effects, so recovery plans must reinforce the importance of maintaining physical health through regular and nutritionally balanced meals, adequate rest, and physical exercise. Because relapse specialists have found that patients are prone to relapse when they deprive themselves of food or rest, they should be specifically advised to avoid becoming too hungry or too tired. They also should be informed that certain foods (e.g., extracts) and medicines (e.g., cough syrups, painkillers) contain alcohol or narcotics and could jeopardize recovery by triggering a physiological reaction. They should therefore be encouraged to tell their health care providers (physicians, dentists, pharmacists, etc.) of their disorder.

Emotional Well-Being

Cognitive-behavioral clinicians have recognized that feelings and thoughts influence behavior (Dimeff & Marlatt, 1998). In the early stage of recovery, when the primary focus is on making behavioral lifestyle changes, the effect of emotions on behavior is critical. Cognitive-behavioral therapy utilizes specific techniques to explore positive and negative consequences of continued use, self-monitoring of substance cravings, high-risk situations, and the development of strategies to address such cravings and situations (U.S. Department of Health and Human Services, 1998). For instance, anger, frustration, loneliness, and depression are emotions often associated with relapse. Thus "HALT" is an AA and treatment slogan that advises individuals in recovery not to get too *h*ungry, *a*ngry, *l*onely, or *t*ired. Patients need to be taught how to control or address these emotions. For example:

> Jane is recovering from an opiate addiction. She is a single mother of three children and is unemployed. She receives Temporary Assistance for Needy Families and is supposed to receive child support from the children's father, but it often does not arrive. She has difficulty making ends meet; she feels that she would be able to pay her bills on time if she received her child support payments on time. She is frequently threatened with eviction, her phone is turned off, and her oldest child was just arrested and placed on probation. She reports she is too busy

with her children to go to NA meetings and rationalizes her isolation in her home as her attempt to stay away from her old using friends.

Jane needs to understand the importance of connecting to other women in recovery by attending 12-step programs and receiving sponsorship. Her isolation needs to be reframed in a way that demonstrates the risks associated with that behavior. Her anger toward her children's father and the associated financial problems must be identified as real problems but not as excuses for escaping into drug use. Case management services that would link her with community resources can aid her in gaining a feeling of control when she previously felt powerless. Case management also can link her with community programs for her children so that she can have more time available to attend 12-step meetings and develop recovery networks.

Euphoric emotions, such as joy and happiness, are also associated with relapse in that they often indicate a false sense of accomplishment and excitement, referred to as the "pink cloud." Recovery plans need to address emotional health and stabilization through the use of self-help groups, aftercare groups, family treatment, situational counseling, case management, and other follow-up interventions.

Use of Self-Help Groups

It is difficult to scientifically assess the effectiveness of 12-step programs because of methodological and sampling problems associated with research on anonymous programs (van Wormer, 1995). However, existing research indicates that AA participation does predict a reduction in drinking and is highly correlated with positive psychosocial outcomes (Kownacki & Shadish, 1999). Twelve-step participation, in combination with formal drug treatment, produces higher rates of abstinence than either formal treatment or 12-step programs alone (Fiorentine & Hillhouse, 2000).

Many practitioners and patients also observe a positive correlation between the quality of 12-step program involvement and the quality of recovery and therefore view involvement in a 12-step program as a basic component of a relapse prevention plan. In recent years several psychometric instruments have been developed to identify a client's involvement in AA, completion of steps, and the adoption of values encouraged by AA (Allen, 2000). These instruments include the Step Questionnaire, Brown–Peterson Recovery Progress Inventory, Alcoholics Anonymous Affiliation Scale, and Alcoholics Anonymous Involvement scale (AAI). For example, the Step Questionnaire consists of 21 questions using a 7-point Likert scale ranging from "strongly disagree" to "strongly agree," and is designed to reveal individuals' acceptance of the first three steps of AA (Allen, 2000; Gilbert, 1991). The Brown–Peterson Recovery Progress Inventory consists of 53 items and is designed to measure progress in AA (Brown & Peterson,

1991). The Alcoholics Anonymous Affiliation Scale consists of nine items that focus on AA-related experiences (Humphreys, Kaskutas, & Weisner, 1998). The AAI consists of 13 items designed to measure participation in AA—that is, how well an individual is "working the program" (Tonigan, Miller, & Connors, 1998).

Monitoring 12-step program attendance is necessary but not sufficient to assess recovery. In addition to monitoring attendance by asking about the number of meetings attended, the topics of the meetings, and what they liked about the meetings, it is equally as important to assess the quality and level of patient involvement in the program. To help patients effectively use these groups, workers need to be familiar with the philosophy and structure of 12-step programs (see Spiegel & Fewell, Chapter 6, this volume), and to recommend the following guidelines for patients and their families:

- Attend meetings on a regular basis (several times per week).
- Attend meetings at different locations before deciding which to attend regularly.
- Attend a variety of different types of meetings (e.g., speaker, discussion, step, big book).
- Develop a close, confidential relationship with someone who is in recovery and has been in the program for at least 2 years (i.e., a sponsor).
- Work the program steps and respect the traditions.

Even though 12-step programs are more prevalent, there are a variety of other self-help and other types of support groups for substance abusers. Some of these distinguish themselves by addressing issues that 12-step programs do not address or by focusing on issues that are appropriate only for some individuals. For instance, Women for Sobriety (WFS) is a self-help support group designed specifically for women. Self Management and Recovery Training (SMART Recovery) is an abstinence-based self-help group that utilizes cognitive-behavioral principles. There are also self-help groups for substance abusers who are Jewish; these groups are specifically designed to offer participants a way to link their Judaism to their ongoing recovery. Some of these groups are meant to complement 12-step groups rather than replace them. Hundreds of self-help support groups may be found on the Internet at *www.open-mind.org/support.htm*.

Use of Aftercare Groups

Another important component in relapse prevention is participation in aftercare groups, which usually exist under the auspices of the primary intensive treatment facility that provided the rehabilitation. These groups aid members in negotiating the transition from structured treatment to unstructured community living, providing continuity between the rehabilitation and the continuing care phases of treatment. Research identifies the need for aftercare programs and their potential for reintegrating recovering drug users into the community (Coughey, Feighan, Cheney, & Klein, 1998). A significant percentage of individuals who complete inpatient substance abuse treatment do not attend recommended aftercare sessions upon discharge (Peterson, Swindle, Phibbs, Recine, & Moos, 1994), whereas individuals who complete outpatient substance abuse treatment are more likely to attend aftercare sessions (McKay, Alterman, McLellan, & Snider, 1994). However, regardless of preceding treatment, attrition rates in aftercare treatment are high (Lash, 1998; McKay et al., 1994).

To be most effective, aftercare groups should meet for 2 years. During early recovery (3–5 months after the rehabilitation phase), meetings should be held weekly; as recovery progresses, the frequency of meetings gradually decreases.

Aftercare groups focus on problem situations and emotional and behavioral reactions to life without alcohol or drugs. These groups typically develop strategies and responses to troubling situations that may present obstacles to continued recovery for patients. For example, many patients who have been in a structured treatment program (either as inpatients or outpatients) have difficulty maintaining a life in the community that does not include alcohol or other drugs. This difficulty is particularly likely when family celebrations, such as weddings, holiday gatherings, or graduations, include alcohol or other drugs. The aftercare group provides the opportunity to discuss each individual's predicament, anticipate reactions, and develop a strategic plan for handling the situation.

Alumni Groups

Alumni groups are typically gatherings planned by the primary intensive treatment provider for patients who have completed the rehabilitation phase of treatment in that program. Due to recent cuts in funding for drug-user treatment (Coughey et al., 1998) and limitations set by managed care companies (Frances & Miller, 1998), there is a shortened length of stay in treatment. As a result, alumni groups are hosted primarily by inpatient programs, where individuals have spent longer amounts of time together. These groups may hold picnics, holiday parties, retreats, and other weekend activities. They provide opportunities to socialize and reminisce with those who were in treatment groups together. These groups provide not only alcohol- and drug-free social activities but also opportunities for people to support one another and to serve as sponsors or role models for more recent clients. Alumni groups are equally important (although not as common) for patients treated in intensive outpatient programs. Of course, patients whose primary intensive treatment did not include a group modality would not have an alumni group.

Family Treatment

Family therapy is a part of most successful substance abuse treatment programs and is considered an essential element in relapse prevention (Heath & Stanton, 1998). It is important to elicit the help of significant others to motivate recovering substance abusers to adhere to treatment requirements and maintain treatment gains following discharge (DeCivita, Dobkin, & Robertson, 2000). Treatment professionals observe that recovery seems to be sustained best when patients' significant others are both supportive of the recovery process and themselves actively involved in the treatment process (Brooks & Rice, 1997). There are 12-step programs (such as Al-Anon and Nar-Anon) designed specifically for family members and others concerned with or affected by the disorder. (Again, see Spiegel & Jewell, Chapter 6, this volume).

It is important for social workers assisting patients in recovery to encourage the involvement of family members (Seilhamer, 1995). Even though family members may not be identified as the primary patient, they certainly may have an effect on the client's recovery—either by providing support or presenting obstacles. For example, Bob, whose story was related earlier, recently completed primary intensive treatment as an outpatient. His wife was not involved in the family treatment program. During treatment, Bob self-diagnosed himself as an alcoholic and an addict and accepted that appropriate continued treatment would include total abstinence. His wife was happy that Bob had benefited from treatment, but she did not understand the importance of abstinence and therefore suggested that he could drink as long as he controlled it. Not realizing that Bob may not be able to control his drinking, she unwittingly undermined his recovery plan.

Individual Counseling

In addition to aftercare groups, some patients may need individual aftercare counseling. As with aftercare groups, the focus of individual counseling during early recovery is on relapse prevention. This type of recovery counseling should specifically address (Dodes & Khantzian, 1998; NIDA, 1999):

- High-risk drinking and drug-using situations.
- Behavioral and psychological triggers to use.
- Patient strengths and resources for dealing with such situations.

- New responses to old situations.
- Other familial, legal, psychological, vocational, or educational obstacles to recovery.

For example, Mary, a flight attendant recovering from alcoholism, had an irregular work schedule that caused her to miss several aftercare group meetings. In addition, she had a job that included serving alcoholic drinks. This aspect of her work was a threat to her recovery unless she learned specific techniques, such as cue exposure (el-Guebaly & Hodgins, 1998), and maintained involvement with 12-step programs and recovery support systems to help her recognize and control her psychological triggers. Individual counseling in conjunction with the aftercare group was particularly helpful during her early recovery phase. Individual counseling also may be necessary to address any unresolved personal issues, such as domestic violence or sexual abuse, that might be a direct threat to recovery.

Social Well-Being

As previously indicated, the maintenance of positive treatment effects often requires new and different responses to old and comfortable situations. Such changes in life, both in style and in approach, are essential to recovery. Therefore, the patient's recovery plan needs to address housing, healthy hobbies, new friends, and employment and work relationships.

Housing

Inappropriate housing (i.e., an environment that does not support and reinforce abstinence and recovery) or lack of housing are major factors in relapse. Therefore it is critical that social workers help patients realistically assess their living situation and secure appropriate housing. For patients who are homeless, this may mean recovery residences, also referred to as halfway houses or quarter-way houses; these are transitional group homes specifically designed for recovering patients who need a supportive drug- and alcohol-free living environment. Patients with unsupportive home environments may need to move in temporarily with supportive friends or relatives. However, no community is immune to the presence of substances. Therefore, a geographic move does not guarantee a drug-free environment.

Hobbies

Most patients in early recovery report that they have idle time; this is the block of time they had previously filled with substance use and all it entailed. Therefore a recovery plan should include alternative activities to fill that time (Alcoholics Anonymous, 1975; Ott & Tarter, 1998). Social workers may need to help patients select a hobby and develop a strategy for regular involvement.

Friends

Situations in which the newly recovering individual becomes lonely or is around other substance users present a high risk for relapse (Margolis & Zweben, 1998). However, most substance abusers report that they have few friends or very few friends who do not use substances. Social workers need to (1) educate patients about the importance of not becoming too lonely, (2) help them develop strategies for dealing with old friends, and (3) help them develop the skills for making new ones. Among other benefits, involvement in a self-help program can provide a new, ready-made social network. It is important to keep in mind that not all people attending self-help groups are abstinent. Therefore, clinicians need to help patients identify and associate with those who are in recovery or do not use or abuse substances.

Employment and Work Relationships

Employment, job performance, and quality of work relationships affect recovery. A 1997 National Treatment Improvement Evaluation Study (NTIES) found more favorable treatment and employment outcomes among individuals who completed their treatment programs (U.S. Department of Health and Human Services, 1997). Employment is also important to a well-balanced life. To the extent that unemployment promotes an unstructured lifestyle or one conducive to substance use, it is an obstacle to recovery. On the other hand, if a patient is employed, the threat of job loss due to a decline in job performance may be an impetus for recovery and therefore an aid in the prevention of relapse. Jobs may be stressful and overwhelming. Due to recent welfare reform work requirements, the need to obtain and maintain employment may be a new and frightening experience for some individuals. Such emotions are likely triggers for relapse and should be monitored. Thus, it is important for clinicians to assess the role that employment may play in the recovery process.

In addition, job performance and the quality of relationships with coworkers often serve as a barometer for the quality of recovery. To minimize the risk of relapse, clinicians need to inquire about the nature and quality of the patient's work and work relationships. Job performance and relationships with coworkers will likely improve as recovery advances. Individuals who are unable to obtain employment may benefit from doing volunteer work.

Spiritual Well-Being

Patients' beliefs and sources of inspiration are important to personal growth. Many individuals undergo life-altering spiritual transformations during recovery that lead to sustained abstinence. Recovering individuals describe this new spirituality as providing them "with a source of energy and sustenance that enables them to 'live life on life's terms,' " and offers a constant source of comfort and reassurance in their lives (Lesley, Fullilove, & Fullilove, 1998, p. 330). A patient's spirituality may or may not include organized religion. *Spirituality* refers to beliefs about a source of inspiration outside the self. In a study of individuals in outpatient programs, researchers found that recovering individuals had a significant increase in spirituality, regardless of their participation in 12-step programs (Borman & Dixon, 1998). This finding supports the importance of addressing spirituality openly in treatment.

Alcoholics Anonymous and other 12-step programs perceive substance abuse as a disorder that affects the patient's spiritual well-being; they therefore include a focus on spirituality. In addition to becoming involved in 12-step programs, patients should be encouraged to participate in activities that they find inspiring and uplifting. Obviously, the specific activities will be determined by each patient's own values; we find that they typically include daily readings, meditation, or daily affirmations.

Toxicology Screening

In some circumstances, the treatment plan (especially in the outpatient context and during the continuing care phase of treatment) may include periodic toxicology screening to verify abstinence. Monitoring abstinence through toxicology screens helps to assure that treatment efforts are serving a therapeutic end rather than enabling the individual to continue substance use under the guise of apparent recovery (Committee on Alcoholism and Addictions, 1998).

To be most effective, such testing should occur randomly. Although hair and nail analyses are not intrusive, they are not used as frequently as urinalysis and blood analysis. The use of nails to monitor drug use lacks validation (Palmeri, Pichini, Pacifici, Zuccaro, & Lopez, 2000); the use of hair analysis is not typically used but has been found to be efficacious in detecting the presence of controlled substances (Ricossa, Bernini, & DeFerrari, 2000). Urinalysis is usually preferable to blood testing because it is less intrusive and less expensive. Urinalysis is used to detect use of drugs other than alcohol, whereas breath analysis is usually used to detect alcohol use. Both types of analysis determine the presence of the substance in the body but do not specify the degree of impairment. Should either of these tests yield a positive result, a more sensitive test should be given to confirm this finding.

Pharmacological Interventions

Certain medications have been found to be effective in the treatment of substance use disorders. Cravings for a substance (especially during the early abstinence stage) are a threat to ongoing abstinence. In addition to the psychosocial strategies previously discussed, medications such as naltrexone (ReVia), which decreases craving for alcohol, and methadone and LAAM (Stimmel, 1999), both opiate replacement therapies, have been effective in the treatment of opiate addiction (NIDA, 1999). Disulfiram is a relapse prevention medication that is self-administered, and like naltrexone, works best when there is a significant other who monitors the daily administration to ensure compliance (Committee on Alcoholism and Addictions, 1998). Studies show that the best treatment outcomes are obtained when these pharmacological approaches are combined with psychosocial forms of treatment (Miller & Smith, 1997).

A RELAPSE PREVENTION MODEL: USE OF CASE MANAGEMENT

Repetitive relapse need not be a part of substance use disorders. Research has shown that the rate of relapse can be reduced with systematic treatment planning and the clinical management and coordination of such care (McLellan et al., 1999; Siegal et al., 1997). Case management models are therefore receiving increasing attention from those involved in the treatment of people with substance use disorders.

   Case management, in its broadest form, is a system of managed service delivery. It may or may not include fiscal management, but it always includes clinical management of client services. The functions of case management vary with different populations and service systems. In the treatment of people with substance use disorders, a balanced service system model is the type most frequently used. This model includes client outreach, accurate problem assessment, case planning, matching clients with the appropriate level of care, advocacy, and structured follow-up (McLellan et al., 1999; Siegal et al., 1997). Case management is very similar to the traditional social casework model of study, diagnosis, and treatment. However, unlike traditional caseworkers, case managers are usually not treatment providers themselves; instead they coordinate, advocate, and broker needed services on behalf of clients. In some instances they also may be responsible for negotiating and reviewing specific costs of client services. The case management model is particularly effective for relapse prevention, which requires a coordinated process of treatment delivery at each stage of treatment and recovery.

Structured Follow-Up

The follow-up component of the case management process is probably one of the most important; yet it is the component least often provided (Bellenir, 1996). Too often treatment professionals spend considerable time getting the patient into treatment and developing treatment and/or recovery plans, only to provide minimal follow-up to ensure compliance and ongoing assessment.

The point of follow-up intervention is to provide support and guidance that reinforce the maintenance of positive treatment effects (Miller, 1989). Follow-up is a form of insurance; it provides patients with the support that is critical throughout the recovery process and it provides social workers with a way to assess patients' ongoing needs and obstacles to recovering.

The specific nature of follow-up should be determined near the end of the rehabilitation phase and incorporated into the recovery plan that is part of discharge planning. Ideally, the social worker is actively involved in this discharge planning process in addition to performing the extended follow-up.

The frequency of follow-up visits should be mutually agreed upon by worker and patient and determined by the patient's compliance with the recovery plan. Most treatment professionals recommend that follow-up continue for approximately 2 years, at a minimum (Older & Searcy, 1990). Furthermore, it is recommended that compliance with the recovery plan and indicators of a healthy recovery be evidenced for 1–2 months before follow-up sessions are decreased. For instance, if a patient who has been seen weekly is following his or her recovery plan and appears to be in recovery, worker and patient should continue to meet weekly for at least once a month before agreeing to decrease the frequency of meeting (Gray, 1989). The following frequency schedule is suggested: weekly sessions for the first 3–4 months, bimonthly sessions for the next 4–6 months, monthly sessions for the next 6–12 months, and quarterly or semiannual sessions for the last 12–24 months (Gray, 1989; Older & Searcy, 1990). However, the actual frequency should be determined by an assessment of the patient's compliance with the recovery plan and the degree to which he or she is bonding with self-help groups and appropriately using other support resources.

Unfortunately, due to funding cuts for drug treatment (Coughey et al., 1998) and reductions in treatment allocations due to managed care restrictions (Frances & Miller, 1998), clinicians oftentimes are not the decision makers when it comes to establishing an aftercare timeframe. The task for clinicians is to stay current with treatment research and use the most efficacious treatments available within the timeframe they are allotted. However, the need for structured follow-up has been recognized by the largest managed behavioral health care company in the United States, which has recently implemented a new "Targeted Case Management" program for clients receiving mental health services. In this program, case managers are assigned to facilitate communication between patients, therapists, physicians, and family members in hopes of identifying factors associated with decompensation and frequent hospitalizations of individuals and to develop plans to prevent additional decompensations and relapses. A major component of this plan is structured telephone and in-person follow-up. Such follow-up services have been found to decrease the number of hospitalizations by half. It is likely that most managed care companies will ultimately follow such a model, as opposed to continuing the current micromanagement of the service delivery system.

Use of Clinical Instruments

Clinical instruments can help clinicians assess their patients' relapse risks and recovery plan compliance. Examples of some of these instruments are included in the appendix of this chapter.

CONCLUSION

Relapse prevention is a crucial component of substance abuse treatment. This chapter has provided an overview of the basic components and clinical approaches that aid in the prevention of relapse. Although specific techniques vary, most treatment practitioners agree on the need to employ a comprehensive, holistic treatment philosophy that addresses clients' biological, psychological, social, emotional, and spiritual needs.

In order to assess these needs throughout the treatment and recovery process, case management that includes extended structured follow-up is critical. Because relapse continues to be prevalent in people undergoing substance abuse treatment, and because much remains unknown about what works for which patients and what mechanisms are absolutely necessary in order for patients to maintain long-term recovery, continuing systematic study and clinical research are vital in helping clinicians unravel this complicated and mysterious phenomenon.

APPENDIX 7.1.
CLINICAL INSTRUMENTS FOR RELAPSE PREVENTION

National Clearinghouse of Alcohol and Drug Information

NCADI provides several of the instruments and relapse prevention workbooks and publications mentioned below. They can be ordered at: 800-729-6686 or www. health.org/pub.

Relapse Prevention: Clinical Report Series (1994)

This report series reviews general strategies for preventing relapse and describes four specific approaches in detail.

Relapse Prevention Package (1993)

This skill development package examines two effective relapse prevention models, the Recovery Training and Self Help (RTSH) program and the Cue Extinction model.

Inventory of Drinking Situations

The IDS is a situation-specific measure of drinking that can be used to identify a client's high-risk situations for alcoholic relapse. It serves as a treatment-planning tool by profiling a client's areas of greatest drinking risk. Administration can be via paper and pencil or computer-interactive software. The 50-page User's Guide describes the development of the IDS and its use in clinical and research settings, presents reliability and validity information and normative data, and provides guidelines for use in both manual and computer formats.

> Addiction Research Foundation
> Department 897
> 33 Russell Street
> Toronto, Ontario M5S 2S1, Canada

Situational Confidence Questionnaire

The SCQ-39 is a situation-specific measure of efficacy expectations that is designed to assess a client's perceived ability to cope effectively with alcohol. Administration can be by paper-and-pencil questionnaire or computer-interactive software. The 45-page User's Guide describes the development of the SCQ and presents guidelines for clinical and research applications. Reliability and validity data are summarized, and normative data are provided. They can be obtained from:

Addiction Research Foundation
Department 897
33 Russell Street
Toronto, Ontario M5S 2S1, Canada

Step Questionnaire

The Step Questionnaire measures how well individuals adhere to steps 11 and 12 of Alcoholics Anonymous. Questions regarding step 11 measure prayer and meditation practices, and questions pertaining to step 12 measure activities related to assisting other persons with alcoholism.
   Contact:

Stephanie Carroll, PhD
California School of Professional Psychology Berkeley/Alameda
1005 Atlantic Avenue
Alameda, CA 94501

Alcoholics Anonymous Affiliation Scale

The AAAS is a 9-item scale that measures AA-related experiences such as working with a sponsor and reading the literature. Data are available on the norms of several samples that differ in gender, ethnicity, and treatment setting. The scale can be obtained from:

Lee Ann Kaskutas, PhD
Public Health Institute
Alcohol Research Group
2000 Hearst Avenue, Suite 300
Berkeley, CA 94709-2176
510-642-5208
alcresgp@arp.org

Brown–Peterson Recovery Progress Inventory

The Brown–Peterson Recovery Progress Inventory assesses spirituality in addiction treatment and follow-up. For more information, see Brown and Peterson (1991).

Alcoholics Anonymous Involvement Scale

The AAI measures involvement in Alcoholics Anonymous. For more information, see Tonigan, Miller, and Connors (1998).

REFERENCES

Alcoholics Anonymous. (1975). *Living sober.* New York: Alcoholics Anonymous World Services.

Allen, J. (2000). Measuring treatment process variables in Alcoholics Anonymous. *Journal of Substance Abuse Treatment, 18,* 227–230.

Allsop, S., Saunders, B., & Phillips, M. (2000). The process of relapse in severely dependent male problem drinkers. *Addiction, 95*(1), 95–106.

Annis, H., & Davis, C. (1989). Relapse prevention. In R. Hester & W. Miller (Eds.), *Handbook of alcoholism treatment approaches: Effective alternatives* (pp. 170–182). Boston: Allyn & Bacon.

Bellenir, K. (1996). *Substance abuse sourcebook.* Detroit, MI: Omnigraphics.

Borman, P., & Dixon, D. (1998). Spirituality and the 12 steps of substance abuse recovery. *Journal of Psychology and Theology, 26,* 287–291.

Brooks, C., & Rice, K. (1997). *Families in recovery: Coming full circle.* Baltimore: Brookes.

Brown, H. P., & Peterson, J. H. (1991). Assessing spirituality in addiction treatment and follow-up: Development of the Brown–Peterson Recovery Progress Inventory. *Alcoholism Treatment Quarterly, 8,* 21–50.

Committee on Alcoholism and Addictions. (1998). *Addiction treatment: Avoiding pitfalls—a case approach.* Washington, DC: American Psychiatric Association Press.

Coughey, K., Feighan, K., Cheney, R., & Klein, G. (1998). Retention in an aftercare program for recovering women. *Substance Use and Misuse, 33,* 917–933.

Daley, D. C., & Raskin, M. S. (Eds.). (1991). Treating the chemically dependent and their families. Newbury Park, CA: Sage.

DeCivita, M., Dobkin, P., & Robertson, R. (2000). A study of barriers to the engagement process of significant others in adult addiction treatment. *Journal of Substance Abuse Treatment, 29,* 135–144.

Dimeff, L., & Marlatt, A. (1998). Preventing relapse and maintaining change in addictive behaviors. *Clinical Psychology: Science and Practice, 5,* 513–525.

Dodes, L. M., & Khantzian, E. J. (1998). Individual psychodynamic psychotherapy. In R. J. Frances & S. I. Miller (Eds.), *Clinical textbook of addictive disorders* (2nd ed., pp. 479–495). New York: Guilford Press.

Dolan, J., & Olander, C. (1990, Summer). Grantmakers and the war on drugs. *Health Affairs,* pp. 202–208.

el-Guebaly, N., & Hodgins, D. (1998). Substance-related cravings and relapses: Clinical implications. *Canadian Journal of Psychiatry, 43,* 29–36.

Fiorentine, R., & Hillhouse, M. (2000). Exploring the additive effects of drug misuse treatment and twelve-step involvement: Does twelve-step ideology matter? *Substance Use and Misuse, 35,* 367–397.

Frances, R. J., & Miller, S. I. (1998). *Clinical textbook of addictive disorders* (2nd ed.). New York: Guilford Press.

Gilbert, F. S. (1991). Development of a "steps questionnaire." *Journal on Studies of Alcohol, 52,* 353–360.

Gorski, T. (1980, November/December). Dynamics of relapse. *EAP Digest,* pp. 16–21, 45–49.

Gorski, T. (1986). Relapse prevention planning: A new recovery tool. *Alcohol Health and Research World, 11*(1), 6–11.

Gray, M. (1989). Case management. U.S. Department of Health and Human Services, *Drug abuse curriculum for employee assistance professionals* (pp. 1–94). Washington, DC: U.S. Government Printing Office.

Gray, M. (1995). The effects of managed behavioral health care on substance abuse detoxification. *Social Work in Health, 21*(2), 71–81.

Green, L., Fullilove, M., & Fullilove, R. (1998). Stories of spiritual awakening: The nature of spirituality in recovery. *Journal of Substance Abuse Treatment, 15,* 325–331.

Heath, A. W., & Stanton, M. D. (1998). Family-based treatment: Stages and outcomes. In R. J. Frances & S. I. Miller (Eds.), *Clinical textbook of addictive disorders* (2nd ed., pp. 496–520). New York: Guilford Press.

Humphreys, K., Kaskutas, L., & Weisner, C. (1998). The Alcoholism Anonymous Affiliation Scale: Development, reliability, and norms for diverse treated and untreated populations. *Alcoholism: Clinical and Experimental Research, 22,* 974–978.

Humphreys, K., Moos, R., & Cohen, C. (1997). Social and community resources and long-term recovery from treated and untreated alcoholism. *Journal of Studies on Alcoholism, 58,* 231–238.

Kownacki, R., & Shadish, W. (1999). Does Alcoholics Anonymous work? The results from a meta-analysis of controlled experiments. *Substance Use and Misuse, 34*(13), 1987–1916.

Lash, S. (1998). Increasing participation in substance abuse aftercare treatment. *American Journal of Drug and Alcohol Abuse, 24,* 31–36.

Lesley, L. G., Fullilove, M. T., & Fullilove, R. E. (1998). Stories of spiritual awakening: The nature of spirituality in recovery. *Journal of Substance Abuse Treatment, 15,* 325–331.

Ludwig, A. (1988). *Understanding the alcoholic's mind.* New York: Oxford University Press.

Margolis, R., & Zweben, J. (1998). *Treating patients with alcohol and other drug problems: An integrated approach.* Washington, DC: American Psychological Association.

Marion, T., & Coleman, K. (1991). Recovery issues and treatment resources. In D. C. Daley & M. S. Raskin (Eds.), *Treating the chemically dependent and their families* (pp. 100–127). Newbury Park, CA: Sage.

Marlatt, A., & George, W. (1984). Relapse prevention: Introduction and overview of the model. *British Journal of Addiction, 79,* 261–273.

McKay, J., Alterman, A., McLellan, A., & Snider, E. (1994). Treatment goals, continuity of care, and outcome in a day hospital substance abuse rehabilitation program. *American Journal of Psychiatry, 151,* 254–259.

McKay, J., McLellan, A., Alterman, A., Cacciola, J., Rutherford, M., & O'Brien, C. (1998). Predictors of participation in aftercare sessions and self-help groups following completion of intensive outpatient treatment for substance abuse. *Journal of Studies on Alcohol, 59,* 152–162.

McLellan, A., Arndt, T., Metzer, D., Woody, G., & O'Brien, C. (1993). The effect of psychosocial services in substance abuse treatment. *Journal of the American Medical Association, 269,* 15.

McLellan, A., Hagan, T., Levine, M., Meyers, K., Gould, F., Bencivengo, M., Durrell, J., & Jaffe, J. (1999). Does clinical case management improve outpatient addiction treatment? *Drug and Alcohol Dependence, 55*, 91–103.

Miller, N., & Smith, D. (1997). The integration of pharmacotherapy and nonpharmacotherapy. *Journal of Addictive Diseases, 16*, 51–64.

Miller, W. (1989). Follow-up assessment. In R. Hester & W. Miller (Eds.), *Handbook of alcoholism treatment approaches: Effective alternatives* (pp. 81–89). New York: Pergamon.

Moore, B. A., & Budney, A. J. (2003). Relapse in outpatient treatment for marijuana dependence. *Journal of Substance Abuse Treatment, 25*(2), 85–89.

National Institute on Drug Abuse (NIDA). (1999). *Principles of drug addiction treatment* (NIH Publication No. 99–4180). Washington, DC: U.S. Government Printing Office.

Older, H., & Searcy, E. (1990). Assuring the continued recovery of EAP clients through post-treatment aftercare. *EAPA Exchange, 20*(6), 22–24. Arlington, VA: Employee Assistance Professionals Associations.

Ott, P. J., & Tarter, R. E. (1998). Comprehensive substance abuse evaluation. In R. J. Frances & S. I. Miller (Eds.), *Clinical textbook of addictive disorders* (2nd ed., pp. 35–70). New York: Guilford Press.

Palmeri, A., Pichini, S., Pacifici, R., Zuccaro, P., & Lopez, A. (2000). Drugs in nails: Physiology, pharmacokinetics and forensic toxicology. *Clinical Pharmacokinet, 38*(2), 95–110.

Peterson, K., Swindle, R., Phibbs, C., Recine, B., & Moos, R. (1994). Determinants of readmission following inpatient substance abuse treatment: A national study of VA programs. *Medical Care, 32*, 535–550.

Price, R. K., Risk, N. K., & Spitznagel, E. L. (2001). Remission from drug abuse over a 25–year period: Patterns of remission and treatment use. *American Journal of Public Health, 91*(7), 1107–1113.

Prochaska, J. O., DiClemente, C. C., & Norcross, J. C. (1992). In search of how people change: Applications to addictive behaviors. *American Psychologist, 47*, 1102–1114.

Ramanathan, C., & Reischl, T. (1999). Innovative approaches to predicting and preventing addiction relapse. *Employee Assistance Quarterly, 15*, 45–61.

Ricossa, M., Bernini, M., & DeFerrari, F., (2000). Hair analysis for driving license in cocaine and heroin users: An epidemiological study. *Forensic Science International , 107*(1–3), 301–308.

Schmitz, J., Oswald, L., Jacks, S., Rustin, T., Rhoades, H., & Grabowski, J. (1997). Relapse prevention treatment for cocaine dependence: Group vs. individual format. *Addictive Behaviors, 22*, 405–418.

Seilhamer, R. (1991). Effects of addiction on the family. In D. C. Daley & M. S. Raskin (Eds.), *Treating the chemically dependent and their families* (pp. 172–194). Newbury Park, CA: Sage.

Siegal, H., Rapp, R., Li, L., Saha, P., & Kirk, K. (1997). The role of case management in retaining clients in substance abuse treatment: An exploratory analysis. *Journal of Drug Issues, 27*, 821–831.

Stimmel, B. (1999). Heroin addiction and methadone maintenance: When will we ever learn? *Journal of Addictive Diseases, 18*, 1–4.

Substance Abuse and Mental Health Services Administration, Office of Applied

Studies. (2002). *National Survey of Substance Abuse Treatment Services (N-SSATS): Data on substance abuse treatment facilities* (USDHHS Publication No. 03-3777). Rockville, MD: Author.

Tonigan, J. S., Miller, W. R., & Connors, G. J. (1998). Alcoholics Anonymous Involvement (AAI) scale: Reliability and norms. *Psychology of Addictive Behaviors, 10,* 75–80.

United States Department of Health and Human Services (USDHHS). (1996). *Counselors' manual for relapse prevention with chemically dependent offenders.* Technical Assistance Publication No. 17, Rockville, MD.

United States Department of Health and Human Services (USDHHS). (1997). *The National Improvement Evaluation Study: The persistent effects of substance abuse treatment—one year later.* Center for Substance Abuse Treatment, Rockville, MD.

United States Department of Health and Human Services (USDHHS). (1998). *A cognitive-behavioral approach: Treating cocaine addiction.* Rockville, MD: National Institute on Drug Abuse.

van Wormer, K. (1995). *Alcoholism treatment: A social work perspective.* Chicago: Nelson Hall.

Washton, A. (1989). *Cocaine addiction: Treatment, recovery, and relapse prevention.* New York: Norton.

PART III

Intervention with Abusers of Different Substances

Despite the fact that most substance abusers in today's world tend to use a combination of drugs, the treatment field is still "specialized": Treatment settings and approaches focus on clients who abuse a particular substance. Part III examines the current treatment approaches offered to individuals with alcohol, opiate, and stimulant abuse problems.

The author of Chapter 8 describes the history of treating individuals with alcohol problems and identifies assessment issues and the broad range of current treatment approaches for this population. In the next chapter, the authors provide a brief history of opiate use and then describe the treatment modalities available to opiate-addicted adults, particularly methadone maintenance, and the role of social workers in such programs. The authors of the final chapter in Part III, Chapter 10, focus on the treatment of stimulant dependence. After a brief discussion of the history and current status of stimulant dependence in the United States, the authors provide an integrated multimodal approach addressing biological, psychological, and social factors that are important in the assessment process and that have an impact on the individual during treatment of stimulant-related problems.

Each of the following three chapters provides ample case examples to illustrate the basic assessment issues and effective treatment approaches when dealing with alcohol-, opiate-, and stimulant-abusing clients in a variety of treatment settings.

CHAPTER 8

Treatment of Alcohol Problems

Philip O'Dwyer

Programs designed to treat alcohol problems usually reflect the prevailing thinking of the time. In recent years the treatment of alcohol problems that experienced such enormous expansion in the 1980s saw its contraction in the 1990s. Lengthy inpatient rehabilitation gave way to a preference for outpatient care. Traditional self-help and disease model programs now compete with variety of innovative strategies that are both brief and solution focused. The revolutionary changes in health care in the United States have also had a marked impact on the treatment delivery system for clients who have problems associated with alcohol.

This chapter describes the key features in the development of treatment approaches for people with alcohol problems, provides a general introduction to prevailing practices, and discusses the implications of current trends for clinical effectiveness.

BRIEF HISTORY OF ALCOHOLISM TREATMENT

The use and misuse of alcohol has troubled society throughout history. Religious groups often held that alcohol was an instrument of the devil and should be prohibited. Drunkenness was widely believed to reflect moral weakness. Attempts in the late 18th century by Thomas Trotter, Benjamin Rush, and others to understand habitual drunkenness as a disease and a public health issue had limited appeal (Rush, 1785/1943). By the end of the 19th century temperance movements arose to keep the temperate people temperate. Their efforts culminated in the Volstead Act of 1919, which ushered in prohibition and which remained the nation's dominant response

171

to alcohol until its repeal in 1933. Efforts at treatment were minimal and few researchers even considered the topic worthy of study (Milam & Ketchum, 1981).

In 1935 two problem drinkers, Bill Wilson and Dr. Bob Smith, having failed to achieve sobriety on their own and regarded as hopeless by the treatment community of their time, decided to help each other. The success of their self-help led to the founding of Alcoholics Anonymous (AA). This movement of recovering people adhered to a relatively simple philosophy that is crystallized in 12 steps and amplified in what is called the Big Book (Alcoholics Anonymous, 1976). For the next 30 years, AA became the principal source of help for those considered to have problems with alcohol. It was free of charge and had only two requirements for participation: a willingness to accept one's disease and a commitment to anonymity. The role of a Higher Power as the ultimate source of help in recovery is featured prominently in AA. While most members considered their higher power to be God, others felt free to substitute the power of the group or any other notion their personal philosophy dictated. Over time AA spread throughout the country and its influence grew. When professional treatment emerged, AA involvement became a strong feature of the treatment enterprise (Anderson, 1981).

THE GOLDEN AGE OF TREATMENT

The Hughes Act of 1970 initiated substantial funding for the treatment and research of alcohol problems. Private insurance carriers soon followed the lead of Congress. The result was the rapid growth of a treatment system and the development of performance standards for clinicians. The Joint Commission for the Accreditation of Healthcare Organizations (JCAHO) accredited treatment facilities and held them accountable for delivering quality services. Public sentiment and disclosures by prominent individuals that they had received treatment converged to make the 1980s the golden age of treatment for people with alcohol problems (O'Dwyer, 1993).

The dominant treatment philosophy in most treatment facilities became the Minnesota model (Engelman, 1989) whose popularity was due, in part, to its vigorous promotion by the Hazelden Foundation (although this approach has been refined since its inception at Willmar State Hospital in Minnesota in the early 1950s). The model blends professional services and the 12 steps of AA. The counselors were usually individuals recovering from alcohol problems; they provided didactic lectures and integrated the principles of AA with individual and group therapy interventions. Initially these counselors were required to have at least a high school education and at least 5 years of sobriety (Laundergan, 1982).

The Minnesota model operates on several assumptions:

1. The client population is homogeneous—all have the same disease.
2. Alcohol problems represent a primary disease that is progressive and to which many of its victims are genetically predisposed.
3. The disease is characterized by loss of control over alcohol and denial of its negative consequences.
4. People recovering from alcohol problems should be part of the interdisciplinary treatment staff.
5. The 12 steps of AA are the pathway to recovery.
6. Education about the effects of alcohol on physical, psychological, and spiritual domains is essential.
7. Alcohol abuse is also a family disease; thus family members also require education and treatment.
8. Individual, group, and family therapy are necessary elements of the recovery process.
9. Clients must attend 12-step-based self-help groups while in treatment and continue the practice for life.

From the perspective of this model, all alcohol problems have a similar etiology, generally believed to be a disease entity that is amenable to a singular treatment approach. These programs were established in residential centers and inpatient settings where clients remained for 21–28 days and often longer. Clients were steeped in recovery language, AA, and the disease concept of alcohol abuse. The Minnesota model later developed into a continuum of care (Anderson, 1981), as evolved versions of the approach emerged: Several days of medically managed detoxification came to precede admission to inpatient rehabilitation, and aftercare services followed it.

THE NEW DECISION MAKERS

In recent years, the mechanisms by which a person with alcohol problems accesses treatment has become carefully controlled. Payers, whether using public funds or a commercial insurance, have established management systems to protect their interests. Only the client who is personally paying for treatment can have a strong voice in the level and extent of care undertaken. Essentially, providers of treatment compete with each other for contracts with managed care systems. In return for referrals, treatment providers agree to accept specific fees and meet specific standards of practice. In addition, before beginning treatment they must obtain preauthorization by describing the client's individual needs to a case manager and outlining the therapeutic goals and objectives to be pursued. Moreover, case managers employed by managed care companies must approve the level of care and the length of treatment provided to the client.

This process is enormously time consuming; it also limits clinicians' treatment options. Managed care constraints have made it too difficult for some clients to access the more expensive levels of care that they may need. Some companies have reduced access to residential care to two opportunities per lifetime. This constraint seems unwise, given that individuals who suffer from alcohol problems—and their families—are high consumers of health care dollars. In the long run, having untreated alcohol-dependent individuals who have no access to essential services may prove to be far more costly to society (O'Dwyer, 1984).

On the positive side, the clinician who has to present a client's clinical condition to a case manager must develop good clinical and verbal skills in order to make an accurate assessment of the client's needs and to recommend a treatment plan that is defensible. Moreover, overuse of expensive treatments is prevented, and the client and clinician together become accountable for appropriate use of health benefits. Consequently, clients who were serial users of treatment in the past or who tended to move from program to program now find limits placed on their options (Rawson, Obert, & Marinell-Casey, 1992).

RANGE OF TREATMENT SETTINGS
FOR PEOPLE WITH ALCOHOL PROBLEMS

The continuum of care for people with alcohol problems has several components: detoxification, residential care, outpatient counseling, and the halfway house setting. In addition, family therapy and AA participation usually are considered important components of treatment.

Detoxification

Alcohol withdrawal can be life threatening and often requires careful medical management. Detoxification strategies are based on the client's history of past withdrawal and the current clinical status. Laboratory studies that include blood alcohol level are usually conducted. Careful medical intervention is required for individuals who have a history of seizures or delirium tremens, especially when combined with elevated blood pressure, rapid pulse rate, and agitation. Librium or phenobarbital are frequently used to ease withdrawal discomfort. A high, or loading, dose may be given initially and tapered over time. A drug screen is extremely important in order to avoid oversedation in clients who may have other sedating drugs in their system. Currently, the criteria for acute care admission are stringent, and intoxication alone is insufficient to justify inpatient detoxification.

The avoidance of recurrent use of alcohol is seldom achieved by detoxification alone, whether it is provided in an acute case setting or on an outpatient basis (Skinner, 1988). Therefore, if relapse is to be prevented, additional treatment strategies are usually required.

Residential Care

Although their numbers have declined dramatically and their length of stay has been reduced to about 7 days, residential treatment facilities remain an important part of the continuum of care for clients dependent on alcohol. In the 1980s, residential facilities (or "rehab" centers) accounted for the bulk of all alcoholism treatment (Goodwin, 1991). Today they treat only a small proportion of the alcohol-dependent population. As private insurance coverage has swung in the direction of outpatient treatment, residential facilities are used mainly by those who can afford to pay for their own treatment, or those who are more severely affected and medically compromised and whose care is more likely to be supported by public funds.

Once admitted to the rehabilitation center, clients are expected to follow a rigid daily schedule. Most facilities are highly structured and include, among their daily activities, morning meditation, educational films, didactic lectures, AA meetings, individual and group counseling, recreational activities, family counseling, and occupational therapy. The pace of treatment tends to be rapid due to the shortened length of stay.

The risk of relapse is high following discharge from residential care, and assisting clients to effectively maintain sobriety is often difficult. Consequently, emphasis is placed on developing a clear and workable aftercare plan and facilitating a solid introduction to self-help groups. Typically, before the client is discharged, a schedule of AA meetings to be attended is developed and connection with outpatient counseling is established. Clients who participated in outpatient therapy *and* attended 12-step meetings have been shown to have better outcomes than those who attended only one, or neither, of these treatment modalities (Ouimette, Moos, & Finney, 1998).

The optimal length of stay in residential treatment settings remains controversial. In an extensive review of the literature on this question, Miller and Hester (1986) concluded that there was no advantage to longer and more intensive treatment programs. In a study comparing a 4-week with a 6-week residential treatment program for people with alcohol problems, no significant outcome advantages to the longer program were found (Trent, 1998). The severity of the disorder, rather than a fixed program length, should determine duration of treatment.

Outpatient Treatment

Current outpatient treatment programs for alcohol problems are distinguished in terms of intensity. So-called intensive outpatient treatment consists of daily treatment encounters ranging from 4 to 6 hours per day, for a period of 2 or more weeks. The clinical content of these programs is similar to that provided in residential settings. In the early 1990s these programs were seen as offering a less expensive alternative to residential care while providing a condensed version of its content. Recently, however, the use of intensive outpatient programs has declined in favor of traditional outpatient treatment coupled with AA involvement. Like residential care, intensive outpatient treatment tends to be reserved for those whose recovery may be unlikely in a less structured level of care.

Moos, Finney, Federman, and Sushinski (2000) found that the overall duration of a client's participation in treatment is more significant than the intensity. The authors proposed that after residential treatment, the provision of outpatient therapy sessions twice per month is cost effective for the less impaired clients; more impaired clients may require more frequent outpatient sessions. Their research also indicated that clients who experienced severe substance abuse disorders derived better outcomes when treated in treatment centers specializing in the treatment of addictions, as opposed to those treated in general medical or mental health centers.

Traditional outpatient alcoholism treatment usually consists of individual and/or group therapy offered once each week for about 12 weeks. An extensive array of treatment approaches is currently offered in different settings. Miller (1995) identified 25 approaches, including social skills training, motivational enhancement therapy, cognitive therapy, behavioral contracting, marital and family therapy, aversion therapy, and relaxation therapy.

One treatment approach that has captured increasing clinical and research interest is that of cognitive-behavioral coping-skills training (CBST). Unlike other cognitive skill-training approaches that focus directly on behaviors and environmental cues for drinking, this approach does not focus exclusively on clients' drinking; instead, it addresses other life areas that may contribute to their alcohol consumption. This approach assumes that excessive alcohol use often results from an individual's inability to cope with life stress (Longabaugh & Morgenstern, 1999). Therefore, clients are helped to improve their cognitive and behavioral skills to better manage their life stressors. Clients may receive anger management training, relaxation training, behavioral marital therapy, or other similar interventions tailored to clients' specific needs.

Denial and *minimization* are significant issues for clients with alcohol problems, and recovery is often influenced by their ability to accept that they have an alcohol-related problem. External pressure on an individual to embrace treatment often triggers resistance. One way of addressing this issue is to use a variant of the Johnson Institute Intervention (Johnson, 1986), which was developed specifically for use in an outpatient treatment setting. The original Johnson model focused on getting an individual into residential treatment and consisted of bringing together the significant people in the person's life and educating them about the disease and the process of recovery. The person with the drinking problem was then included in a session and the drinking behavior confronted in a kind but firm manner that hopefully dissolved the denial and convinced the person to enter treatment.

Ino and Hayasida (2000) have applied this general strategy to clients who were already in treatment for alcohol abuse or dependence. In this model, family members are invited to the treatment center to provide positive verbal statements of encouragement to the client. The goal is to encourage the client to participate fully in the treatment process (Ino & Hayasida, 2000). However, unlike in the Johnson Intervention model, no ultimatum is given by the family. Ino and Hayasida found that patients exposed to this approach before their discharge from treatment had significantly better abstinence rates and higher follow-up participation.

This finding is consistent with the work of Miller (1995), who advocates the use of motivational enhancement therapy as part of the treatment process. This method proposes that a clinician focus on individual intervention with the client, helping the client to become clearly aware of the adverse consequences of drinking—and thereby increasing his or her motivation not to drink. The incorporation of motivational interviewing is a response to the widespread observation that clients who have addiction problems often lack internal sources of motivation to change and will not necessarily change because someone else thinks that they need to do so.

A major national study compared the use of CBST, motivational enhancement therapy, and 12-step facilitation therapy (Mattson et al., 1998). This study, frequently referred to as Project MATCH, found significant positive outcomes for each treatment approach. This finding suggests that, as a general proposition, all these treatments for clients with alcohol problems are effective. However, the incorporation of 12-step facilitation treatment approach into outpatient groups resulted in slightly more favorable results. (This approach assisted clients in their understanding of AA and required them to participate in AA meetings.) This finding suggests that clients should be introduced to the self-help philosophy as outlined in the 12 steps and 12 traditions of AA. Ideally, treatment should attempt to weave 12-step thinking with clinical counseling strategies. AA seems to add a spiritual dimension to treatment that assists clients in finding meaning in their lives. This sense of meaning may have eluded them in the past and contributed to their abuse of alcohol.

Halfway House

Some clients who are homeless or live in socially unstable environments experience a continuous threat to their recovery, especially in the early stage. The halfway house is a facility in which they can live for a modest fee and be closely monitored in a chemical-free environment. It is called "halfway house" because it represents a midpoint between the structure of residential care and the freedom of living at home. Clients are free to go to work or attend school and participate in AA meetings. Some clients also attend individual or group counseling in the community while living in the halfway house.

Use of Acupuncture

The use of acupuncture for medical and psychological problems in China and other Far Eastern societies extends back to distant history. The use of this procedure is currently common in many alcohol abuse treatment settings. Despite its promise, Swedish scholars found that those who received acupuncture as part of outpatient therapy reported no significant difference in craving level or consumption reduction than the control group (Sapir-Weise, Berglund, Frank, & Kristenson, 1999). There was a slight but nonsignificant positive finding that males who received acupuncture did remain in treatment longer than the control subjects.

Relapse Prevention

The relapse prevention approach is a significant element of treatment; much of it relies on the work of Gorski, who developed the concept of protracted alcohol withdrawal syndrome (PAWS) (Gorski & Miller, 1982). This model identifies 37 warning signs of relapse. For almost 20 years, treatment programs utilized this model without the scientific support usually required of such a popular strategy. Finally, Miller and Harris (2000) operationalized the 37 signs of impending relapse and tested their reliability and validity. They concluded that the confidence treatment providers have placed in PAWS has been justified. The authors suggested that the relapse warning signs could be clustered under one general factor, which they called "demoralization/depression." They found that lower levels of relapse risk existed among clients who exhibited a sense of meaning in life, honesty, hope, low levels of emotional negativity, stable eating and sleeping patterns, clear thinking, the absence of self-pity, and a sense of peace and stability (Miller & Harris, 2000). These data can guide treatment providers in preventing relapse by carefully assessing clients for depressed mood and a sense of hopelessness. When these issues are identified, clients may need psychiatric intervention in conjunction with treatment for alcohol problems. Although the use of psychotropic medications with clients who have addiction problems must be judiciously implemented, prevention of relapse may require such a measure. Individuals who feel discouraged and negative about life often will use alcohol as a medication to relieve these feelings. However, such temporary relief only intensifies the negative mood disturbance because of the depressant properties of the alcohol. (See also Gray and Gibson, Chapter 7, this volume.)

Family Treatment

Because it is commonly known that alcoholism can have devastating effects on the family (Straussner, Weinstein, & Hernandez, 1979), many treatment facilities include the family in the treatment process. O'Farrell and Feehan (1999) have identified three different family perspectives used in the treatment of alcoholism. The first is the *family disease approach*, which asserts that the entire family suffers from this disease and its members are frequently referred to as "codependents." This approach makes extensive use of Al-Anon, and family education focuses on the disease concept of alcoholism. The client and family are usually treated separately.

The second model is the *family systems approach*, in which the focus is on the entire family as a system. All family members participate in the therapeutic process, as the roles, alliances, and communication patterns that support drinking in the family are examined. Changes in the family system are suggested in order to support the client's sobriety.

Both client and family also receive treatment together in the third model, which is focused on a *behavioral approach in which abstinence is rewarded*. A reward system is implemented that reinforces positive family interactions, and family members offer verbal acknowledgment whenever they observe a desired behavior in the client. Such positive reinforcement tends to ensure that the desired behavior continues.

PREVENTION OF ALCOHOL PROBLEMS

In recent years numerous efforts have been made to prevent the spread of alcohol problems. Dangerous drinking patterns on college campuses throughout the country have captured national attention, and most institutions of higher learning have developed specific strategies to curb binge drinking. Despite this phenomenon of heavy alcohol consumption, most college students do not go on to develop alcohol dependence; rather, they normalize their alcohol use without intervention (Bennet et al., 1999). However, Vik, Culberson, and Sellers (2000) found that almost 66% of college students who drank heavily did not recognize the need to reduce their drinking, despite adverse consequences in their lives and evidence of growing tolerance to alcohol. Thus, in spite of intense preventive education, denial of problems related to alcohol abuse tends to obscure the need to alter drinking behavior in many young people.

When individuals who are dependent on alcohol come to acknowledge their drinking problems, it is important that formal treatment and/or AA involvement occur as soon as possible. It has been shown that such clients will have better outcomes than those whose treatment is delayed (Timko, Moos, Finney, Moos, & Kaplowitz, 1999). Therefore, physicians and other health care professionals who encounter clients with obvious alcohol problems should encourage these drinkers to embrace treatment promptly.

ASSESSMENT CONSIDERATIONS

The Institute of Medicine Report to Congress (1990) stressed the importance of developing a thorough assessment of each client. Such an assessment should evaluate several areas of functioning, not only chemical use. This approach to assessment implies that alcohol problems exist on a continuum of impairment and suggests that, as a result, some clients may need intensive treatment, whereas others may benefit from brief intervention, and still others may respond well to preventive efforts. Careful assessment enables the clinician to design a treatment plan that corresponds to each client's level of impairment. Exclusive focus on people whose behavior meets the DSM-IV-TR criteria for alcohol dependence overlooks the needs of clients who are alcohol abusers. Although not dependent on alcohol, these individuals do experience significant problems because of their alcohol consumption, including car accidents, health problems, and other injuries, as well as a host of occupational and family issues.

The first step in making an assessment is to conduct a biopsychosocial history. The key elements to be evaluated are discussed in the following material.

Alcohol Use

To evaluate the client's use of alcohol, the clinician should begin with current consumption level, including amount consumed in the past 48 hours. In order to assess the need for detoxification, the clinician should observe the client's behavior and note any past history of withdrawal. Clients who have experienced withdrawal seizures, delirium tremens, or hallucinations may need to be detoxified under medical management. When other medical complications exist, hospitalization may be warranted. Life-threatening symptoms are the usual criterion for hospital detoxification.

Past history of alcohol consumption needs to be elicited in order to obtain information needed to make a DSM-IV-TR diagnosis. Questions should focus on loss of control over alcohol, increased tissue tolerance to alcohol, physical withdrawal symptoms, and social disruption associated with alcohol consumption. Clinically significant impairment suggests a diagnosis of alcohol dependence. An alternative diagnosis may be that of alcohol abuse. Criteria for abuse include maladaptive patterns of consumption that may interfere with work, driving, or family functioning. Additional useful information might include relapse history, prior treatment attempts, family history of addictive problems, level of denial, and attitude toward AA.

Two widely used diagnostic instruments for assessing alcohol problems are the Michigan Alcohol Screening Test (MAST; Skinner, 1979) and the Substance Abuse Subtle Screening Inventory–3 (SASSI-3; Lazowski, Miller, Boye, & Miller, 1998).

Psychological and Emotional History

Important psychological and emotional areas to evaluate include current psychological symptoms, history of emotional problems, identification of relatives with any emotional disturbance, current or past use of prescribed medications, suicidal potential, and history of psychological, physical, or sexual abuse. It is also important to identify the client's strengths. A clear picture of psychological functioning is often impossible to obtain until about 1 month of sobriety has occurred, because the effect of alcohol itself may be misperceived as the source of an observed emotional problem.

Family of Origin and Childhood History

Assessment of early family experience should focus on the client's relationships with parents, stepparents, and/or siblings. Knowledge of family dynamics and ethnocultural factors (Straussner, 2001) is often essential in treating this population.

Social History

Areas of the client's social history that should be explored include level of education, employment, current relationships, marriages, children, peer groups, spiritual orientation, current living arrangements, financial status, and social skills.

Physical Health Assessment

The physical health evaluation is usually conducted by a physician or physician's assistant. It may contain a review of systems, an alcohol/drug screen, and other laboratory studies including liver enzyme and bilirubin levels.

Based upon all these data, the clinician develops a tentative treatment plan. The proposed plan should include the goals and objectives of treatment and the level of care recommended.

CLINICAL KNOWLEDGE AND SKILL

In order to provide effective treatment for clients who have alcohol problems, clinicians need to have substantial knowledge in the following areas:

- Withdrawal signs and symptoms
- Pharmacology of alcohol and psychoactive drugs
- Medical consequences of alcoholism
- Interpreting diagnostic laboratory studies
- Psychological dynamics, including the role of denial
- Use and interpretation of diagnostic assessment instruments
- DSM-IV-TR diagnostic categories
- Models and techniques of alcoholism treatment
- The theory and practice of crisis counseling
- The philosophy and steps of AA
- Relapse prevention
- Ethnocultural awareness
- Familiarity with relevant research

Having achieved mastery of these areas, the effective clinician needs to develop skills through which this knowledge is expressed. These skills include:

- Communicating a nonjudgmental disposition
- Developing an effective therapeutic relationship
- Facilitating the client's self-diagnosis
- Motivating the client and his or her family to participate in treatment
- Practicing in interdisciplinary teams
- Maintaining a coherent clinical record
- Utilizing computer technology
- Communicating effectively with managed care organizations
- Treating special populations, such as adolescents, women, and older adults

A CLINICAL VIGNETTE

While acknowledging that each client is unique, the following case reflects an amalgam of male alcohol-dependent individuals and illustrates some of the commonly occurring features.

John Jones is a 46–year-old white middle-class client who sought treatment at an outpatient substance abuse clinic for help with his excessive drinking after being arrested for drunk driving for the third time.

Mr. Jones had already called his insurance carrier to obtain authorization for the intake session. A traditional biopsychosocial history was conducted, and a multidimensional range of information was generated about the client's clinical status. Mr. Jones was in no acute distress and presented no signs of withdrawal. He appeared to be bright and capable of insight.

The assessment revealed that Mr. Jones had begun his drinking career when he was 16 years old. At that time he consumed a six-pack of beer on weekends. By the age of 20 he was drinking at least three nights per week at the rate of 8 beers per night. By 30 years of age he was consuming up to 10 beers each day. This level of consumption continued until 1 week ago, at which time he was arrested while driving under the influence of alcohol.

Although he had attended AA in the past in compliance with court orders after his first two arrests, Mr. Jones felt that he had "nothing in common with these people" and that he was "drinking because of job stress and marriage problems." His score on the MAST and his SASSI-3 profile indicated a high probability of a substance dependence disorder. He had made no significant effort to discontinue his alcohol consumption in the past, and his current participation in treatment is the result of legal and family influences. Mr. Jones seemed depressed and defensive in his emotional functioning; he denied engaging in any suicidal ideation. He stated that he was currently on medication for elevated blood pressure, but denied any history of drug or medication abuse.

Mr. Jones described his father and two uncles as "heavy drinkers." His childhood was described as non-nurturing. He was the middle child of five, raised in a rigid family in which he felt "unloved and unimportant." His school performance was poor, despite his intellectual abilities, and he dropped out at the beginning of the 12th grade.

Mr. Jones has been married to his wife Mary for the past 16 years, and they have two sons. He has been experiencing financial stress due to legal fees, court costs, and missing work as a result of "hangovers." He claimed that Mary was also "a heavy drinker," although, when interviewed later, she claimed that she "only drank to help tolerate his drinking."

Mr. Jones was given a physical examination; the findings included enlargement of the liver and substantially elevated liver enzymes; his blood pressure was slightly elevated, despite the use of medication. Mr. Jones was prescribed Antabuse (disulfiram), which he was to begin taking once his liver enzymes normalized. He was also prescribed ReVia (naltrexone) to curb his craving for alcohol.

His diagnosis and initial treatment plan indicated the following:

- *Problem*: Alcohol dependence, 303.90, with physiological dependence.
- *Goal*: Total abstinence from alcohol.
- *Objectives*: (1) Participate in a motivational enhancement group; (2) understand the disease concept of dependence on alcohol; (3) learn the medical consequences of excessive alcohol use; (4) understand the process of recovery; (5) correct cognitive distortions about addiction; (6) identify personal relapse triggers; (7) develop two relapse prevention strategies for each trigger; (8) learn the philosophy and 12 steps of AA; (9) attend five AA meetings each week; (10) actively participate in group and individual therapy; (11) participate in family education and joint sessions with his wife at a later time.
- *Level of care*: It was recommended that Mr. Jones pursue these and other objectives in an intensive outpatient treatment program, which would consist of 4 hours of treatment each day, for 3 weeks. Mrs. Jones will be further evaluated for alcohol problems and a separate plan developed. Once a stable recovery process is in place, the related issues of job stress and marriage problems will be addressed. After 1 month of complete abstinence, his mood will be reevaluated and the issue of the "non-nurturing" childhood explored. Following intensive outpatient care, it is expected that regular outpatient counseling would continue and be approved by the managed care company.

It is important to note that as the treatment process unfolds, new information may emerge that requires changes to this treatment plan. Therefore, it is essential that the treatment staff remain flexible and willing to make changes in a timely manner.

CONCLUSION

Current clinical practice in the treatment of alcohol problems has become less intuitive and more scientifically based. Pressure to accomplish more in less time has resulted in a growing emphasis on effective clinical research, and the growth of managed care has increased accountability. In order to provide effective treatment for individuals with alcohol problems, clinicians need to learn how to make accurate assessments and develop specific treatment objectives and measurable treatment plans.

Treatment in the years ahead is likely to reflect greater influence of research, as more randomized clinical trials are conducted. The challenge is how to make use of these findings in a way that still provides humane and caring treatment for individuals suffering from the impact of alcohol abuse and dependence.

REFERENCES

Alcoholics Anonymous. (1976). *Alcoholics Anonymous* (3rd ed.). New York: Alcoholics Anonymous World Services.

Anderson, D. (1981). *Perspectives on treatment: The Minnesota experience.* Center City, MN: Hazelden Foundation.

Bennett, M., McCrady, B., Johnson, V., & Padina, R. (1999). Problem drinking from young adulthood to adulthood: Patterns, predictors and outcomes. *Journal of Studies on Alcohol, 60,* 605–614.

Emerick, C., Tonigan, J., Montgomery, H., & Little, L. (1993). Alcoholics Anonymous: What is currently known? In B. McCrady & W. Miller (Eds.), *Research on Alcoholics Anonymous: Opportunities and alternatives.* New Brunswick, NJ: Rutgers Center on Alcohol Studies.

Engelman, J. (1989). Minnesota treatment revolution. *Hazelden Update, 7,* 3–5.

Goodwin, D. (1991). Inpatient treatment of alcoholism: New life for the Minneapolis plan. *New England Journal of Medicine, 325,* 804–806.

Gorski, T., & Miller, W. (1982). *Counseling for relapse prevention.* Independence, MO: Herald House–Independence Press.

Ino, A., & Hayasida, M. (2000). Before-discharge intervention method in the treatment of alcohol dependence. *Alcohol: Clinical and Experimental Research, 24,* 373–376.

Institute of Medicine. (1990). *Broadening the base of treatment for alcohol problems.* Washington, DC: National Academy Press.

Johnson, V. (1986). *Intervention: How to help someone who doesn't want help.* Minneapolis, MN: Johnson Institute Books.

Laundergan, J. (1982). *Easy does it: Alcohol treatment outcomes, Hazelden and the Minnesota model.* Minneapolis, MN: Hazelden Foundation.

Lazowski, L. E., Miller, F. G., Boye, M. W., & Miller, G. A. (1998). Efficacy of the Substance Abuse Subtle Screening Inventory–3 (SASSI-3) in identifying substance dependence disorders in clinical settings. *Journal of Personality Assessment, 71*(1), 114–128.

Longabaugh, R., & Morgenstern, J. (1999). Cognitive-behavioral coping-skills therapy for alcohol dependence: Current status and future directions. *Alcohol Research and Health, 23,* 78.

Mattson, M., Del Boca, F., Carroll, K., Cooney, N., DiClimente, C., Donovan, D., Kadden, R., McRee, B., Rice, C., Rychtarick, R., & Sweben, A. (1998). Patient compliance in Project MATCH: Session attendance predictors and relationship to outcome. *Alcoholism: Clinical and Experimental Research, 22,* 1328–1339.

Milam, J., & Ketchum, K. (1981). *Under the influence.* New York: Bantam.

Miller, W. (1995). Increasing motivation for change. In R. Hester & W. Miller (Eds.), *Handbook of alcoholism treatment approaches and effective alternatives* (2nd ed., pp. 89–104). Boston: Allyn & Bacon.

Miller, W., & Harris, R. (2000). A simple scale for Gorski's warning signs for relapse. *Journal of Studies on Alcohol, 61,* 759–765.

Miller, W., & Hester, R. (1986). Inpatient alcoholism treatment: Who benefits? *American Psychologist, 41,* 794–805.

Moos, R., Finney, J., Federman, E., & Sushinski, R. (2000). Specialty Mental healthcare improves mental out comes: Findings from a nationwide program to monitor the quality of care for patients with substance use disorders. *Journal of Studies on Alcohol, 61,* 704–713.

O'Dwyer, P. (1984). Cost-effective rehabilitation: A process of matching. *EAP Digest, 4*(2), 33–34.

O'Dwyer, P. (1993). *Alcoholism treatment facilities.* In S. L. A. Straussner (Ed.), *Clinical work with substance-abusing clients* (pp. 119–134). New York: Guilford Press.

O'Farrell, T., & Feehan, M. (1999). Alcoholism treatment and the family: Do family and individual treatments for alcoholic adults have preventive effects for children. *Journal of Studies on Alcohol, 13,* 125– 129.

Ouimette, P., Moos, R., & Finney, J. (1998). Influence of outpatient treatment and 12 step group involvement on one year substance abuse treatment outcomes. *Journal of Studies on Alcohol, 59,* 513–522.

Rawson, R., Obert, J., & Marinell-Casey, P. (1992). Perspectives in managed care: Let's prove that treatment works. *Addiction and Recovery, 12,* 1.

Rush, B. (1943). An inquiry into the effects of ardent spirits upon the human body and mind, with an account of the means of preventing and remedies for curing them. *Quarterly Journal of Studies on Alcohol, 4,* 325–341. (Original work published 1785)

Sapir-Weise, R., Berglund, M., Frank, A., & Kristenson, H. (1999). Acupuncture in alcoholism treatment: A randomized outpatient study. *Alcohol and Alcoholism, 34,* 629–635.

Skinner, H. (1979). A multivariate evaluation of the Michigan Alcohol Screening Test. *Journal of Studies on Alcohol, 40,* 831–844.

Skinner, H. (1988). *Toward a multiaxial framework for the classification of alcohol problems* [Position paper]. Washington, DC: Institute of Medicine.

Straussner, S. L. A. (Ed.). (2001). *Ethnocultural factors in substance abuse treatment.* New York: Guilford Press.

Straussner, S. L. A., Weinstein, D., & Hernandez, R. (1979). Effects of alcoholism on the family system. *Health and Social Work, 4*(4), 112–127.

Timko, C., Moos, R., Finney, J., Moos, B., & Kaplowitz, M. (1999). Long-term treatment careers and outcomes of previously untreated alcoholics. *Journal of Studies on Alcohol, 60,* 437–447.

Trent, L. (1998). Evaluation of a four versus six week length of stay in the Navy's alcohol treatment program. *Journal of Studies on Alcohol, 59,* 270–279.

Vik, P., Culberson, K., & Sellers, K. (2000). Readiness to change drinking among heavy drinking college students. *Journal of Studies on Alcohol, 61,* 674–680.

CHAPTER 9

The Treatment
of Opiate Addiction

Ellen Grace Friedman
Robin Wilson

Opiates are a classification of drugs that includes opium, morphine, heroin, codeine, and synthetic opiates such as methadone. Opiates have been used throughout history for therapeutic purposes, such as the alleviation of physical pain, as well as for pleasure. Widely known for their addictive potential, heroin, morphine, and other opiate use remain widespread today. Heroin is both the most abused and the most rapidly acting of the opiates (Committee of Methadone Program Administrators [COMPA], 1999). Since narcotic abuse is illegal and therefore often hidden, it is difficult to know the exact number of people who abuse or are addicted to opiates. It is estimated that there are 980,000 people who are addicted to heroin in the United States (Centers for Disease Control and Prevention [CDC], 2002). Following is a brief history of opiate use, a description of treatment modalities available to adults who are opiate addicted, and a discussion of the role of social workers in addiction treatment programs.

A BRIEF HISTORY OF OPIATE ADDICTION

Opiates were used for medical purposes in the American colonies as early as the 1700s. In the early 1800s, two opium alkaloids, morphine (1805) and codeine (1832), were isolated from the opium poppy, increasing the number of available opiates (Winn, Chester, May, & Sutton, 1967). Radical changes in the extent of opiate use resulted from two events in the

1800s: the invention of the hypodermic needle and the Civil War. The hypodermic needle, invented in 1843, was brought to the United States in 1856. The needle allowed opiates, notably morphine, to be injected directly into the veins, thereby increasing the strength and speed of the drug. During the Civil War opiates were widely administered to soldiers wounded in battle or suffering from dysentery. After the Civil War ended, there were many medically addicted soldiers: "A term prevalent at the time, 'soldier's illness,' actually meant opiate addict" (Winn et al., 1967, p. 18).

During the 1800s, the use of opiates was not generally offensive to public morals. Opium, the most widely used opiate, was taken orally, smoked, or used in suppository form, and morphine was taken orally, rectally, or hypodermically. In 1898, heroin was first synthesized, and, because its addictive potential was not fully understood, it was used to detoxify persons addicted to morphine.

Medical and public opinion of opiate use began to shift around 1900. Many physicians recognized opiate use as a problem, and legislation was enacted. The first federal attempt to control opiate use came in 1909, "with an act that prohibited the importation of opium, its preparations and derivatives, except for medical purposes" (Winn et al., 1967, p. 22). The Harrison Act of 1914 further attempted to control the production and distribution of opiates through the imposition of an occupational tax on all persons dealing in opiate drugs. Whereas prior to the Harrison Act, physicians were allowed to distribute opiates to maintain addicted persons, court decisions following the act prohibited this distribution. Many physicians were arrested for prescribing opiates (Brecher et al., 1972), and soon most physicians stopped treating addicted people altogether. Although passage of the Harrison Act did not stop opiate use, it did change the nature of the users. Before the Harrison Act, women represented the majority of heroin and morphine users; afterward, the sex ratio changed greatly, and estimates during the 1960s indicated that males outnumbered women among known addicted individuals by five to one or more (Brecher et al., 1972).

By 1920, more than 1.5 million "victims of the drug habit" were reported (Newman, 1971, p. xvii). "Cut off from both legal drugs and clinic assistance [and] unable to break their habits, addicts turned to an underworld market that had been only a minor source of supply previously" (Winn et al., 1967, p. 23). According to Brecher and colleagues (1972), "as a result, the door was opened wide to adulterated, contaminated, and misbranded black-market opiates of all kinds" (p. 47).

In the early 1950s, the American Medical Association and the American Bar Association issued reports urging that the government reevaluate its opiates policy. In 1962, the Supreme Court, in *Robinson v. California*, ruled that criminal conviction for addiction to opiates violated the Eighth and Fourteenth Amendments (Chavkin, 1990). These events helped bring about the present era, in which medical intervention has once again become an accepted treatment for opiate-addicted individuals.

TREATMENT APPROACHES

There are several treatment options for opiate addiction, including: medically supervised inpatient detoxification, medically supervised inpatient rehabilitation, therapeutic community, drug-free outpatient and community-based treatment, 12-step/self-help groups, methadone maintenance, methadone to abstinence, and the use of long-acting methadone LAAM (levo-alpha-acetyl-methadol) and, more recently, buprenorphine (National Institute on Drug Abuse [NIDA], 2000).

Inpatient Detoxification and Medically Supervised Withdrawal

Opiate-dependent individuals require detoxification as a first step in treatment. Detoxification, which is the process of freeing the addicted person's body from physiological dependence on drugs, can be done either during an inpatient hospitalization or on an outpatient basis under medical supervision. Although the time needed for detoxification varies, it is seldom longer than 5 days. During the detoxification process, patients receive services such as individual, group, and family counseling and education about the disease of addiction. They also may receive counseling that focuses on relapse prevention and recovery strategies, developing abstinent support systems, and aftercare planning to assure a supportive transition to the next level of care.

Therapeutic Communities

The first therapeutic community (TC) in the United States, Synanon, was started in California in 1958. When the TC movement began, most residents were opiate abusers (DeLeon, 1994). Currently, many residents are polysubstance dependent. TCs use a highly structured residential setting and peer influence to help individuals with addictions change their lifestyles, beliefs, and behaviors (Tims, DeLeon, & Jainchill, 1994). Many of the staff members are graduates of these TCs. Residents are resocialized to assume responsibility for themselves, and privileges are given in accordance with their willingness to conform, learn, and participate in the program. Residents of TCs are gradually prepared to reenter the outside community or become incorporated permanently into its structure (DeLeon, 1994). More recently, a variety of TCs has emerged to serve the special needs of mentally ill chemical abusers (MICAs) and women—two groups that have not done well in the traditional, highly structured and confrontational TC settings.

Drug-Free Outpatient Programs

Drug-free outpatient programs use individual, group, and family counseling techniques, and include psychoeducational material, relapse prevention counseling, motivational interviewing and cognitive-behavioral groups (NIDA, 2000). Programs frequently hold on-site 12-step meetings and then help clients transition to community-based self-help groups. The purpose of outpatient programs is to assist recovering addicted individuals in developing drug-abstinent lifestyles while remaining in the community. Since welfare reform was enacted, outpatient programs have increased their vocational efforts because substance abuse providers are now required to assist patients obtain work and secure their economic self-sufficiency. The goals of outpatient treatment programs, therefore, include assisting patients in obtaining the necessary skills and attitudes to become economically self-sufficient as well as to maintain abstinence from drugs.

12-Step Programs

The 12-step model of treatment for opiate addition is based on the principles and practices of Alcoholics Anonymous (AA), which offers peer-led meetings in the community (see Spiegel & Jewell, Chapter 6, this volume). Opiate-addicted persons can attend Narcotics Anonymous (NA) meetings, where they, too, are granted total anonymity, may participate as much or as little as they choose, and have a shared goal of abstinence from opiate use. The 12-step meeting is also a forum that provides a drug-abstinent social context whereby members learn to listen, communicate, and support each other. Nar-Anon is a 12-step program that is available for family members of individuals with opiate addiction.

During the past few years, 12-step meetings for methadone patients, Methadone Anonymous (MA), have been developed at a number of methadone programs. The goal of MA is to obtain abstinence from opiates and other chemicals, including alcohol. Because methadone maintenance is recognized as a treatment, MA members may continue its use as long as they participate in a treatment program (McGonagle, 1994). Many methadone maintenance treatment program patients who have attended AA and NA have felt stigmatized in these programs because of their ongoing use of methadone. In contrast, MA provides a forum that allows them to speak freely, not only about their addiction, but also about their experiences in methadone treatment.

Methadone Treatment

Methadone is a long-acting synthetic opiate, developed in Germany during World War II as a synthetic painkiller (Rosenbaum, 1982). In the early 1960s, Drs. Vincent Dole and Marie Nyswander of Rockefeller University opened the first methadone maintenance treatment program at Beth Israel Hospital in New York City to research the therapeutic value of methadone maintenance. Although methadone had been used in the United States since 1948 to detoxify opiate-addicted individuals, the concept of maintaining addicted persons on it was new (Rosenbaum, 1982).

Dole and Nyswander postulated that methadone maintenance could relieve what they believed was the metabolic disorder created by chronic addiction to opiates. Reports of their findings demonstrated that addicted persons maintained on methadone quickly stopped using opiates, and methadone was hailed as the "Cinderella drug" that many believed could quickly solve the opiate problem (Newman, 1971, p. xiv). Methadone was credited with the ability to save lives, eliminate criminal behavior, and totally eliminate drug craving. In 1967, methadone programs became publicly funded, and in 1968 the American Medical Association endorsed the use of methadone as a maintenance treatment.

Government funding allowed for a tremendous growth in the number of methadone patients in the 1960s and 1970s. The number of patients enrolled in methadone maintenance treatment programs increased from 25,000 in 1971 (Rosenbaum, 1982) to 135,000 in 1976 (Bourne, 1976). Today, it is estimated that over 179,000 persons receive services in methadone treatment facilities across the United States. In New York alone, methadone treatment is used by 43,000 individuals and is the most widely used therapy for heroin addiction throughout the state (COMPA, 1999).

LAAM Treatment

LAAM is a long-acting synthetic opiate that can block the effects of heroin for up to 72 hours, with few side effects, when taken orally (NIDA, 2000). Briefly tried as a treatment modality in the 1970s, LAAM has resurfaced in response to the growing demand for opiate treatment.

Patients on LAAM are medicated three times per week, due to LAAM's long-acting effect, and therefore have no need for daily medication or for take-home medication, as is true for methadone users. This is an advantage for patients who do not meet the requirements for a reduced methadone pickup schedule and wish to come to the clinic less often in order to meet employment, educational, or family obligations. Moreover, with fewer patients attending the clinic daily, additional treatment slots become available. Although some patients are attracted to the idea of LAAM because of the reduction in clinic visits, the use of LAAM is not for everyone. Some patients are ineligible because of their medical condition, whereas others who are in crisis or emotionally unstable may not benefit from the resulting decreased daily structure and increased free time (Finn & Wilcock, 1997)

Buprenorphine Treatment

Buprenorphine, a semisynthetic opiate derivative, is another medication used in the treatment of opiate addiction. Some of the advantages of buprenorphine include reduced heroin use and cravings, less toxicity than other medications, and mild withdrawal symptoms (Johnson et al., 2000). Physicians are able to prescribe buprenorphine in their private offices or at substance abuse programs after receiving special training. Doctors who prescribe buprenorphine are required to provide patients with referrals to treatment programs, where they can receive counseling and other social services.

THERAPEUTIC USES OF METHADONE

Currently, methadone is used in several different ways. In an inpatient setting, methadone is used to detoxify persons addicted to heroin by first substituting for heroin and then lowering the methadone dose until the patient is drug free. A major criticism of this form of treatment is that detoxification alone, without a motivation to change and without adequate follow-up care, is often ineffective and results in a high relapse and readmission rate.

Methadone is also used for prolonged detoxification over a period of years, during which the addicted person is offered psychosocial rehabilitation, vocational assistance, and crisis management. Such gradual reduction in methadone dosage allows time for the person's body to adjust; it also allows the patient to address important issues that could lead to relapse before completely tapering off the methadone. Such prolonged detoxification can be accomplished in a traditional methadone maintenance treatment program or in a methadone-to-abstinence program. In the methadone-to-abstinence treatment, the patient is accepted by the program with the explicit understanding that he or she will gradually taper off methadone.

The most common use of methadone, however, is as a long-term treatment, referred to as *methadone maintenance*. In this model, patients remain in treatment indefinitely and receive ongoing counseling, medical assistance, and vocational services. Tapering from methadone is voluntary and neither encouraged nor discouraged. The particular value of this long-term modality is that patients, after stabilizing on methadone, have the opportunity to receive counseling and support while working on their social and vocational goals without experiencing opiate craving or withdrawal. The areas of concern for many methadone patients are securing housing, improving family relationships, developing an abstinent social network, resolving crises without relapsing, and engaging in educational or vocational endeavors that will support their abstinence and increase their self-esteem.

In spite of the growth of methadone programs, controversy still exists about the legitimacy of this treatment approach. As noted by Cooper (1989), "some of the antagonism towards this form of treatment results from personal bias and prejudice regarding this patient population, which is perceived by some to be composed largely of antisocial or weak persons unable to give up their self-destructive behavior" (p. 1664).

Supporters and critics of methadone maintenance cite various advantages and disadvantages of this model (CDC, 2002). Some of the cited advantages include:

- At sufficient doses, methadone successfully blocks the craving for heroin; therefore taking additional opiates has no euphoric effect.
- Methadone can be taken orally, eliminating the risk of getting and transmitting diseases through use of needles (e.g., cellulitis, hepatitis, thrombophlebitis, HIV infection, and AIDS).
- Methadone has an extended duration of 24–36 hours, whereas heroin lasts only 6–8 hours. This means that as long as methadone is taken daily, patients will not experience withdrawal.
- Methadone is devoid of serious side effects, although, as with other opiates, constipation and sweating may occur. Impotence, sleep problems, and loss of libido, which have been reported as side effects, can be easily corrected by dose adjustment.
- Methadone is a cost-effective treatment. According to the federal government, the average cost to society over a 6-month period is $21,000 for an untreated addicted person, $20,000 for an imprisoned addicted individual, and only $1,750 for methadone maintenance (Harvard Mental Health Letter, 1995).
- Patients attend methadone clinics according to schedules based on their progress in treatment. Therefore, patients who are most in need of supervision and care are required to attend most often.
- Making clinic visits to pick up methadone brings patients into contact with health care professionals, thereby providing them with prompt access to medical and social services as well as addiction counseling.
- Methadone reduces crime, improves health status, and helps opiate-dependent individuals attain productive lifestyles. The success of the use of methadone maintenance in reducing crime, death, disease, and drug use is well documented (Appel et al., 2001).

Critics of methadone maintenance cite the following disadvantages:

- Methadone is addictive, so its use substitutes one drug addiction for another.
- When used by pregnant women, methadone is transmitted to unborn children, who are born addicted and may have to be detoxified.
- Methadone programs do not really treat addicted persons and help them to change; they only make them more comfortable.

A TYPICAL METHADONE
MAINTENANCE TREATMENT PROGRAM

The operations of methadone maintenance treatment programs (MMTPs) are bound by the federal Drug Enforcement Agency as well as by state regulations. Treatment programs that operate in hospital settings are also accredited under the Joint Commission on Accreditation of Hospitals. These overseeing agencies place many conditions on MMTPs and regulate the maximum allowable dose of methadone, duration of treatment, clinic visit scheduling, and staffing patterns.

Admission to a program is based on interviews with designated staff, including the program physician, as well as a urine test to determine current drug use. To be admitted for treatment, applicants must be at least 18 years old and must demonstrate a minimum of a 1-year history of opiate addiction. Opiate dependence can be demonstrated by "track marks," the scar tissue that forms after the skin is punctured during drug use, and by prior treatment, hospital, or prison records. The urine test demonstrates current opiate use and reveals any other drugs that the applicant may be using.

MMTPs are either freestanding or hospital affiliated. Programs are typically staffed by a physician, an administrative supervisor, nurses, and counselors, as well as other professionals such as social workers, vocational counselors, and HIV specialists. Some programs also employ physician's assistants and nurse practitioners.

All patients receive a complete physical examination upon admission and, in some states, such as New York, every year thereafter. Following state regulations, the methadone dose is determined by the physician, who adjusts it according to the patient's need, withdrawal symptoms and cravings have ceased.

Progress in rehabilitation is measured by absence of substance abuse, length of time in treatment, responsibility in handling the take-home methadone, absence of criminal activity, and productive use of time. Drug abuse is measured by patient's self-report, physical appearance, analysis of randomly collected urine samples, and physical examinations.

Frequency of individual and group counseling sessions is determined on a case-by-case basis. Initially, patients see an addiction counselor at a minimum of twice a month, and then, after they are stable and progressing in treatment, on a monthly basis. Individual counseling provides a forum for patients to address their drug abuse and explore personal concerns and vocational potential at the same time that they are developing their ability to remain drug free and moving into productive and fulfilling lives.

Group counseling sessions provide an important arena in which to explore personal and shared concerns. Recent advances in the understanding and treatment of addiction have led to the development of groups that offer specifically tailored cognitive-behavioral therapy, motivational interviewing, relapse prevention, and other state-of-the-art approaches (NIDA, 2000). Regardless of the theoretical framework, clinic groups provide support, constructive socialization, development of problem-solving skills, and drug education. Additionally, many MMTPs offer parenting classes and vocational and educational groups.

Consistent with the concept of maintenance is the option for patients to taper off from methadone voluntarily. This is most often done on an outpatient basis, although some patients choose to complete the last stages of a methadone taper in an inpatient setting. After patients taper, some programs offer continued counseling support. An advantage to remaining in treatment after tapering off methadone is that patients can be followed closely and quickly restabilized on methadone, should they relapse and begin to abuse opiates again.

Whereas critics of methadone maintenance treatment cite the inability of these programs to curb the alcohol and cocaine abuse of many of the clients, proponents praise it as a valuable form of harm reduction. The harm reduction approach offers a set of practical strategies and meets drug users "where they are at" as a way of reducing the harm associated with their drug use (see Seiger, Chapter 3, this volume). Methadone maintenance is a particularly important harm reduction strategy, given that patients enrolled in this treatment engage in fewer high-risk behaviors, such as needle sharing and criminal acts (Ball & Ross, 1991). While the ultimate goal of treatment—that patients completely stop their abuse of all substances—is maintained, harm reduction recognizes that a patient may relapse many times and may engage in other drug use along the way. Every step patients take toward their recovery, such as using fewer drugs or lesser amounts of any given drug, reduces the harm to themselves and others.

TREATMENT NEEDS OF METHADONE PATIENTS

Despite the fact that methadone patients come from all walks of life and all ethnic groups, their common history of chronic opiate use, often beginning during their adolescence, creates serious emotional, health, social, and vocational problems—which, in turn, creates common treatment needs.

Many opiate-addicted individuals entering MMTPs display serious social dysfunction. A majority of patients comes from emotionally and financially impoverished backgrounds. As a result of both their backgrounds and their "drug lifestyle," many opiate-addicted individuals have been unable to develop social and vocational skills. At the same time, many face racial prejudice as well as society's negative stereotyping of all addicted persons.

Individuals with opiate addiction frequently have not completed high school and lack the skills necessary for employment. Those who have been able to secure employment during their addictions often have unstable work histories, having lost jobs because their work adjustments were poor or because their addictions became known to their employers. Most patients in methadone maintenance treatment need vocational assistance to develop the skills they need to become employable; they also need to learn how to find and keep jobs (Harvard Mental Health Newsletter, 1995).

Addicted persons often have criminal histories due to conviction for possession of drugs or as a result of having committed crimes to support their drug habits. Once they become involved in criminal lifestyles and have police records, legitimate employment options become limited. Most patients with both addiction and criminal histories have learned to be tough and street savvy. Survival on their terms takes precedence over playing by the rules and functioning successfully in the "straight world." Although enrollment in methadone maintenance treatment reduces criminal activity (Ball & Ross, 1991), many patients need help to establish social support systems that reinforce drug abstinence, vocational achievement, and healthy ways of relating.

Moreover, in the process of becoming addicted and maintaining their addictions, which leads to increasingly self-destructive behavior, many individuals lose the support of their family members and become entrenched in dysfunctional relationships with other addicted people (Kaufman, 1994). The loss of family and other meaningful social ties increases their sense of shame and alienation. Many opiate-using women become involved in relationships fraught with battering and abuse; some have lost custody of their children due to their drug involvement. These experiences further increase their sense of worthlessness and disenfranchisement (Straussner & Zelvin, 1997).

Studies of the family dynamics of addicted persons have described inconsistent, overindulgent, or rejecting mothers and passive and absent fathers (Kaufman, 1994). Research into the family-of-origin histories of methadone patients indicates that many experienced abuse or neglect as children, and one-third came from substance-abusing homes (New York State Division of Substance Abuse Services, 1987). Several studies estimate that between 40 and 75% of adolescent and adult women who abuse alcohol and other substances have been neglected or sexually abused (Karageorge & Wisdom, 2001; Smyth & Miller, 1997). An understudied area is the prevalence of sexual abuse in the histories of opiate-addicted men.

It is not surprising that many people who are addicted to opiates feel hopeless about themselves and about the possibility of changing their life. Childhood memories of loss and pain and adult experiences of isolation and humiliation underlie the pervasive low self-esteem that plagues the opiate-addicted individual. The veneer of arrogance these individuals often present is used defensively to hide their underlying feelings of worthlessness. Treatment planning in MMTPs must take into account the low self-esteem of patients. Cultural issues also need to be recognized (Straussner, 2001). Treatment needs to provide consistency, support, and reassurance, as well as specific strategies for changing attitudes and lifestyles.

Patients are resocialized through the process of adjusting to program policies and procedures that reward responsibility, drug abstinence, and progress toward economic self-sufficiency. The rewards for demonstrated abstinence, including reduction in clinic visits and the granting of methadone to take vacations, can be useful in helping to motivate patients to change. MMTPs frequently provide the first successful interaction an opiate-addicted person has with a social service agency.

The following vignette portrays a typical patient:

George was 29 years old at the time he applied for methadone maintenance treatment. He was fearful that without the stability of methadone, his opiate use would destroy his family life, his job, and his health. Two drug-addicted siblings had died from complications due to AIDS.

George was born in Puerto Rico and came to New York City at age 6. His father left home when George was 3 years old, and he was raised by his mother and stepfather. George was the youngest of five siblings. He does not remember his father but states that his stepfather was an alcoholic who physically abused him and his mother. George began using marijuana and alcohol at age 13 and heroin at age 14. He dropped out of school at this time and began hanging out on the streets. George realized that he was addicted at age 15 when he first experienced withdrawal. He had tried to detoxify three times, twice in a hospital and once on his own. Upon admission to methadone maintenance treatment, George was supporting his addiction by work as a street vendor and by robbery.

George was living with a woman who did not abuse drugs, with whom he had two children. His legal history included five convictions, two for robbery and three for loitering and drug possession. At the time of program admission, George was on probation.

During the first year of methadone maintenance treatment, George abused cocaine and alcohol. However, he continued to work, and his family life improved. His counselor saw him at least once a week for support. Although referred to the cocaine abuse group and Alcoholics Anonymous (AA), George refused to attend. When offered testing for the HIV virus, he agreed and tested negative. Initially he was guarded and shared little information with program staff. After his counselor repeatedly initiated discussions about the presence of cocaine in his urine, George finally admitted to his alcohol and cocaine problem. With the help of his counselor, George then detoxified from alcohol and began to attend 12-step MA groups at the methadone program. After 3 years in treatment, George requested educational services in order to earn his high school diploma.

George has been in treatment for 5 years and remains on methadone maintenance. He works full time now and no longer abuses any drugs or alcohol. He has completed probation and has not been arrested since enrolling in the MMTP. Individual weekly counseling, once used primarily to support his drug abstinence, now focuses on helping him raise his children, improve his relationship with his family, and upgrade his employment. He continues to attend clinic groups to support his abstinence from cocaine and alcohol. George believes that his enrollment in methadone maintenance has provided him with the support he needs to keep his family together.

Health Issues

Many methadone patients report minor and major illnesses upon admission and after beginning treatment. Many illnesses are related to prior drug use, whereas others are due to poor self-care. Regular health screenings and frequent contact with medical staff help detect illnesses and support the engagement of patients in appropriate medical treatment.

Today many methadone patients are infected with the HIV virus and tuberculosis; dual infection with HIV and tuberculosis results in an acceleration of both diseases (Snyder et al., 1999). Many methadone maintenance patients also suffer from the hepatitis C virus, which is often transmitted via injection (Novick, 2000). Because of the fear of AIDS and hepatitis C, many drug users have changed their route of drug taking from injection to snorting or sniffing opiates.

Most MMTPs today provide HIV testing and counseling, as well as counseling on safer sex. MMTPs often work collaboratively with agencies that provide support services for patients who become too ill to attend a program. The following case illustrates the care given to one such patient.

Susan is a 37-year-old Jewish woman who has been enrolled in methadone maintenance treatment for 6 years. She is married to a man who is also in methadone treatment, and they live together in a cheap hotel. Susan's brother had adopted her 11-year-old son during the time that Susan was abusing drugs. After a year in methadone treatment, Susan took the HIV test; she was positive for the virus. Three years later, Susan's condition worsened and she was diagnosed with AIDS while hospitalized. Until this diagnosis, Susan had refused to take antiretroviral medication to slow the progression of her illness. She also continued to abuse cocaine and avoided counseling. When Susan became ill, her counselor visited her at the hospital and suggested that she join the women's group and a group for HIV-positive patients at the clinic once she felt better. Susan agreed and became an important and well-liked member of the groups.

With the encouragement of her counselor and members of the group, Susan agreed to take medication. She continues to suffer from AIDS. Her counselor supported Susan in reaching out to her estranged family, and gradually she has been able to resolve her relationship with her brother and son. Susan now faces the challenge of living with a chronic, life-threatening illness, but now she knows that she has the resources—help and support from program staff and her peers.

TREATMENT NEEDS OF POLYSUBSTANCE-DEPENDENT PATIENTS

Patients who are polysubstance-dependent individuals are addicted to more than one drug. Frequently, polysubstance abuse precedes entry into methadone maintenance treatment. It is not unusual for patients applying for treatment to report that in addition to their addiction to heroin, they are also abusing marijuana, cocaine, and/or alcohol (Kaplan, Sadock, & Greeb, 1994). Opiate addicts are vulnerable to inhalant and amphetamine abuse, which also has increased in the past 5 years (Center for Substance Abuse Treatment, 2002). Another route to polysubstance abuse and addiction is through mixing drugs together to increase the high or to mitigate withdrawal symptoms. For example, patients report the use of Valium, alcohol, and heroin to decrease the withdrawal symptoms following crack cocaine use, or the use of Elavil to feel less depressed.

Since the beginning of the crack cocaine epidemic, there has been a dramatic rise in the number methadone maintenance clients addicted to cocaine. Alcohol abuse is another serious problem for some methadone patients. Alcohol impacts on the effectiveness of methadone and makes it difficult to ensure that the patient is receiving the correct dose. Because methadone can block only opiates and cannot impede the effects of alcohol, cocaine, or other substances, abuse or dependence on these substances must be treated separately. Such treatment may include detoxification followed by rehabilitation and ongoing work on recovery toward abstinence.

Many methadone patients vigorously deny polysubstance abuse because they feel ashamed of their multiple addictions, are unwilling to stop using other drugs, and/or fear the loss of program privileges. Clients' abuse of, or dependency on, other substances is usually revealed through history taking, client appearance, self-report, urine screenings, or physical examinations. Individual and group counseling are used as first steps to help these patients overcome their denial and fear so that they can effectively utilize available services.

Patients with polysubstance abuse problems need medical evaluations to determine if inpatient drug detoxification is required. If patients require hospitalization, arrangements can be made by the MMTP to facilitate admission. If patients do not require, or are unwilling to accept, inpatient treatment, they are encouraged, or may even be mandated, to attend daily activity or educational groups at the methadone program or in the community. Referrals to mental health services are made, as needed.

Because opiate dependency is recognized as a chronic condition, relapse does not mean failure (Newman, 1989). It is equally important to recognize that secondary drug use may continue as a vestige of the addictive lifestyle, which is difficult to relinquish. The case of Bill provides an example of how MMTPs work with patients who use other drugs.

Bill is a 53-year-old Italian American man who has been in methadone maintenance treatment for 15 years. For 12 years he worked as a doorman. When his mother died 3 years ago, Bill began to drink heavily and lost his job a year later. He lives with Gloria, a 38-year-old woman who is also enrolled in a methadone program. They dated for 10 years and have lived together for 8 years. Bill had been very dependent on his mother throughout his life. He was an only child whose father was killed in an accident when Bill was 6 months old. His mother never remarried, and Bill lived with her until she died. When his mother died, Bill was grief-stricken and overcome with loneliness. He began to drink for solace, and his drinking quickly got out of control.

Efforts to assist him with his drinking problems and grief were unsuccessful until Bill lost his job and Gloria threatened to leave him. Once Bill was willing to accept assistance, his counselor referred him for inpatient alcohol detoxification, followed by daily attendance at AA meetings. During his detoxification from alcohol, Bill's methadone dosage remained stable, and Gloria began to attend Al-Anon meetings in order to understand his addiction and receive support for herself.

FEMALE METHADONE PATIENTS

Research on the characteristics and treatment needs of women with opiate addiction has been hampered by the fact that, until recently, most studies used male cohorts. Studies indicate that the addicted woman is, in some ways, different from her male counterpart (Kaufman, 1994; Straussner & Zelvin, 1997). Women who have opiate addiction have lower self-esteem than men who have opiate addiction (National Institute of Drug Abuse, 1979). Recent studies of women on methadone indicate that they are at high risk for partner violence, HIV, and hepatitis (Gilbert et al., 2000).

Women entering methadone treatment often have few emotional or social sources of support. They are more likely to live alone, to be single parents, or to live with a partner who is abusing drugs (New York State Division of Substance Abuse Services, 1987). This means that opiate-addicted women in treatment often require more support and social services from their programs than do their male counterparts.

Among the special service needs of these women are support groups, gynecological and prenatal care and education, as well as assistance in locating day-care facilities for children. To help female patients, methadone programs also must work to eliminate the sex-role stereotyping in counseling that is detrimental to their rehabilitation process (Hser, Anglin, & Booth, 1987). The following case illustrates the kind of help given to a female patient.

Matilda is a 51-year-old African American woman with a 34-year history of heroin and cocaine addiction. Matilda entered her current MMTP after she relapsed following 4 years of abstinence. Over the course of treatment, Matilda disclosed the abusive nature of her relationship with her common-law husband of 17 years, with whom she has a 10-year-old son. With encouragement from her addiction counselor, she engaged in individual and family therapy with her son in a nearby mental health clinic. Matilda was able to leave the abusive relationship after 2 years of treatment.

Following this separation, Matilda was motivated to complete her Work Experience Program (WEP) assignment as part of the Welfare to Work initiative. Although Matilda had almost completed high school and attended a fashion institute in her younger years, drugs had become a way of life that left no room for vocational development and achievement. As part of her recovery, her vocational counselor helped her to obtain her GED and begin night school to learn computer science.

Matilda was able to give up cocaine once she had stabilized on methadone, started acupuncture treatment, and began attending cocaine groups at the MMTP. After 5 years of methadone treatment, Matilda is now on a 3-day pickup schedule; she works full time at a bank and also takes care of her son. Some of the contributing factors to Matilda's success were the methadone, which stopped her opiate craving, her strong desire to survive and progress, her concern about her son, and the unconditional support of her addiction counselor and her psychotherapist.

CHILDREN OF METHADONE PATIENTS

The majority of opiate-addicted women in treatment is of childbearing age, and most have children. Since many women enrolled in methadone maintenance treatment have suffered from inadequate parenting, there is concern about how these women parent their own children. A wide range of issues can affect parenting for substance-abusing women, which affects them as well as their children, including victimization, child maltreatment, parental substance abuse, mental health problems, low self-esteem and stigmatization, family systems issues, substance abuse during pregnancy, and social and economic resource deficits (Smyth & Miller, 1997).

The physical, social, and mental health needs of the children of methadone-maintained parents are of great concern to methadone program staff. During pregnancy, program physicians and social workers monitor the health of the expectant mothers. Pregnant patients are given information about drug interactions, encouraged to use prenatal services regularly, and taught what to expect during and after delivery. Women of childbearing age are encouraged to have their HIV status checked, since HIV infection can be passed on to the fetus. Medication (AZT) is available to reduce the risk of transmission of the HIV virus (Friedman, 1997).

Studies of women in MMTPs indicate that these women have better pregnancy outcomes when compared with heroin-addicted women or addicted persons who take methadone on the streets (Chavkin, 1990). Pregnant women are not encouraged to taper from methadone during their pregnancy, out of concern for the unborn fetus and the potential that the mother may return to opiate and other drug use. They are counseled about the likelihood that their infants will be born addicted to methadone and will need to be detoxified at birth. They are also given relevant information about child protective service laws. Although these laws mandate the reporting of children born addicted, they clearly indicate that no case is to be reported if the mother is taking a legally prescribed medication, such as methadone (Straussner, 1989).

When a parent is unable to provide for the well-being of his or her child and is unwilling to accept assistance, the case must be reported to the state child protective service bureau. After a methadone program reports the case, help is offered to patients to assist them in making the necessary changes to keep or (re)establish custody of their children.

CURRENT ISSUES AFFECTING
OPIATE ADDICTION TREATMENT

Opiate addiction treatment programs have expanded their services to meet emerging client needs. Current services offered to opiate-addicted persons include assessment and treatment of health issues and vocational services to move patients toward economic self-sufficiency.

HIV/AIDS, Hepatitis, and Related Conditions

At a time of limited resources, the health and social service needs of patients remain staggering. As indicate previously, MMTPs serve many patients who are HIV+ and/or infected with hepatitis C. Offering HIV counseling and testing services on site and providing education to patients about hepatitis as well as HIV/AIDS are necessary parts of methadone maintenance treatment today. These needs have necessitated additional staff training, increased staffing, and, at times, a refocusing of the treatment to address the patient's medical condition.

Welfare Reform

Welfare reform has made an indelible mark on the recovery process for opiate-addicted people in treatment, bringing into sharper focus the need for programs to provide comprehensive vocational services. From the onset of the Personal and Work Opportunity Reconciliation Act, signed into law by President Clinton on August 8, 1996, individuals in drug and alcohol treatment who applied for public assistance must be evaluated for their ability to work (Legal Action Center, 1998). Because federal assistance to families has a 5-year lifetime limit, patients must develop work skills to be able to support themselves and their families within that timeframe.

Since many methadone patients are supported by public assistance, programs have been challenged to assist patients to move quickly toward self-sufficiency by developing their work skills. This new demand has required that programs revisit their mission and redirect their focus. Welfare reform has reinforced the role of MMTPs in educating, guiding, and supporting patients to engage in treatment, develop vocational/educational skills, and become socialized for entry into the workplace. Currently methadone programs offer vocational assistance from the first day of treatment and closely monitor not only patients' progress in treatment but also their ability to work. Without the support of their methadone program, many patients would be unable to meet the demands of welfare reform.

THE ROLE OF SOCIAL WORKERS IN OPIATE-TREATMENT PROGRAMS

The role of social workers in opiate addiction recovery programs varies. Because regulations governing many drug programs do not specify a particular role for social workers, they may be found working in direct practice, as supervisors, or as administrators. Recently, as part of the growing movement of professionalization in the field of substance abuse treatment, more and more social workers are moving into leadership roles in programs that treat opiate-addicted individuals.

Social Workers as Clinicians

Social workers are uniquely equipped to treat opiate-addicted individuals. Trained in biopsychosocial and cultural perspectives, they are knowledgeable about the impact of emotional, cultural, and socioeconomic factors on addicted persons. Social workers are equipped to address the special needs of addicted clients by seeing clients in their psychosocial and socioeconomic contexts, not only in behavioral terms. Furthermore, if a client is in need of psychiatric care, social workers are equipped to assess and refer them (FORUM, 2002). The professional value of providing nonjudgmental service is essential in the treatment of a population that has internalized society's view of addicted persons as weak, antisocial, and self-destructive. Commitment to client self-determination allows social workers to understand, remain objective, and display empathic skills in their work with patients who may remain deviant and self-destructive. Social workers are trained to recognize and treat relapse, child neglect, and HIV illness as human problems to be understood and resolved through care and support rather than taken as signs of moral failure.

Social workers also are trained to assess and intervene with a range of techniques that is useful in working with addicted persons. Individual casework helps patients establish a trusted relationship with a worker who can help them address their problems. Such a relationship enables patients to accept support and develop self-awareness. The worker serves as a positive role model for patients, many of whom have no other positive models in their lives.

Training in group work enables social workers to establish and lead groups that provide patients with the opportunity to overcome social isolation, receive peer support, develop alternatives to drug and alcohol abuse, and develop healthier ways of relating to others. In addition, crisis intervention skills enable social workers to assess situations quickly and to intervene professionally on behalf of patients. Social workers know when and how to enlist community support and how to locate and network with community resources.

Social Workers as Clinical Supervisors

In the role of clinical supervisor, social workers help develop the skills and knowledge base of the counseling staff by providing guidance and direction on the biopsychosocial and strength-oriented approach to patients. Outcome studies have shown that patients improve most when exposed to a positive staff attitude and flexible treatment conditions (Cooper, 1989).

Supervision of counseling staff in addiction treatment programs is a complex task. Many drug treatment programs employ persons in recovery from addiction as well as professional counselors. Counselors who have abused opiates require supervision to address their issues of overidentification and countertransference as well as to develop basic counseling skills. Professionals require supervision to (1) overcome their biases toward persons suffering from addiction, (2) remedy their lack of understanding regarding the addicted person's lifestyle, and (3) increase their understanding of the medical aspects of addiction. Since patients present many different problems and require individualized treatment planning, all counselors need training and supervision to develop their assessment and intervention skills, their knowledge of HIV infection and hepatitis as well as cocaine and alcohol abuse, and their ability to help patients develop self-sufficiency and address such issues as relapse prevention, parenting, and child neglect.

The following are two vignettes describing how social workers may function as clinical supervisors.

Jeffrey was a 43-year-old African American counselor with a history of opiate addiction. He came to supervision feeling overwhelmed and angry about the amount of work he had to do. At first, he was angry with his social work supervisor and the system. During many discussions with the social work supervisor, Jeffrey came to understand that he was most upset with his patients for not getting better, as he had, and for making him feel devalued. He also recognized that his patients' resistance induced feelings of worthlessness in him and aroused fear that his performance as a counselor would be judged by whether or not his patients recovered quickly. The supervisor helped Jeffrey to recognize the differences between his patients and himself, to reframe his work to develop more realistic expectations of himself, and to become less angry and more empathic.

Doris was a white middle-class social worker assigned to help patients who were HIV infected or AIDS diagnosed. She felt frustrated that patients were rejecting her help and discouraged that they refused to speak with her about their feelings and fears. With the help of her social work supervisor, Doris began to understand that her unspoken demand that patients speak about their illness every time they met was the reason some patients avoided her. Additionally, the supervisor assisted Doris to recognize her middle-class values and how they affected her expectations of her clients. She redefined her work to allow her patients greater autonomy and began to establish relationships in which patients felt free to talk about their various interests and concerns. As Doris learned to be more flexible in her approach to her work, much of her patients' mistrust dissipated, and they began to reach out for her help.

Social Workers as Administrators

As administrators, social workers can help create programs that meet federal and state regulations, maximize staff utilization, and improve client care. By assessing the strengths and problems in the agency, social workers are able to create a cooperative, respectful, and creative environment for staff and patients. As administrators, social workers are able to (1) develop new programs for patients, (2) network successfully with other service providers, and (3) facilitate methadone patients' access to care in the community by sensitively and skillfully explaining patients' dynamics and needs to other professionals and funding sources. The following is an example of how a social work administrator may function in his or her role.

> Since becoming the administrator of an MMTP 2 years ago, Betty had established a social work student unit in her program. In addition to training students, this unit provided work satisfaction and professional growth for her social work staff and helped to increase the number of professionals who were knowledgeable about drug abuse treatment. She worked to develop in-service group training for line staff and created a group program at the agency. In response to the staff complaints of feeling overwhelmed, Betty worked to eliminate unnecessary paperwork and to streamline existing systems. She was able to arrange for the clinic to close for 2 hours each week to give staff the opportunity to catch up on paperwork and thereby raise morale.
>
> Because of her training in social work, Betty worked closely with other service providers and was able to explain the treatment needs and dynamics of methadone patients to them and assuage their fears and their resistance to treating these patients. This process increased the opportunities for patients to receive mental health and other treatment in the community. Betty also obtained grants to meet the vocational and social service needs of program patients.

CONCLUSION

Opiate addiction is a complex, biopsychosocial illness. Because the use of opiates involves mental and physical health issues and social consequences, different programs are available to meet the unique needs of those who suffer from opiate addiction. Outpatient programs, therapeutic communities, MICA programs, and MMTPs have each demonstrated their efficacy in the treatment of opiate-addicted persons. Social workers can and do play a vital role in understanding the dynamics of, and in the provision of treatment to, individuals addicted to opiates.

REFERENCES

Appel, P. W., Joseph, H., Kott, A., Nottingham, W., Tasiny, E., & Habel, E. (2001). Selected in-treatment outcomes of long-term methadone maintenance treatment patients in New York State. *Mt. Sinai Journal of Medicine, 68*(1), 55–61.

Ball, J. C., & Ross, A. (1991). *The effectiveness of methadone maintenance treatment: Patients, programs, services, and outcome.* New York: Springer-Verlag.

Bourne, P. (1976). Methadone maintenance. In *Overview of substance abuse* (pp. 161–172). New York: Narcotics and Drug Research Inc.

Brecher, E. M. and the Editors of *Consumer Reports.* (1972). *Licit and illicit drugs.* Boston: Little, Brown.

Center for Substance Abuse Treatment. (2002, July). *Using buprenorphine for office-based treatment of opiate addiction.* Rockville, MD: CSAT SAMHSA.

Centers for Disease Control and Prevention (CDC). (2002). Methadone maintenance treatment. In *IDU/HIV Prevention.* Atlanta: Author.

Chavkin, W. (1990). Drug addiction and pregnancy: Policy crossroads. *Public Health and the Law, 80*(4), 77–94.

Committee of Methadone Program Administrators (COMPA). (1999). *Regarding methadone and other chemotherapies.* New York: Author.

Cooper, J. (1989). Methadone treatment and the acquired immunodeficiency syndrome. *Journal of the American Medical Association, 262*(12), 1664–1668.

DeLeon, G. (1994). Therapeutic communities. In M. Galanter & H. D. Kleber (Eds.), *Textbook of substance abuse treatment* (pp. 447–464). Washington, DC: American Psychiatric Association Press.

Finn, P., & Wilcok, K. (1997). Levo-alpha-acetyl-methadol (LAAM): Its advantages and drawbacks. *Journal of Substance Abuse Treatment, 14*(6), 559–564.

FORUM. (2002, Fall). *Social workers in MMTs.* Chicago: Author.

Friedman, E. (1997). The impact of AIDS on the lives of women. In S. L. A. Straussner & E. Zelvin (Eds.), *Gender and addictions: Men and women in treatment* (pp. 197–222). Northvale, NJ: Aronson.

Gilbert, L., El-Bassel, N., Rajah, V., Foleo, J., Frye, V., & Richman, B. (2000). HIV, HCV, and partner violence: A conundrum for methadone maintenance programs. *Mt. Sinai Journal of Medicine, 67*(5–6), 452–464.

Harvard Mental Health Newsletter. (1995). *Treatment of addiction* (Part 3), *12*(4), 1.

Hser, Y., Anglin, M., & Booth, M. (1987). Differences in addict careers. *American Journal of Drug and Alcohol Abuse, 13*(4), 253–280.

Johnson, R. E., Chutuape M. A., Strain E. C., Walsh S. L., Stitzer M. L., & Bigelow, G. E. (2000). A comparison of leveomethadyl acetate, buprenorphine, and methadone for opioid dependence. *New England Journal of Medicine, 343*(18), 1290–1297.

Kaplan, H. I., Sadock, B. J., & Greeb, J. A. (1994). *Synopsis of psychiatry* (7th ed.). Baltimore: Williams & Wilkins.

Karageorge, K., & Wisdom, G. (2001). *Physically and sexually abused women in substance abuse treatment: Treatment services and outcomes*. Rockvillle, MD: National Evaluation Data Services, Center for Substance Abuse Treatment.

Kaufman, E. (1994). *Psychotherapy of addicted persons*. New York: Guilford Press.

Legal Action Center. (1998, October). *Welfare as we know it now*. New York: Author.

McGonagle, D. (1994). Methadone Anonymous: A 12 step program. *Journal of Psychosocial Nursing, 32*(10), 5–12.

National Institute of Drug Abuse. (1979). *Addicted women, family dynamics, self-perceptions and support systems* (USDHEW Pub. No. 80-762). Washington, DC: U.S. Government Printing Office.

National Institute on Drug Abuse (NIDA). (2000, July). *Principles of drug addiction treatment* (NIH Publication No. 0004180). Rockville, MD: Author

Newman, R. (1971). *Methadone maintenance in the treatment of narcotics addiction*. New York: Academic Press.

Newman, R. (1989, October 31). Unpublished letter to the editor. *Medical Journal of Australia*.

New York State Division of Substance Abuse Services. (1987). *Parents in methadone treatment and their children*. Albany, NY: Author.

Novick, D. M. (2000). The impact of hepatitis C virus infection on methadone maintenance treatment. *Mt. Sinai Journal of Medicine, 76*(5–6), 437–443.

Rosenbaum, M. (1982). Getting on methadone: The experience of the woman addict. *Contemporary Drug Problems, 11*(1), 113–114.

Smyth, N. J., & Miller, B. A. (1997). Parenting issues for substance-abusing women. In S. L. A Straussner & E. Zelvin (Eds.), *Gender and addictions: Men and women in treatment* (pp. 123–150). Northvale, NJ: Aronson.

Snyder, D., Paz, E. A., Mohle-Boetani, J., Fallstaf, R., Black, R., & D. Chin. (1999). Tuberculosis prevention in methadone maintenance clinics. *American Journal of Respiratory and Critical Care Medicine, 160*, 179–185.

Straussner, S. L. A. (1989). Intervention with maltreating parents who are drug and alcohol abusers. In S. Ehrenkranz, E. Goldstein, L. Goodman, & J. Seinfeld (Eds.). *Clinical social work with maltreated children and their families* (pp. 149–177). New York: New York University Press.

Straussner, S. L. A. (Ed.). (2001). *Ethnocultural factors in substance abuse treatment*. New York: Guilford Press.

Straussner, S. L. A., & Zelvin, E. (Eds.). (1997). *Gender and addictions: Men and women in treatment*. Northvale, NJ: Aronson.

Tims, F. M., DeLeon, G., & Jainchill, N. (Eds.). (1994). *Therapeutic communities: Advances in research and application* (NIDA Research Monograph No. 144). Washington, DC: U.S. Government Printing Office.

Winn, M., Chester, A., May, M. Jr. & Sutton, M. R. (Eds.). (1967). *Drug abuse: Escape to nowhere*. Philadelphia: Smith, Kline, & French.

Witkin, G., & Griffin, J. (1994). The new opium wars. *U. S. News and World Report, 117*, 39–44.

CHAPTER 10

Treatment of Stimulant Dependence

David M. Ockert
Armin R. Baier
Edgar E. Coons

The abuse of stimulants presents a problem of enormous scope and proportion from social, psychological, and medical perspectives. Psychomotor stimulants include cocaine (in the form of powder, *freebase*, or *crack*) and the amphetamines (including amphetamine/*speed*, methamphetamine/*ice*, and crystal methedrine/*crank*). The devastating effects of these substances affect every age group, including the unborn. In many cases the consequences of stimulant abuse are psychosis, brain damage, and death.

Why, then, do stimulant abusers run such risks? One answer is that stimulants produce an intense pleasure during early phases of dependence that strongly reinforces any behaviors necessary to allow continued use. This immediate, reinforcing euphoria is more powerful in controlling behavior than is the realization that, in the long run, chemical dependency can impair—and may even destroy—life.

Complex political, economic, and psychosocial factors determine what substances are used and abused in society today. An analysis of the influence of the political and economic climate on the drug problem is beyond the scope of this chapter. Nevertheless, this climate exists and must be understood by treatment professionals, as well as policymakers, in order to design effective strategies for prevention as well as for early intervention and treatment.

The purpose of this chapter is to present the history and current status of stimulant dependence in the United States; to emphasize the need for an understanding of an integrated multimodal approach that addresses stimulant-related biological, psychological, and social factors that have an impact on the individual in both assessment and treatment; and to present a case study of such an approach to assessment and treatment.

HISTORY AND EPIDEMIOLOGY

For centuries the people of South America have chewed the leaves of the coca plant to obtain a mild stimulant effect, apparently without any resulting dependence. Cocaine, the chief active ingredient in the leaves of the coca plant, was first isolated in alkaloid form in 1844 (Brecher & the Editors of *Consumer Reports*, 1972). During the latter half of the 19th century, those European and American physicians and pharmacists aware of its stimulant effect began to use cocaine medicinally in various elixirs and tonics (such as the original form of Coca-Cola) and for the treatment of catarrhs (in snuff-like powdered form). Sigmund Freud and other physicians used cocaine, injected under the skin, to treat depression and chronic fatigue. However, they soon discovered that daily use could cause full-fledged symptoms of mental disturbance similar to those seen in delirium tremens (Brecher et al., 1972; Jones, 1953).

Recreational use of cocaine in the United States, which began around 1890, was legally restricted in 1914 with the passage of the Harrison Act (Courtwright, 1991). As cocaine use declined, amphetamines, a large group of synthetic stimulants that includes methamphetamine and crystal Methedrine, was marketed in the United States. Although restricted, amphetamines were easily found on the black market, and their use steadily increased following World War II. Despite further attempts to restrict illegal sale, the use of a nonsanctioned amphetamine (speed) increased explosively during the 1960s. By the 1970s successful police action against illegal manufacture and sale of amphetamines had led to a resurgence of cocaine importation and use (Brecher et al., 1972).

During the 1970s cocaine, used intranasally, began replacing amphetamine use. At this time, cocaine was judged to be a relatively safe, nonaddicting, euphoriant agent (Greenspoon & Bakalar, 1980). This perception was reinforced by reports from two national commissions on drug abuse, which concluded that amphetamines cause substantial morbidity but that cocaine does not (Gawin & Ellinwood, 1988; National Commission on Marijuana and Drug Abuse, 1973; Strategy Council on Drug Abuse, 1973). This erroneous conclusion, and the popular notion that cocaine is safe, derived in large part from the fact that cocaine dependence results in mostly psychological, rather than physical, withdrawal symptoms (Gawin & Ellinwood, 1988).

By the late 1970s cocaine also was being used in a smokable form (freebase or base) which proved to have the greatest dependence liability of all drugs. The introduction of *crack* (a smokable form of cocaine similar to freebase but diluted with an inert filler and sold in small, inexpensive quantities) resulted in a rapidly escalating number of cocaine users during the 1980s. (In the Western United States, crack was originally called *rock*.) Amphetamine use again increased in the 1980s with the emergence of *ice*, a smokable form of methamphetamine. Originally abused primarily in Hawaii and the Western Southwestern states, by the mid-1990s, methamphetamine abuse had begun spreading to the Midwestern and Southern regions (National Institute on Drug Abuse [NIDA], 2000).

The 1998 National Household Survey on Drug Abuse (NIDA, 1999a) reported that the number of cocaine users reached its peak at 3% of the U.S. population in 1985, reduced to 0.7% of the population in 1992, and has remained relatively the same since then. However, it also reported that the number of *frequent* cocaine users (0.3% of the population in 1997) showed a significant increase over that figure for 1991, comparable to the increase in new users of cocaine in the early 1980s. The survey also found higher rates of use among certain segments of the population—young adults ages 18–25, black and Hispanic individuals, those in large metropolitan areas, those living in the Southern and Western United States, and unemployed persons. Since household surveys of illegal drug use contain inherent methodological problems that call into question their reliability and validity, these data must be viewed guardedly in order to avoid underestimating the full extent of the abuse of stimulants.

EFFECTS OF STIMULANTS

A neurobehavioral theory of stimulant dependence rests on an understanding of the neurochemical impact these drugs have on the brain and the resulting effect on behavior. This section discusses stimulant dependence in terms of neurobehavioral theory as a bridge to understanding the neurobehavioral model of assessment and treatment of stimulant dependence (Rawson, Obert, McCann, Smith, & Scheffey, 1989).

Neurochemical Impact of Stimulants

Although the behavioral and physiological effects of cocaine and the amphetamines are similar, they are structurally dissimilar and show significant differences in their operation at the level of the nerve cell (NIDA, 2000). One significant difference is the duration of action: Cocaine has a half-life (i.e., the time required for half the amount of a substance introduced into the body to be broken down or eliminated by natural process), and thus a duration of euphoria, of less than 45 minutes, whereas amphetamines have a half-life up to eight times longer (Galanter & Kleber, 1994). Consequently, intranasal cocaine use is characterized by readministration of the drug at intervals of 10–20 minutes, causing rapid and frequent mood changes.

Compared with methamphetamine users, cocaine users are more likely to use in binges, spend more on drugs, and drink more alcohol. Methamphetamine users, on the other hand, are more likely to be female, use daily, use marijuana, and exhibit more severe medical and psychiatric problems (Rawson et al., 2000). However, when amount and duration of cocaine use are comparable to high-dose amphetamine use, the psychological and behavioral effects of each are indistinguishable (Galanter & Kleber, 1994).

At the heart of the neurobehavioral model is the recognition that the highly complex set of behaviors required by humans to function effectively are assembled and maintained by reinforcement contingencies. Certain brain mechanisms that mediate pleasure and its reinforcing quality are required to support this process. These are the mechanisms that are affected by substances of abuse in ways that lead to problems of drug dependency.

What are these ways? One of the reinforcement mechanisms in the brain manufactures and utilizes the biochemical *dopamine*. This dopamine mechanism is normally activated by behaviors that bring the individual in contact with needed goals and, as such, serves to signal pleasure that those behaviors are appropriate to survival and should be continued in the present and/or made note of for future use, should the needs arise again. However, when this dopamine reinforcement mechanism is artificially activated by stimulants, its pleasures may reinforce ongoing behaviors that are not necessarily relevant to survival and may even interfere with goal-appropriate behaviors or be actively maladaptive—such as social withdrawal or even patently antisocial acts.

The dopamine system also seems to be involved in mediating the *cross-priming dependencies* frequently observed between stimulants. For example, research has identified a dopamine avenue by which nicotine use predisposes the individual to a susceptibility to cocaine recidivism (Wise, 1988). Similar cross-priming interactions between cocaine and alcohol have been suggested (for a general review, see Carlson, 2001). This mechanism explains the fact that a client with a history of dependence on one substance can also have a history of dependence on many other substances. Polysubstance abuse raises the question of whether the proclivity for becoming chemically dependent to *any* substances of abuse is an inherited psychological or neurophysiological characteristic, or whether it is the early addiction to one substance that biases the system toward susceptibility to other substances. Whatever the answer, it seems that many of the reinforcements involved in stimulant substance dependence share a dopamine mediator mechanism in the brain that can be activated by a broad class of substances of abuse.

The manner in which the dopamine mechanism is activated differs for different classes of substances and is reflected in the pattern of response to repeated use of these substances. Repeated opiate substance abuse, for example, leads to the development of tolerance, in which higher and higher doses are required to induce pleasure and to prevent highly unpleasant withdrawal effects from cessation of use. By contrast, repeated cocaine use leads to an increased sensitization of the dopamine mechanism, so that the rewards and euphorias induced by its activation are heightened (of course, thereby, increasing the desire and cravings to use the drug). However, cocaine use also sensitizes a compensatory mechanism that damps down the dopamine mechanism when cocaine is not in use, so that the user experiences unpleasant feelings, including dysphoria and a decreased ability to experience pleasure, until cocaine use is resumed (Hyman, 1996). Thus, unlike opiate addiction, cocaine dependency does not require increased dosages but, rather, more frequent usage to obtain relief from the negative anhedonic effects of abstinence.

Cocaine is a highly effective reinforcer: Studies of primates that were provided with unlimited access to cocaine, food, and water show that they were most likely to select cocaine repeatedly over food and water, even to the point of death (Pollin, 1984). The reinforcing effects of cocaine appear to be directly proportional to the rapidity of onset of euphoria. Administering cocaine intravenously and inhaling freebase or crack are more reinforcing routes of administration than intranasal use and incur a greater vulnerability for dependence. Two to five years of snorting cocaine may be required for dependence to develop; however, smoking freebase or crack, which allows for diffusion and absorption in the large pulmonary area, shortens the time required to develop dependence to mere weeks (Gawin & Ellinwood, 1988). High-dose use produces disinhibition, impaired judgment, feelings of grandiosity, impulsiveness, and hypersexuality (Gawin & Ellinwood, 1988).

A most alarming effect of regular use of all stimulants is increased incidence of psychotic behaviors: hallucinations, delusions of persecution, mood disturbances, and repetitive behaviors (NIDA, 1998). A psychotic reaction caused by the use of stimulants usually subsides with abstinence. However, the exposure to stimulants appears to produce long-term changes in the brain that make the person more likely to display psychotic symptoms if he or she takes the drug again, even months or years later (Sato, 1986).

Medical Complications of Stimulants

Stimulants can cause cardiovascular and respiratory consequences, such as arrhythmia, heart attack, chest pains, and respiratory failure. For example, cocaine users have been found to have heart attacks 24 times more frequently than nonusers (Siegel et al., 1999). Stimulants are also known to cause neurological injury, including acute or persistent headaches, seizures, strokes, and coma (Galanter & Kleber, 1994; NIDA, 1999b). Route of administration (smoked, orally ingested, injected, or snorted) can also lead to various medical conditions, such as nosebleeds, chronic nasal irritation, loss of smell, bowel gangrene, and endocarditis, among others, due to cut off circulation (Galanter & Kleber, 1994; NIDA, 1999). Prolonged use predisposes some users to Parkinsons's disease (McCann et al., 1998). Furthermore, stimulant use during pregnancy has been reported to be a contributing factor in neonatal complications, including premature delivery, low birth weight, smaller head circumference, and shortness in body length (Chasnoff, 1991).

Impact/Effects of Stimulant Use and Dependence

Stimulant use progresses through a series of phases. In the introductory phase, the positive aspects of use outweigh the negative. During episodes of initial use, increases in energy, sexual function, status, confidence, work output, popularity, thinking ability, and euphoria are reported. At this point, the negative aspects are due mainly to the financial cost and the drug's illegality. As dependence on stimulants develops, the negative aspects increase in the form of vocational disruption, relationship problems, and financial crises. There may be temporary relief from depression and lethargy; in this phase euphoria occurs only on initial administration. As dependence further intensifies, nosebleeds, infections, financial jeopardy, relationship disruption, family distress, and impending or actual job loss may result. Finally, only momentary relief from depression and fatigue is experienced. In the final stages, weight loss, seizures, impotence, severe depression, paranoia, psychosis, loss of family and loved ones, unemployment, bankruptcy, isolation, and even death are likely consequences (NIDA, 1999; Rawson et al., 1989).

Stimulant Abstinence

When a stimulant abuser discontinues use, weeks or months of stimulant abstinence are required for pleasure mechanisms, made tolerant by drug use, to begin to readjust their lowered responsiveness to levels adequate for maintaining stable and optimistic moods. *Stimulant abstinence syndrome* refers to the physical and psychological symptoms that the dependent person experiences following the initiation of abstinence from cocaine or other stimulants. Stimulant abstinence proceeds through three stages: crash, withdrawal, and extinction.

Crash

The crash is an extreme exhaustion that immediately follows a binge and can continue in lessened form for up to 15 days. Initially there is intense depression, agitation, and anxiety. Severe depression is often accompanied by suicidal ideation, which can manifest itself at any time from 1 to 8 hours after abstinence is initiated. Over the first few hours, the craving for stimulants is supplanted by a craving for sleep. This craving often leads to the use of benzodiazepines, sedatives, opiates, marijuana, or alcohol to reduce agitation and induce sleep. Prolonged hypersomnolence (excessive sleep) and, during brief awakenings, hyperphagia (excessive eating) may follow. After hypersomnolence ends, some residual dysphoria may linger (American Psychiatric Association, 1994; Galanter & Kleber, 1994; Gawin & Kleber, 1986a; Miller, Gold, & Smith, 1997; Ockert, Coons, Extein, & Gold, 1985).

Withdrawal

Withdrawal symptoms are the opposite of stimulant effects, as decreased energy limits ability to experience pleasure (American Psychiatric Association, 1994; Galanter & Kleber, 1994; Miller et al., 1997). Clinical observations have shown that the protracted abstinence period can be subdivided into distinct phases: (1) an early "honeymoon phase" (10–45 days following initiation of abstinence) characterized by overconfidence, inability to initiate change, episodic cravings, and alcohol use; (2) the "wall" (45–120 days into abstinence), characterized by an intense and often sudden onset of increased anhedonia, mood swings alternating between intense agitation and depression, thoughts of relapse justification, and cognitive rehearsal; and (3) the "adjustment phase" (120–180 days into abstinence), characterized by vocational dissatisfaction, relationship problems, and lack of goals (Obert et al., 2000; Rawson et al., 1989).

Extinction

As the cues (or "triggers") associated with the craving for stimulants cease to be satisfied by the production of a euphoric state, the intensity and frequency of the craving are gradually diminished and anhedonic fatigue and dysphoria recede. Despite the fact that cravings may be diminished, however, renewed cravings can occur months or years after the withdrawal period (Gawin & Kleber, 1986a).

ASSESSMENT

Stimulant dependence requires a comprehensive initial assessment. The history of a client's drug use is necessary to establish the severity of the drug dependence and the consequent disruption in biopsychosocial areas of his or her life. Other important variables are age of onset, duration of drug use history, and dosage.

In addition to medical and psychosocial assessment, the clinician might find it helpful to use an instrument such as the *Addiction Severity Index (ASI)*, which is a structured interview designed to assess the severity of adjustment problems in medical, legal, psychiatric, drug abuse, alcohol abuse, employment, and family areas (McLellan, Luborsky, Woody, & O'Brien, 1980).

Historical and Current Drug Use

A complete history of all drug and alcohol use (licit and illicit use, age of onset, and the span of time that drugs have been used) is necessary to begin an assessment. It can generally be assumed that the higher the dose and the longer the period of either chronic or binge use, the more biopsychosocial problems will have been incurred. Periods of extensive multiple drug use are of particular importance.

An important aspect of assessment is to determine which drug is the primary substance of abuse and which drugs are secondary. Stimulants can be either primary or secondary. When stimulants are primary, the route of stimulant administration will affect the pattern of use of other drugs. For example, cocaine snorters and users of amphetamines (either in crystalline or pill form) typically use alcohol, benzodiazepines, marijuana, or sedative–hypnotics. Those who inject stimulants may use a mixture of stimulants and opiates injected simultaneously ("speedball"). Crack, freebase, and "ice" smokers are more likely to discontinue simultaneous or independent abuse of other drugs, but are likely to use sedating drugs (such as large amounts of alcohol) to self-medicate the acute effects of the stimulant crash. In time, however, this ameliorating use of sedating intoxicants may develop into a new dependence (Gawin & Ellinwood, 1988). Secondary use of stimulants typically occurs among severe alcoholics or opiate-dependent persons in order to increase alertness and to offset the sedating effects of the primary intoxicant.

Severity of Use

An essential first question in an assessment is whether the client believes that the current use of stimulants constitutes a problem. It is extremely common for stimulant users to believe that, because their use is not daily but rather follows a weekly or biweekly binge cycle, they are not "addicted" and consequently do not need therapeutic intervention. It is useful at this point to elicit from the client a description of any biopsychosocial dysfunctions and to evaluate the extent to which the client can attribute problems in living directly to drug use. It is often most clinically useful to explore the individual's reasons for seeking treatment as a means to understand the level of the individual's awareness in this regard.

There are four basic questions to use in determining the severity of stimulant use. How it is taken? How much is taken? When? Where?

How Is the Stimulant Administered?

Briefly restated, clients may be using stimulants in a variety of forms and methods: loose cocaine or "crank" (used intranasally); stimulants in pill form (taken orally); cocaine or other crystalline amphetamine cooked with water (intravenously injected); and freebase, crack, or "ice" (smoked). As indicated, intravenously injected cocaine, freebase, crack, and "ice" have a more immediate and powerful impact on the entire brain and are more likely to result in daily administration than intranasal use (Galanter & Kleber, 1994).

How Much Stimulant Is Used?

Cocaine in loose form is sold in grams or fractions of a gram. An eighth of an ounce ("eightball") is considered a very high dose if all of it is consumed within 24 hours, regardless of the mode of administration. However, if smoked in freebase form, it creates a more potent, acute event. Cocaine amounts in crack vary, depending on the amount of additives. Crack is usually sold in relatively inexpensive amounts packaged in vials or bags, which provide approximately two brief euphoric events ("rushes") per vial or bag. The use of 10–40 vials of crack in a period of 1–3 days would be considered a high dose. Amphetamines in pill or smokable form provide effects of varying degrees and duration, depending on the dosage.

When Are Stimulants Used?

Use typically begins as a weekend or party event. As dependence increases, use is likely to be determined more by availability and financial resources than by any other factors. "Payday habits" are extremely common, and compulsive, uncontrolled use increases as binges become more intense and frequent.

Where Are Stimulants Used?

During the introductory phase, stimulants are usually used at parties, on special occasions, and at gatherings of friends or coworkers. With continued use, there is a tendency for people to use drugs in isolation or in more impersonal locations, such as "crack houses."

By gathering all this basic information, the clinician can more accurately assess the severity of the problem and determine the appropriate treatment plan.

History of Attempts at Abstinence

As with any assessment of substance abuse, it is important to ascertain the client's previous attempts to terminate use and to determine the extent of success or failure. This will involve an assessment of what made periods of abstinence possible, including previous treatments, changes in life circumstances (e.g., a new job), and external threats (e.g., pending bankruptcy, arrest, homelessness, job loss, divorce), as well as an assessment of the client's subjective experience of attempts at abstinence (e.g., does the client believe that attempts are doomed to failure?).

Psychological Assessment

As discussed above, stimulant abuse can cause certain psychological symptoms: depression, agitation, paranoid delusions and hallucinations, suicidal ideation and attempts, violent impulses, and such cognitive dysfunctions as loss of concentration and memory. It is essential that all of these possible symptoms be explored; generally the more severe the symptoms, the more progressed is the stimulant dependence. Stimulant users are likely to progress from paranoid delusion to auditory, then visual, hallucinations during intoxication, and finally to hallucination and delusion even when not intoxicated.

Since these symptoms of stimulant abuse are similar to symptoms of psychopathology that is *not* related to the use of intoxicants, assessment of underlying psychopathology is crucial. Treatment approaches that focus exclusively on drug use and neglect the relevance of social–psychological pathology are bound to fail and may even reinforce dysfunctional drug-using behavior (Galanter & Kleber, 1994). Findings suggest that persons with affective disorders and residual attention-deficit disorders (formerly termed "hyperactivity") are overrepresented among the drug-abusing population (Gawin & Ellinwood, 1988; Weiss, Mirin, Michael, & Sollogub, 1986).

The use of stimulants to self-medicate depression has been posited since Freud cited the drug's antidepressant activity in 1884 (Weiss et al., 1986). The evidence for this hypothesis comes from several areas: (1) the profound euphoria induced by cocaine (Resnick & Resnick, 1985; Weiss et al., 1986); (2) the ability of cocaine, like antidepressant drugs, to increase noradrenergic activity in the central nervous system (Blanken & Resnikov, 1985; Weiss et al., 1986); and (3) the pharmacological similarity of cocaine to amphetamines, which have been used effectively in the treatment of some depression (Brecher et al., 1972). There are several reports of termination of stimulant use by patients with affective disorders after psychotropic medication appropriate to their psychopathology was administered (Gawin & Ellinwood, 1988; Khantzian, Gawin, Kleber, & Riordan, 1984; Weiss & Mirin, 1986).

Distinguishing stimulant-induced symptoms from symptoms of underlying pathology is not simple or straightforward under any circumstances, and in some cases it may not be possible until the client has remained drug free for a significant period following termination of acute stimulant withdrawal. However, time and circumstantial factors can make distinctions of symptom causes somewhat more reliable. The age of onset is the most obvious factor: Are the symptoms premorbid; that is, did they exist prior to the use of a stimulant? It is necessary to note that prior use of other intoxicants, such as alcohol, marijuana, or tranquilizers, can also be a cause of depression. Similarly, symptom occurrence that is seasonal or periodic might indicate seasonal affective disorder or cyclical or recurrent affective disorder. Specific onset or increase in symptoms following a significant life crisis or the onset of a major stressor might signal the existence of a reactive depression or posttraumatic stress disorder. Finally, symptoms that occur during extended periods of abstinence from stimulants are more likely to be non-stimulant-related.

Any assessment must, of course, take into account the client's personality development and any personality dysfunction. Such issues in regard to stimulant use are not significantly different from those presented by other substances of abuse and need not be discussed at length here. The emotional development of substance abusers is often arrested, in certain respects, at the age of onset of use (Kleber & Gawin, 1987), and any other developmental inhibitions, such as serious problems resulting from unresolved separation–individuation (Resnick & Resnick, 1985), are likely to be exacerbated by stimulant use. These factors may point to important considerations in determining a client's ability to tolerate life stressors in the absence of stimulants and/or ability to handle treatment in group settings.

It is worthwhile to note here that Resnick and Resnick (1985) found that compulsive cocaine users commonly have an Axis II diagnosis of borderline or narcissistic personality disorder. Clients exhibiting characteristics of borderline personality disorder may require a more restrictive treatment environment in order to limit the negative impact of impulsivity. Narcissistic clients may require a less confrontational treatment environment in order to avoid excessive narcissistic injury.

Sexual behavior in relation to stimulant use is of particular importance in the psychological evaluation (Washton, 1989). Many clients state that sexual arousal appears to increase during the euphoria of initial stimulant use. Accordingly, sexual activity may trigger the thought of stimulant use. Indiscriminate sexual activity and extended periods of sexual involvement often result from stimulant use and must be addressed as a treatment issue. Moreover, the exchange of sexual favors for stimulants is a common feature within the stimulant-using population. Because sexual activity is indiscriminate, clients may be at greater risk of contracting sexually transmitted infections, including HIV and hepatitis; this at-risk behavior necessitates further assessment and counseling. In addition, indiscriminate sexual activity often leads to an experience of shame, which should be explored in the course of treatment.

Medical Evaluation

Medical evaluation is necessary for a number of reasons. First, chronic stimulant use causes many physical injuries; some of the most common are scar tissue on the heart muscle, arrhythmia, and high blood pressure. Liver damage is possible with use of multiple drugs. Alcohol has long been known to be hepatotoxic, as are substances used to "cut" cocaine and heroin in order to increase volume. These injuries may need to be addressed in treatment. Second, other medical causes need to be eliminated as competing explanations for stimulant-related symptoms. Elevated liver enzymes, for example, may cause fatigue and nausea, which might otherwise be viewed as symptoms of depression. High body temperatures can cause mental states that can also be symptoms of psychopathology, such as hallucinations and disorientation. Elevated blood sugar serum levels can cause mood swings not unlike those caused by the stimulant abstinence syndrome. Furthermore, many illnesses have been shown to be accompanied by depression. This alone might make the allure of stimulants all the more compelling. In order to proceed with the assessment and make appropriate treatment choices (psychotherapeutic and/or pharmacological), the clinician must have adequate information. Finally, indiscriminate sexual behavior associated with stimulant use requires the medical evaluator to order tests for all the sexually transmitted diseases.

An evaluation of current physical status should include a blood chemistry profile (liver enzyme levels, white blood cell count, etc.), tests for sexually transmitted diseases, an electrocardiogram (EKG) to determine heart rhythm, and an electroencephalogram (EEG) to assess brain wave activity.

Assessment of Social, Legal, and Employment Areas

The assessment requirements regarding the social, legal, and employment issues that accompany stimulant abuse are basically identical to those accompanying any other substance abuse. Several aspects of stimulant abuse, however, do have a specific effect on these areas and need to be addressed here.

As discussed earlier, stimulant dependence can develop rapidly (especially when the stimulant is smoked). Consequently, it is not unusual for stimulant smokers to present a long list of losses at intake: the irreparable loss of all savings, assets, housing, employment, and extended family support networks—indeed, the basic necessities of life—within the period of a year or, in extreme cases, within a period of months. This desperate state of affairs not only places the client in individual crisis but also may have disastrous effects on many of the client's significant others.

Thus prompt and complete assessment of the status of the client's family and social networks is crucial. At the time of assessment, the client's family may be so dysfunctional, overburdened with crises, and/or on the brink of dissolution that immediate intervention may be necessary to secure the continuation of family life. This kind of crisis intervention is especially important because the significant others may be the only available source of external limits on the client's stimulant use (e.g., by controlling the client's income, cashing the client's paycheck, etc.). Immediate intervention also may be necessary to prevent or encourage the removal of children from the client's care.

Legally, clients often find themselves facing prosecution for illegal acts (especially buying, selling, and/or possessing illegal substances; theft; prostitution), committed under the influence of the stimulant, which they could not conceive of doing when not using drugs. Clients may be extremely reluctant to divulge information they experience as shameful. Care must be taken to elicit such information in a nonjudgmental manner, so that appropriate use can be made of it in treatment.

Illustration of Assessment

The following case history exemplifies the assessment process with a typical stimulant-abusing client.

> Louis, a 30-year-old married school maintenance worker, set up an appointment at an outpatient chemical dependency treatment facility after reading an advertisement in the local Yellow Pages. At the intake session, he stated that he was seeking help because he was spending too much money on cocaine and that, although he felt his cocaine use was not all that severe, the urge to use it was increasing. He did not identify alcohol or any other drug as a problem.
>
> However, a thorough history of drug use revealed that from ages 14–19 he had smoked marijuana daily. Upon his entry to the Marines at age 19, he began drinking one or two pints of rum every other day, a habit he continued after discharge from the service at age 24. At age 25, he began to snort cocaine occasionally with drinking buddies in the neighborhood. At age 28, his alcoholic father passed away, causing Louis to become depressed and to stay indoors for 2 weeks, during

which time he drank steadily. His next paycheck was spent entirely on cocaine and crack, which he tried then for the first time and liked immensely. His biweekly payday became the occasion for increasingly lengthy crack binges with neighborhood drug-abusing acquaintances. Alcohol use began to take on a new pattern, increasing at the start of the crash following each crack binge and continuing heavily (2 pints of rum per day) through the week following the binge. To this pattern, Louis added heroin, which he had snorted five times in the year prior to the intake, each time to alleviate the effects of the cocaine crash.

At the time of intake Louis was using approximately 10–15 $10 containers of crack per weekend (postpayday) binge, and he occasionally used one or two containers on other days if he had sufficient cash. Louis managed to give rent and food money to his wife before he set off to meet his drug-abusing acquaintances at the local grocery, which sells crack under the table. This group had become his sole social outlet. They usually smoked their crack in someone's automobile or apartment. Louis's cousin, who also had a severe crack problem, had recently been arrested while purchasing drugs on the street. Louis felt it could just as well have been him, and he was afraid that he would be the next to be arrested.

Louis had first sought treatment from the local Veterans Administration hospital 6 months earlier. He was treated in the inpatient alcohol rehabilitation program for 15 days and discharged with the instruction to participate in community Alcoholics Anonymous meetings. He began using cocaine and alcohol again 1 week after discharge. This was the only period of voluntary abstinence he had experienced since the onset of alcohol use.

At the time of intake, Louis had not used cocaine for 5 days but had been drinking from two beers to two pints of rum daily. He was very talkative, joking occasionally, but more often restless in his seat and apparently somewhat agitated. He denied feeling depressed and stated that he was always tense or anxious. He admitted being quick to anger but never violent or suicidal. He had no prior history of psychiatric treatment. He stated that he had always been restless as a child and that his 9-year-old son had recently been diagnosed as hyperactive. He described his mother as having been "depressed a lot." In the previous year Louis had become aware that he had an increasingly difficult time concentrating and that he was sometimes confused when attempting to make a decision. Although he was able to fall asleep after drinking in the evening, his sleep was short and he woke often during the night. He reported a lifelong problem with sleep disturbance. He denied having hallucinations but admitted to mild paranoid delusions (e.g., falsely assuming that the police were at the door) during cocaine use.

Louis was evaluated by a physician at the outpatient facility and was found to have no current medical illness or physical dysfunction. Accordingly, physical illness was ruled out as a source of his symptoms.

In Louis's case, his primary drug of abuse, alcohol, had taken a secondary position to cocaine over the course of several years. Louis's crack use had reached a severe level, a fact that he attempted to minimize. His symptoms of agitation, low tolerance for frustration, sleep disturbance, and mild confusion are typical of the crash from heavy crack use. Because of his history of continuous drug and alcohol use, there was no period of adult life with which to accurately compare his present symptoms. There may have been indications in his personal and family history of psychiatric problems, but the intake history alone was insufficient to distinguish any possible psychiatric factors he may have had from his drug symptoms.

TREATMENT

Based on research as well as clinical treatment of stimulant-dependent clients, it is apparent that an integrated multimodal approach addressing each patient's drug-related social, psychological, and biological problems is needed. This treatment approach relies on a joint consideration of neurochemical and psychosocial mechanisms. The most effective treatment plan for such clients is based on each client's therapeutic needs and ability to function at each stage of the stimulant abstinence syndrome: initiation of abstinence/crash, the honeymoon phase, the wall phase, and, finally, the adjustment phase. The case of Louis, discussed above, is used later to illustrate the application of a multimodal approach in the context of these phases.

Before the phases of treatment are discussed, it is important to note that the modalities of treatment—medical, psychological, and social—need to be addressed in different ways, depending on the needs of a particular client at a particular phase in treatment. The treatment approach with each client depends on an ongoing assessment of his or her ability to master each phase of treatment. One treatment professional needs to be responsible for coordinating the treatment priorities of a client, as problems and assets change throughout the treatment process. Medication, physical exercise, individual behavioral as well as cognitive and insight-oriented psychotherapies, group therapy, family and couple sessions, and community resources are all tools that can be combined in a dynamic, strategic array that is uniquely suitable to the individual client. This individualized approach to a drug-dependency problem requires variations in sequence, frequency, and variety of services delivered.

Initiation of Abstinence/Crash

Treatment can only begin with the initiation of abstinence. Since stimulants produce no medically dangerous withdrawal symptoms, hospitalization is usually unnecessary (Gawin & Ellinwood, 1988). However, hospitalization is recommended for clients who have (1) a history of repeated failed attempts to abstain during the 5- to 10-day crash period; (2) those with severe and unresponsive depression, paranoid delusional thinking, or suicidal ideation or attempts; and (3) those who completely lack a structured living environment.

In many cases, however, clients can weather the crash phase without relapse if they have appropriate treatment support. Treatment should be intensive during this phase, preferably on a daily basis and including additional opportunities for telephone contact, whenever necessary. Individual treatment enables the therapist to conduct an ongoing assessment of the client's relapse potential and to help the client address the myriad individual crises that invariably occur in early abstinence. Initially, treatment interventions should be primarily behavioral in approach: How can the client change his or her behavior to avoid access to, and the opportunity to use, stimulants? It is also important to establish external controls on the client's access to money and free time, if possible.

Group treatment can play an important corollary role by focusing on educational concerns; that is, by remedying the client's lack of knowledge with information on the nature of stimulant dependence, the phases of the stimulant abstinence syndrome, and the behavioral requirements of early abstinence. Another goal of group involvement should be introducing the client to 12-step self-help support groups, such as Narcotics Anonymous (NA) and Cocaine Anonymous (CA). Such meetings may be held within the context of group treatment at the treating facility, and/or clients may be instructed or encouraged to attend such meetings in the community individually or with fellow group members. Certainly, any day during this initial phase that does not contain a scheduled treatment visit ought to include a 12-step meeting.

Family involvement focuses on instructing significant others about the nature of the client's stimulant dependence, especially the compulsive, uncontrolled response to stimulating triggers (e.g., cash or the sight of cocaine and the paraphernalia of use) that users experience. When significant others understand this compulsivity, their defensive condemnation and blame can sometimes be diminished; in addition, they can often be encouraged to provide external sources of control, as appropriate. Crisis intervention and appropriate referral to community assistance also may be indicated.

A significant innovation in treatment during early abstinence is the administration of psychotropic medications to counteract the disruption of neurotransmitter release and reabsorption (Ockert, 1984; Ockert, Extein, & Gold, 1987). This medication stabilizes the client emotionally and decreases the severity of such crash symptoms as insomnia, anxiety, depression, and inability to concentrate, all of which can trigger the conditioned need for more stimulants. Furthermore, by treating despondency and attentional deficits, these medications make clients more accessible to talk therapy. This accessibility is important because such therapy is the principal avenue by which we can best address certain social situations, as well as historical and current emotional factors that often lie at the root of addiction. Medications commonly used range from antidepressants to mood stabilizers and neuroleptics; which drug class is chosen should depend on the signs and symptoms that a patient presents.

The Honeymoon Phase

Between 6 and 15 days into abstinence, clients usually describe a gradual lessening of dysphoric symptoms, begin to feel a sense of returning to "normal," and often express an overconfidence in their ability to remain drug free. This phase is popularly known in 12-step programs as the "pink cloud."

At this point, treatment focus usually shifts markedly. In both individual and group sessions, greater attention must be paid to the various phases of stimulant withdrawal and recovery, especially to the fact that the honeymoon phase is followed by the wall phase and that, without proper preparation, clients are prone to relapse when the change occurs. The cognitively and behaviorally oriented relapse prevention theory of Marlatt and Gordon (1985), among others, is especially appropriate at this stage. Clients need to assess their unique patterns of drug use and begin to fashion a relapse prevention strategy for themselves that allows for the experience of self-efficacy through use of schedules, cognitive preparation, behavioral techniques, and measures of success. Fundamental to this approach is clients' understanding of relapse as a series of events that can, but need not, result in using the drug (Marlatt & Gordon, 1985). In this conception, the process of recovery is an educational one of learning, often by examining one's mistakes, how and when to seek intervention to prevent movement toward drug use. Clients may be asked to contract for behavioral change (especially in regard to participation in 12-step programs, scheduling of leisure and work hours to focus on abstinence, and avoidance of situations with cocaine associations) and to terminate all alcohol and marijuana use. It is best to connect with clients and test urine several times a week to ensure treatment compliance and to intercept relapse behavior at the earliest possible opportunity.

It is essential that clients be encouraged to continue psychotropic medications when indicated, despite (indeed, precisely because of) their mood improvement. This is especially true in light of the often sudden onset of mood swings in the subsequent wall phase and the time lag of several weeks before most psychotropics reach an adequate blood level for depression relief. In addition, whether or not clients are taking medications, regular aerobic activity (such as running, jogging, swimming, or bike riding) should be strongly emphasized at this point. Aerobic activity is very useful in establishing control (or in supplementing the antidepressant medication in establishing control) over the emotional symptoms of the stimulant abstinence syndrome (Siegel, 1985). Sufficient aerobic activity induces the subjective experience of a "second wind" or "runners' high," in which the physical stress of the activity forces the neurochemical system to produce and release more enkephalins (such as endorphins), which in turn counteract, for a short period, the neurochemical deficiencies induced by stimulant dependence.

Family treatment at this phase typically involves continuing education about the phases of recovery (especially the soon-to-be-experienced difficulties of the wall phase). In addition, the stimulant-dependent person is assisted in reorienting to his or her appropriate role in the family system. Other areas of social function are also addressed, especially issues of work performance, dealing with demands for recompense for past behavior (e.g., paying drug debts, handling legal proceedings), and helping children cope with sudden and perhaps unsettling changes in the drug-abusing parent.

The Wall Phase

About 2½ months after the initiation of abstinence, the wall phase commences, usually with the sudden and inexplicable onset of increased anhedonia and mood swings between agitation and low-energy depression. Relapse potential is greatly increased during this phase. Clients begin to express significant frustration and discouragement with treatment. It is important to address the discouragement openly in group and individual sessions (or to elicit its verbal expression if it is being expressed in acting-out behavior) by reemphasizing the biochemical causes of this change in mood. Any misattribution of this phase to personal deficiencies, treatment inadequacies, or fatalistic worldviews must be firmly and repeatedly shown to be incorrect. Instead, the group and individual treatment agenda should readdress the previously discussed relapse prevention concepts and techniques, using specific examples of relapse-oriented behavior that the clients currently present. For example, as clients begin to disclose their seemingly justified failures to attend 12-step meetings, continue their exercise routines, limit the availability of cash, or make scheduled treatment appointments, these events can be cognitively reframed in terms of relapse behavior patterns, and prompt behavioral interventions can be proposed. Efforts should be made to enhance the positive reinforcement of the experience of efficacy by encouraging group recognition of the achievement that will result from the client's behavioral intervention.

The likelihood of actual stimulant use at this stage needs to be addressed in two ways: (1) by initiating cognitive rehearsal of circumstances in which clients are likely to find themselves confronted by opportunities for drug use; and (2) by discussing what needs to be done if such use actually occurs. It is crucial to explain to clients that a slip to drug use means not that further relapse is necessary or justified but rather that immediate return to the treatment environment (a) is the most effective intervention, (b) will prevent further relapse, and (c) will allow them to learn how *not* to make the same mistake in the future. Relapse must be dealt with in a nonjudgmental, nonpunitive manner on the part of both treatment staff and fellow clients.

Psychotropic medication dosages may need to be reevaluated by medical staff if the current dosage does not seem adequate to address the increased depression and other anhedonic symptoms that arise. In addition, conjugal and family counseling may need to be intensified to address increased tensions that result from mood changes and low tolerance of frustration. At this point, significant others need to be informed of the reasons for the changes and the behavioral steps the client needs to take to reassert control over his or her progress in recovery.

The Adjustment Phase

Most clients gradually emerge from the extreme depression of the wall phase somewhere from 120 to 180 days into abstinence. However, the anhedonia often continues as clients become less focused on their uncomfortable moods and increasingly confront the problems they face in living, some of which are self-inflicted by a history of drug use. Clients are often bewildered by the prospect of rebuilding failing marriages, handling vocational dissatisfaction, and learning to establish a drug-free social network and lifestyle.

Group and individual treatment can begin to address underlying emotional issues involving anger, guilt, isolation, boredom, and low self-esteem. It is hoped that by this time, clients will have attained sufficient emotional capacity to undertake an insight-oriented psychotherapy or, in some cases, a goal-oriented one.

Couple and family therapy also may begin to take a more constructive approach, as significant others are required to do less damage control and can establish goals for the future of the family system. Vocational counseling also may be appropriate in some cases.

It is best to continue psychotropic medication protocols through the sixth month of abstinence. At that time, if the psychiatric treatment staff thinks it appropriate, then treatment staff and client can mutually agree to initiate a planned trial off medication to evaluate whether any further depressive condition exists.

Illustration of Treatment

The case of Louis (whose assessment was described previously) illustrates the various stages of treatment and recovery.

Initiation of Abstinence

At the intake Louis did not appear to have any of the factors that would have made an inpatient detoxification necessary. Therefore the assessment team, consisting of the medical director, the clinical director, and the primary individual counselor, established a treatment plan that addressed medical, social, and psychological aspects of the initial phase of recovery. Louis was given a schedule of required appointments for participation in either individual or group treatment during each workday of the first week of treatment.

After a medical evaluation conducted the same day as the intake, he was prescribed an antidepressant. Louis took his initial dose that same evening. His sleep improved somewhat the first night, and by the third day of treatment he was expressing a greater sense of calm and a more positive outlook.

Following intake, Louis met with the social worker who would serve as his individual counselor, and plans were devised to keep him as far as possible from those people, places, and things (especially money) that would make it possible for him to use alcohol or cocaine during the first week of abstinence. At the educational group meeting that he attended the next day, the importance of 12-step programs was stressed and each group member was asked to study a meeting schedule and choose the meetings they would attend prior to the next group session. Louis was asked to give a urine sample at each session for laboratory analysis, and he was told that this procedure would continue during his entire time in the program.

The Honeymoon Phase

In his individual treatment sessions, Louis's counselor focused on discovering the specific details of Louis's drug use, with the goal of identifying behavioral patterns that needed to be changed in order to prevent opportunities to use alcohol and drugs. These included the usual persons, places, and things, as well as certain emotional states or interpersonal interactions, that preceded the actual use. For Louis, this meant learning to identify the sequence of events from the beer at lunch with coworkers, to the trip past his hangout spot on the way to park the car, to the angry interaction with his wife, and finally the escape from the house and the walk to the hangout spot. Ways to intervene behaviorally were discussed, and a plan for implementation was devised and accepted. Louis agreed to keep a written schedule of his daily activities in order to plan in advance the steps he needed to take to avoid drug use. Since his wife had refused to attend a family session, Louis and his counselor discussed ways to communicate with her and to provide materials for her to read to educate her about his drug dependence.

After several weeks Louis, no longer troubled by strong urges to use cocaine, was beginning to feel that he was no longer susceptible to the dangers of further use. He admitted to having had wine at a family gathering and, with much prodding, stated that others felt he had drunk too much. He was resistant to the idea that alcohol might lead him to using cocaine again. Furthermore, he had been inconsistent in attending his NA meetings. The counselors decided to lead a thorough discussion of the dangers of alcohol use during group meetings. Using formal written worksheets and informal discussion, the group began to put alcohol use into the context of a series of events that could lead to relapse. The group helped Louis identify how he himself could intervene, on his own behalf, to prevent further movement toward the use of cocaine. Group members also were asked to account to one another for their plans to attend 12-step meetings and failures to follow through with those plans. Louis's reluctance to attend meetings was partially alleviated by the offer of a group member to take Louis to a favorite NA meeting. Both individual and group sessions also focused on the need to recognize the symptoms of the wall phase, which he was approaching. Louis responded by taking his exercise regimen more seriously, a change for which he received much praise from fellow group members.

Because family treatment was still not agreeable to Louis's wife, family issues were emphasized in individual treatment. In fact, his improved mood and behavior had already begun to create a new sense of harmony at home.

The Wall Phase

In the eighth week of treatment Louis began to cancel every other appointment at the last minute, claiming that, with the approach of the Christmas holidays, his job required additional overtime work. The urine left the following Monday tested positive for marijuana use. When confronted with this information, Louis at first denied the possibility then admitted he had smoked marijuana with his brother-in-law after work on the prior Friday. He attributed this use to the need to be high to escape the frequent quarrels he was having with his wife. On further inquiry, it became clearer that for a week he had been out of sorts, feeling increasingly irritable at work and at home and unable to follow his established schedule for meetings or exercise. He sometimes forgot to take the prescribed antidepressant medication. His individual counselor immediately reemphasized the need for Louis to intervene to stop this movement toward relapse and reacquainted him with the nature of the wall phase and its likely effects. Louis agreed to take further steps to improve his situation, all the while insisting that he had no intention of using cocaine. He subsequently failed to appear for the next group session. Messages were left for him, which he did not return. The counselor finally reached Louis shortly before the next individual session. He stated that he had used cocaine, to which the counselor responded with sympathy and strong invitations to come to the scheduled session. Louis arrived at the session accompanied by his wife. He explained that the previous Friday he had used $20 worth of crack after drinking with friends at his hangout spot. Far from being the ecstatic return to cocaine he had anticipated, his drug experience had been rather painful because of his guilt and disappointment with himself. His wife had refused to talk to him until the previous night, when he told her that he was too ashamed to return to treatment. She had accompanied him to make sure that he did not detour on his way to the session.

Both Louis and his wife were praised for having come in immediately to process this cocaine use, despite any despair or disappointment they might be feeling. The counselor quickly educated them both about the nature of Louis's mood swings, urges, and possibilities for continued abstinence. The relapse was framed as an educational opportunity, a way to discover what mistakes had been made in order to act differently in the future and to avoid further mistakes. Both Louis and his wife expressed some relief on hearing this, and they left with a renewed sense of direction and understanding. An agreement for further couple sessions was made.

In the following group session, Louis was encouraged to describe his experiences to the group in terms that emphasized the learning opportunities it had presented. The group responded favorably.

The individual counselor consulted with the medical staff, and it was decided that an increase in the antidepressant medication dose was appropriate at this time. Louis reported mood improvement within a few days at the increased dose.

The Adjustment Phase

By the middle of the fifth month of treatment, Louis had become less prone to mood swings and much more adept at spotting relapse-related symptoms in order to take steps to prevent drug use. He began to open up in his group about the conflicting emotions he felt toward his ailing father, which stimulated extensive discussions about relationships with older parents and their effects on behavior toward their own children. In individual sessions, Louis became increasingly aware of his underlying feelings of low self-esteem. He and his counselor were able to contract to focus more specifically on this issue over a number of sessions.

A trial period off the antidepressant medication was planned to determine whether further use was needed. Louis showed no signifi-

cant deterioration in mood for a month after the medication was removed, and a mutual decision was made to discontinue it. After two
more couple sessions, Louis's wife had decided not to come in for further meetings, insisting that childcare responsibilities made her participation impossible. Louis was disappointed by her decision, and it was
necessary to deal with his feelings extensively in his individual sessions. He completed the planned treatment program 7 months after he
began it. He continued his involvement with his 12-step program and
also continued to see his individual counselor on an as-needed basis.

CONCLUSION

In the foregoing example, Louis represents just one client among a wide
variety of stimulant abusers, all of whom face considerable odds in the
struggle to achieve and maintain abstinence. Cocaine or other stimulant
abuse simultaneously causes severe biological, psychological, and social
dysfunction. It is necessary, then, to embrace the complexity of this problem by viewing stimulant dependency from a multifaceted and interactive
perspective. This perspective, in turn, demands the creation of an integrated multidisciplinary treatment approach. Such treatment, when designed
to address the various phases of the stimulant abstinence syndrome and
tailored to the needs of the individual, is capable of fulfilling client needs
and effecting better outcomes. Undoubtedly, our understanding of stimulant dependence will increase as our knowledge of neurobiochemistry and
its impact on psychological processes continues to develop. New treatment
methods will consequently incorporate this information to increase the
probability of relapse prevention and to improve the prognosis for recovery from dependence.

REFERENCES

American Psychiatric Association. (1994). *Diagnostic and statistical manual of men-
tal disorders* (4th ed.). Washington, DC: American Psychiatric Association.
Blanken, A. J., & Resnikov, D. C. (1985). *National drug and alcoholism treatment
utilization survey summary report on drug abuse treatment units.* Rockville,
MD: National Institute on Drug Abuse.
Brecher, E. M., & the Editors of *Consumer Reports.* (1972). *Licit and illicit drugs.*
Boston: Little, Brown.
Carlson, N. R. (2001). *Physiology of behavior* (7th ed.). Boston: Allyn & Bacon.
Chasnoff, I. J. (1991). Drug and alcohol effects on pregnancy and the newborn. In N.
S. Miller (Ed.), *Comprehensive handbook of drug and alcohol addiction.* New
York: Marcel Dekker.
Courtwright, D. (1991). The first American cocaine epidemic. *Newsletter of the Co-
caine Crack Research Working Group, 1*(1), 3–5.

Galanter, M., & Kleber, H. D. (1994). *Textbook of substance abuse treatment*. Washington, DC: American Psychiatric Association Press.

Gawin, F. H., & Ellinwood, E. H. (1988). Medical progress: Cocaine and other stimulants. *New England Journal of Medicine, 318*(18), 1173–1182.

Gawin, F. H., & Kleber, H. D. (1985). Cocaine use in a treatment population: Patterns and diagnostic distinction. *National Institute on Drug Abuse Research Monograph Series, 61,* 182–192.

Gawin, F. H., & Kleber, H. D. (1986a). Abstinence symptomatology and psychiatric diagnosis in cocaine abusers. *Archives of General Psychiatry, 43,* 107–113.

Gawin, F. H., & Kleber, H. D. (1986b). Pharmacological treatments of cocaine abuse. *Psychiatric Clinics of North America, 9,* 573–583.

Greenspoon, L., & Bakalar, J. B. (1980). Drug dependence: Non-narcotic agents. In H. I. Kaplan, A. M. Freedman, & B. J. Sadock (Eds.), *Comprehensive textbook of psychiatry*. Baltimore: Williams & Wilkins.

Hyman, S. E. (1996). Addiction to cocaine and amphetamine. *Neuron, 16,* 901–904.

Jones, E. (1953). *The life and work of Sigmund Freud* (Vol. 1). New York: Basic Books.

Jones, R. T. (1985). The pharmacology of cocaine. *National Institute on Drug Abuse Research Monograph Series, 50,* 34–53.

Khantzian, E. J., Gawin, F., Kleber, H. D., & Riordan, C. E. (1984). Methylphenidate treatment of cocaine dependence: A preliminary report. *Journal of Substance Abuse Treatment, 1,* 107–112.

Kleber, H. G., & Gawin, F. H. (1987). Cocaine withdrawal. *Archives of General Psychiatry, 44,* 298.

Marlatt, G. A., & Gordon, J. R. (Eds.). (1985). *Relapse prevention: Maintenance strategies in the treatment of addictive behaviors*. New York: Guilford Press.

McCann, U. D., Wong, D. F., Yokoi, F., Villemagne, V., Dannls, R. F., & Ricaurte, G. A. (1998). Reduced striatal dopamine transporter density in abstinent methamphetamine and methcathinone users: Evidence from positron emission tomography studies with [^{11}C]WIN-35,428. *Journal of Neuroscience,, 18*(20), 8417–8422.

McLellan, A. T., Luborsky, L., Woody, G. E., & O'Brien, C. P. (1980). An improved diagnostic evaluation instrument for substance abuse patients: The Addiction Severity Index. *Journal of Nervous and Mental Disease, 168,* 26—33.

Miller, N., Gold, M., & Smith, D. (1997). *Manual of therapeutics for addictions*. New York: Wiley.

National Commission on Marijuana and Drug Abuse. (1973). *Drug use in America: Problem in perspective: Second report of the National Commission on Marijuana and Drug Abuse*. Washington, DC: National Institute on Drug Abuse.

National Institute on Drug Abuse (NIDA). (1998). Tearoff: Comparing methamphetamine and cocaine. *NIDA Notes, 13*(1).

National Institute on Drug Abuse (NIDA). (1999a). *National household survey on drug abuse: Population estimates 1998*. Washington, DC: U.S. Government Printing Office.

National Institute on Drug Abuse (NIDA). (1999b). *Research report series: Cocaine abuse and addiction*. Retrieved November 20, 2000, at www.nida.hih.gov/Research Reports/Cocaine/cocaine3.html

National Institute on Drug Abuse (NIDA). (2000). *Research report series: Metham-*

phetamine: Abuse and addiction. Retrieved November 20, 2000, at www.nida. nih.gov/Research Reports/Methamph/methamph2.html

Obert, J. L., McCann, M. J., Marinelli-Casey, P., Weiner, A., Minsky, S., Brethren, P., & Rawson, R. (2000). The Matrix model of outpatient stimulant abuse treatment: History and description. *Journal of Psychoactive Drugs, 32*(2), 157–164.

Ockert, D. M. (1984). *A multi-modality drug abuse treatment program for high economic status patients.* Unpublished doctoral dissertation, Columbia University.

Ockert, D. M., Coons, E. E., Extein, I., & Gold, M. S. (1985). Lowered drug abuse recidivism following psychotropic medication. *National Institute on Drug Abuse Research Monograph Series, 67,* 494.

Ockert, D. M., Extein, I., & Gold, M. S. (1987). Posthospital outcome in suburban drug addicts. *Psychiatric Medicine, 3*(4), 419–426.

Pollin, W. (1984). Cocaine pharmacology, effects and treatment of abuse. *National Institute on Drug Abuse Research Monograph Series, 50,* vii.

Rawson, R., Huber, A., Brethren, P., Obert, J., Gulati, V., Shoptaw, S., & Ling, W. (2000). Methamphetamine and cocaine users: Differences in characteristics and treatment retention. *Journal of Psychoactive Drugs, 32*(2), 233–238.

Rawson, R. A., Obert, J. L., McCann, M. J., Smith, D. P., & Scheffey, E. H. (1989). *The neurobehavioral treatment manual: A therapist manual for outpatient cocaine addiction treatment.* Beverly Hills, CA: Matrix Center.

Resnick, R., & Resnick, E. (1985). Psychological issues in the treatment of cocaine abuse. Proceedings of the Committee on Problems of Drug Dependence. *National Institute on Drug Abuse Research Monograph Series, 67,* 290–294.

Sato, M. (1986). Acute exacerbation of methamphetamine psychosis and lasting dopaminergic supersensitivity: -A clinical survey. *Psychopharmacology Bulletin, 22,* 751–756.

Siegel, A. J., Sholar, M. B., Mendelson, J. H., Lukas, S. E., Kaufman, M. J., Renshaw, P. F., et al. (1999). Cocaine-induced erythrocytosis and increase in von Willebrand factor: Evidence for drug-related blood doping and prothrombotic effects. *Archives of Internal Medicine, 159,* 1925.

Siegel, R. K. (1985). New patterns of cocaine use: Changing doses and routes. *National Institute on Drug Abuse Research Monograph Series, 61,* 171–181.

Strategy Council on Drug Abuse. (1973). *Federal strategy for drug abuse and drug traffic prevention.* Washington, DC: U.S. Government Printing Office.

Washton, A. (1989). Cocaine abuse and compulsive sexuality. *Medical Aspects of Human Sexuality, 23,* 32–39.

Weiss, R. D., & Mirin, S. M. (1986). Subtypes of cocaine abusers. *Psychiatric Clinics Of North America, 9,* 491–501.

Weiss, R. D., Mirin, S. M., Michael, J. L., & Sollogub, A. C. (1986). Psychopathology in chronic cocaine abusers. *American Journal of Drug and Alcohol Abuse, 12,* 17–29.

Wise, R. A. (1988). Psychomotor stimulant properties of addictive drugs. *Annals of the New York Academy of Sciences, 537,* 228–234.

PART IV

Assessment and Intervention with Families of Substance Abusers

Working with families of substance-abusing clients has always been one of the major roles of social workers and family therapists. The three chapters in this section focus on working with different family members affected by substance abuse.

The first chapter in Part IV, Chapter 11, considers the family as a whole. The author integrates traditional family therapy concepts and approaches with the specialized issues and interventions applicable to families with a substance-abusing member. In the next chapter, the author discusses how the partner of the alcohol or other drug abuser is affected. The wife, husband, or lover of the substance abuser is seen as an individual with his or her own pain and treatment needs and should be viewed as a primary client who needs and deserves help for his or her own sake. The final chapter in this part, Chapter 13, explores the dynamics of treatment issues when dealing with children of drug and alcohol abusers. Since, as the author points out, the research and clinical literature on young and adult children of alcoholic persons is much more comprehensive than that on children of other drug abusers, this chapter, by and large, focuses on children of alcohol-abusing parents—the largest group of people impacted by parental substance use.

Although the current funding sources tend to limit the services offered to family members of substance-abusing individuals, the authors in this part point out the crucial need for services to be made available to all family members who currently live with, or used to live with, a substance-abusing individual.

CHAPTER 11

Family Treatment
of Substance Abuse

Jeffrey R. McIntyre

It is estimated that 11% of the population of the United States abuses or is addicted to mind- and mood-altering substances. Using the commonly accepted formula that one person's behavior affects between four and six other people, then 126–188 million Americans—45–68% of the population—may be affected by another's substance abuse.

People develop compulsive attachments to mind- and mood-altering substances for a variety of biophysiological, psychoemotional, and social–interpersonal reasons. As a person forms an attachment to a substance and its effects, the partner/spouse develops complex psychological and behavioral ways to control him- or herself and others close to him or her, in an effort to control the substance abuser. Increasing amounts of time, "strategic" planning, and emotional energy are expended in this process. The children also spend time and energy figuring out how to handle their fears and anxiety and how to deal with their parent's behavior "under the influence." Through these subtle and not-so-subtle, covert and overt interactions, codependency and addictive family systems are created (Bepko & Krestan, 1985; Berenson, 1975; Black, 2001; Elkin, 1984; Jackson, 1954; Johnson, 1990; Kaufmann, 1985; McIntyre & Hawley, 1998; Stanton, Todd, & Associates, 1982; Steinglass, Bennett, Wolin, & Reiss, 1987; Straussner, Weinstein, & Hernandez, 1979; Treadway, 1989; Wegscheider-Cruse, 1989).

This chapter provides an overview of the role of addictions in the family process. It describes how addictions to alcohol and other drugs alter

237

family members' interpersonal behaviors and their beliefs about themselves and discusses the factors that are important to include in the assessment and treatment of families with substance-abusing members.

AN OVERVIEW OF THE CHEMICALLY
DEPENDENT FAMILY PROCESS

Substance abuse can serve two different functions: (1) It can be a primary problem that is causing difficulties and conflicts for the individual and the family, and (2) it can also be a symptom of underlying, unmet needs, undeveloped life skills, and unresolved life issues that the substance abuser and her or his family are attempting to take care of through the use of the substance(s). In this systemic view a presenting problem—in this case, one family member's addiction—is understood to be both an attempt by family members to deal with life's needs and challenges and a serious problem for the individual family member (Lankton, Lankton, & Matthews, 1991; McIntyre & Hawley, 1998; D. Treadway, personal communication, June 1980; 1989). For example, the use of a substance can help a person express intimate feelings, such as tenderness and affection or engage sexually; or it can help the person handle conflict and anger by relieving the fear and anxiety about the expression of such emotions. Paradoxically, in relieving or compensating for specific needs or feelings, the substance may also increase them, enhancing or exaggerating the experience of the need because it goes unmet or unsatisfied, blocked by the numbing, analgesic effects of the substance.

The use of a substance also may help a person maintain interpersonal boundaries and experience a temporary sense of self-esteem, power, and self-confidence. Drinking or drugging after work may be a way to relieve stress, to mark a boundary between the day's work and going home, to bond a couple through the ritual use of a substance, or to cope with the anxiety evoked by the intimacy and confusing complexity of family life. Simultaneously, the mood-altering substance may be a way to satisfy the tolerance and craving that is increasingly regulated by the abuser's brain biochemistry in combination with psychological and interpersonal factors (Brick & Erickson, 1998; DuPont, 1997; Ketcham & Asbury, 2000). Over time, alcohol and other drugs are used to solve the problems arising from life, as well as the problems arising from their increasing psychophysiological dependency. What begins as compensatory and pleasurable coping behavior eventually alters an entire family system into one that is regulated by mood-altering chemicals, out-of-control emotional reactions, and powerful feelings of guilt, fear, shame, and despair. This systemic or coevolutionary process eventually involves not only everyone in the nuclear family but also members of the extended family, coworkers, and other people who are involved with various members of the family (Brown & Lewis, 1999; McIntyre & Hawley, 1998; Steinglass et al., 1987).

It is important to remember that few people set out deliberately to develop an addiction or to be a member of a chemically dependent family system. There is not one type or class of family that is more likely to develop an addiction. The impact of chemical dependency on the family usually develops indirectly and insidiously, and the damages from repeated incidents of substance abuse are profound and long-lasting (Brown & Lewis, 1999; Cork, 1969; Jackson, 1954; Straussner et al., 1979).

While intoxicated, in a "wet" state, addicted family members may feel permission, or become habituated, to behave in ways unacceptable to them when sober, or in a "dry" state (Berenson, 1976). Alcohol and other drugs disinhibit cognitive attitudes and beliefs as well as emotional references (i.e., learned experiences that control behavior), giving people a false sense of inflated powers. For example, a person might be more assertive, aggressive, or sexual when drinking or using drugs than when sober. The abuse of alcohol and other drugs disinhibits people in the family system and allows them to behave in new, usually irresponsible, ways. The alcohol or drugs enable the user, the spouse, and/or the children to use the effect of the substances as a cue or trigger to act out, rather than talk out, what they want and need from one another. This pattern results in the development of a limited range of learned responses, family role expectations, beliefs, and "rules" that regulate communications (Berenson, 1992; Black, 2001; Steinglass et al., 1987; Wegscheider-Cruse, 1989).

The family evolves interpersonal processes without responsible negotiation or mutuality, resulting in "power without responsibility" (Elkin, 1984). Communications and responsibility for actions become confused or even lost in an atmosphere of accusations and defensive responses. Trust is destroyed. Without realizing it, family members become dependent on the person's drinking or drug use to say and do things they might not otherwise say or do. The teenage daughter may stay out much later than expected because she knows Mom is home drunk and Dad works late to avoid dealing with his wife's developing addiction. Expectations that family members have of one another to behave in certain ways rigidify "under the influence" into emotional overfunctioning (the codependent members) and underfunctioning (the substance-abusing member), leading to an increasing experience of false and inflated pride in different ways of coping in each family member that defends against feelings of failure (Bepko & Krestan, 1985). Substance abusers may attempt to escape or find relief from their own rigid expectations or the expectations they imagine others have of them. Family members can become as "intoxicated" in their emotional reactivity as the chemically dependent member is in his or her drinking or drug use (Brown, 1988, 1995; Cermack, 1986; McIntyre & Hawley, 1998; Subby & Friel, 1982; Treadway, 1989; Wegscheider-Cruse, 1989).

An adolescent son, for example, may feel hurt about his father's drinking and then act out the anger for other family members, especially his mother. While raging at his father, he finds that his mother quiets him down and indirectly praises him by being oversolicitous or soothing. Without realizing it, the son becomes "intoxicated" by his anger, feeling both pumped up with the adrenaline rush that the anger provides and from the special attention that he is given. He receives positive feedback from his mother, and possibly a sibling or two, for standing up to Dad, which validates him and sanctions his anger in the future. In the same situation, hearing the shouting, other siblings may withdraw into a web of secret fantasies in which they are powerful and "intoxicated" (simultaneously frightened and soothed) in a magical safety they create in their bedroom.

Recursive communication patterns become established. For example, the communications expressed in intoxicated states, even though they might have some truth in them, are split off and defined as less valid by family members than the communications of the sober state. Family members do not take the chemically dependent person's intoxicated communications seriously ("Oh, Dad [or Mom] has just been drinking again"). Paradoxically, this virtual dismissal reinforces the substance abuser's sense of frustration and powerlessness and ensures further use of drugs or alcohol in order to feel "powerful" enough to deliver his or her communication another time (Elkin, 1984; Steinglass et al., 1987). Subsequently, they use drugs or alcohol in order to feel more powerful and more assertive, while the family listens even less and takes the intoxicated communication less seriously. Thus the family's communication in wet states becomes "crazier and crazier," with random declarations, promises, attacks and counterattacks; despair and despondency become "the norm." As a person's addiction and his or her partner's, or parent's emotional responses (e.g., lectures, nagging, anger, despair, sadness) grow more out-of-control in tandem, the family becomes locked into predictable patterns of ineffectively communicating needs and affects. Interactions become simultaneously more exaggerated and constricted, limited to a narrow range of feelings such as sadness, anger, disappointment, frustration, and failure. Contradictions in communication, confusion, and other complicated negative emotional processes take over the cognitive, emotional, interactive, and spiritual life of the family. Shame, fear, and disbelief in people's reliability to do what they say they will do become the normative ground of family life (Fossum & Mason, 1989).

THE PROCESS OF RECOVERY

Recovery is a process with somewhat predictable phases for both the substance abuser and the family, with developmental tasks for the family to learn and master in each phase of recovery (Berenson, 1992; Brown & Lewis, 1999; Horberg & Schlesinger, 1992; McIntyre & Hawley, 1998; D. Treadway, personal communication, June 1980; 1989). However, it is important to view each family's way of handling each stage of recovery as unique, with both the family as a whole and each family member having his or her own psychological and developmental needs. Some families do not follow the phases as described here, whereas others follow them quite predictably. Some families pass through them quickly, others slowly. Issues that are part of the recovery process, such as developing a new identity as a recovering person (Brown, 1985, 1995; Brown & Lewis, 1999), may overlap with the developmental issues that are inherent in the family life cycle, such as parents having to redefine their roles as their children leave home (Carter & McGoldrick, 1998).

The first phase, known as *early recovery* or the transition stage, takes place over the first year or two of recovery. It is marked by the restabilization of biological, psychological, and interpersonal systems that have been disrupted or destroyed over the years. During early recovery, family members need to reestablish relationships and develop trust without the interference of alcohol or drugs. It is important to identify and understand the emotional and interpersonal needs the use of the substance met for the chemically dependent person as well as the whole family. What have family members been able to access through the substance use that they could not meet or satisfy otherwise?

Because this phase involves the transition to new ways of relating, it is painful; there is a profound sense of "groundlessness" and emptiness, of not knowing what to expect (Berenson, 1992). Former patterns of drinking and drugging, which were once reliable and predictable, have disappeared, destabilizing the couple and the family in a variety of new ways. It is a period that has been referred to as "the crisis" (Straussner et al., 1979) or "the trauma" (Brown, 1991, 1995) of recovery and can be as unpredictable and difficult as the earlier years when the addiction was developing (Brown & Lewis, 1999).

The period of *middle recovery* usually ranges from the third to the fifth year. During this phase, some recovering individuals may find themselves increasingly focused on issues of family life, work, and the world around them. Many hope that any underlying problems in the marriage and the family will just evaporate. If acceptable changes do not occur, families may then bring their problems to a therapist. Often they present problems involving symptomatic behavior(s) (e.g., an affair, the development of phobias, eating disorders, behavioral disorders, psychosomatic disorders) with little or no awareness that the recovery from the drinking or drugging is part of the problem. Children may begin to act out or express negative feelings either because they are fed up with their parents' lack of change or because they finally trust the recovering person to handle their feelings.

Their acting out may serve a protective function that brings the family together to address the fears and anxieties that are simmering under the surface (Madanes, 1984).

The fourth or fifth year begins the third phase (Berenson, 1992) of *ongoing recovery* for couples and families (Brown & Lewis, 1999). This phase may bring up a variety of spiritual, philosophical, or value issues. It may include a desire to find a way to express feelings of gratitude for having a chance to live and enjoy life. A recovering person may create ways to be more involved in service to other recovering people. Others in the family may want to be of service to the community. A desire to have more meaningful and intimate relationships within the family may emerge. During this phase, the family is challenged to create an environment in which individual identity and gender and social role expectations are differentiated and supported. Often this task involves developing or expanding a capacity for an "enjoyment in living" and an enjoyment of the process of change as an expected part of life (Lankton & Lankton, 1986; Lankton et al., 1991).

BASIC ISSUES IN ASSESSMENT

Individuals or families requesting treatment present their substance abuse problems either directly or indirectly (D. Treadway, personal communication, June 1980; 1989). In the direct approach the adult requests help with his or her substance use disorder, codependency, or problems attributed to being raised in a chemically dependent family; or help with the drinking or drugging of a spouse/partner, child, or parent. Indirect requests are made by people who do not, or only minimally, connect their problems to the impact of their own or a family member's substance abuse. The indirect requests may come in the form of problems such as depression, the emotional unpredictability of a partner, phobias, specific or generalized anxieties, violence, psychosomatic disorders, marriage/relationship difficulties, or problems with children (e.g., depression, attention-deficit/hyperactivity disorder [ADHD], behavioral misconduct). In these indirect presentations of the addiction, they present the usual issues people present to social workers and family therapists without any reference or connection to the substance abuse. The therapist has to make that connection.

During assessment, a clinician needs to discern the way in which the family is presenting their problems and to begin to create appropriate treatment plans and interventions. To confront an indirect presentation of an addiction problem directly, by being either too "educational" or too confrontational, is to risk creating an unnecessary conflict with the family. The therapist's responsibility is to work diligently to help the family solve their presenting problem(s), using the developing trust the family places in the therapy to begin to discuss how the alcohol or drug use is interfering with the family's effectiveness at solving the presenting problem.

Since a clinician usually receives a request for treatment from one member of a family, the first consideration is how to involve all family members in the assessment and treatment process. A simple strategy is to suggest that the individual invite other family members to attend the first session in order to help create a more comprehensive picture of the family members and how they are working to solve the presenting problem. This is known as the system-building stage (D. Treadway, personal communication, June 1980). How the steps of this stage are accomplished—who first requests help and what he or she has to do and say to get other family members to come to the therapy—provides the therapist with initial assessment data. As other members of the family attend therapy, the therapist focuses on the presenting issues and the interactional and emotional dynamics of the family that are contributing to the creation of the presenting problem.

Children are profoundly affected by parental addictions because of the unpredictability of the behavior of both parents (Black, 2001; Cork, 1969; Moe, 1998; Seixas & Youcha, 1985; Wegscheider-Cruse, 1989). Assessment, therefore, must include a careful evaluation of the children's experience (Hawley & Brown, 1981; Moe, 1998; Zilbach, 1986) and should be presented to parents as a routine component of the assessment process.

It is important to focus on the severity and function of the addiction for the substance-abusing person, for individual family members, and for the family as a whole. In assessing the severity of the impact of the addiction, it is important to determine whether the chemically dependent family member needs be detoxified under medical supervision or can stop using a substance on his or her own. If the substance abuser experiences physiological withdrawal, either inpatient or outpatient medical care will be necessary and should be encouraged. All family members need to be assessed for emotional and behavioral problems, including depression, suicidality, ADHD or ADD (attention-deficit disorder), severe anxiety, and physical or sexual abuse. The assessment process helps the family and the therapist identify the co-evolutionary issues that will need to be addressed during treatment. An effective assessment helps the family begin to develop a narrative of being "in charge" by describing what they experience during the "dry" and "wet" phases of the addiction. Validating family members' stories and connecting the development of problems in the family to development of the addiction problems may naturalize and relieve some of their shame, as well as open them to the possibility of taking charge of their own actions and doing something about the problems, rather than letting the problems control them.

Family assessment also needs to identify the psychological, attitudinal, and behavioral skills the family will need to develop in order to support their substance-free existence (Roberts & McCrady, 2003). The therapist should examine such areas as life-cycle stages, the self in the family system, family-of-origin issues, social and community networks, and communication and emotional processes (S. R. Lankton, personal communication, February 1982; McIntyre, 1981–1992; McIntyre & Hawley, 1998). Such data will aid in formulating goals and protocols for treatment, in making a differential diagnosis, and in distinguishing the effects of the addiction from other developmental issues that need attention (D. Treadway, personal communication, June 1980; 1989). During the assessment process, it is also important to note and acknowledge the capacities, strengths, and resilience family members have developed in response to the chemical dependency (Jacobs & Wolin, 1991; McIntyre & Hawley, 1998; Treadway, 1989).

TREATMENT

Organizing a Treatment Plan

The goal of treatment planning is to produce change; it is a process of interaction between a therapist, or a treatment team, and a family to produce this change. Studies of addiction treatment for individuals (Hester & Miller, 1989) show that plans that are adapted to each person are more effective than generic programming. Similarly, each family needs to be seen as unique, and treatment plans need to be adapted to each family. The therapist focuses on influencing and persuading individual family members and the family as a whole to alter beliefs, behaviors, ways of interacting and communicating, and ways of perceiving and experiencing one another. The goal is to shift specific family interactional patterns, as well as the narrative or story that family members present about their interactions and their problems (Diamond, 2000; M. White, personal communication, June 1994; White & Epston, 1990). An exchange takes place between the way family members present their pain and the way a therapist helps them reframe and transform the pain, utilizing their prior capacities, resources, and abilities to change and solve serious problems (Lankton & Lankton, 1983, 1986).

Contracting

The first step in treatment is to develop a contract with the family. This involves determining the goals of therapy. A family's stated goals—or the changes family members want to effect in their lives—become the primary focus of treatment. Based on the assessment, however, the therapist may have additional thoughts about changes that family members need to make. The therapist may suggest these changes directly, by presenting psychoeducational information or giving direct suggestions, or indirectly, through the use of stories and metaphors (Lankton & Lankton, 1986). The goals and ideas about desired changes must be reviewed throughout treatment to ensure that they are being addressed in a way that suits the family.

During the development of the therapy contract, it is important to communicate that therapy will enhance family members' capacity to experience choices about how they think, talk, and interact with each other, and how to work more effectively together as a family (Lankton & Lankton, 1983). Throughout the assessment and treatment process, the therapist has the right to request that family members do not use drugs or alcohol on the day of the session (or even throughout the whole treatment process).

Because families typically are experiencing immediate emotional and interpersonal pain, a directed, problem-solving approach is usually most effective (Berg & Miller, 1992; de Shazer, 1988, 1994; Grove & Haley, 1993; Haley, 1987; O'Hanlon & Weiner-Davis, 1989; Treadway, 1989). Families rarely seek help for underlying issues. It is useful for the therapist to think in terms of obtaining specific outcomes or solutions (Berg & Miller, 1992; de Shazer 1994; O'Hanlon & Weiner-Davis, 1989. It important to think in terms of steps that family members can take to realize doable actions connected to their goals (O'Hanlon & Weiner-Davis, 1989; Treadway, 1989). Accomplishment of specifically agreed-upon behaviors and action steps can be an effective way for family members to experience self-efficacy, one of the foundational stones of self-esteem. Collaborating with the family to create doable action steps cultivates trust and lays the groundwork for discussing the role drugs or alcohol plays in disrupting a family member's sense of self-efficacy if another member's drug or alcohol use interferes with the therapy.

Treating Direct Presentations

When a family directly seeks help for a substance abuse problem, the first order of business is to create a contract about intended goals. The family may or may not be seeking abstinence. If the severity of physiological dependency is unclear or the denial of substance abuse is strong, then the therapist may introduce a carefully structured, controlled substance use contract. Such a contract is an agreement to limit the use of the substance to a pattern of minimal, random, social use. The contract addresses both the psychological and physiological dependency. Randomizing the substance use allows the clinician join the substance abuser in denial, and helps the abuser determine whether he or she has a substance abuse problem. It is best to recommend that such controlled and randomized drinking or drugging be maintained for a minimum of 3 years to determine genuine remission from addiction. (Such a timeline is completely arbitrary, just as the timeline for cancer remission is completely arbitrary. One is in "remission" from cancer as long as no cancer returns, and one is remission from mood-altering substance addictions as long as no addiction to the substances returns.) Although the person needs to drink or drug in moderation for the rest of his or her life, most alcohol- or other drug-addicted people are comforted by thinking about a 3-year timeline than a notion of *forever*, which arouses more anxiety. Most substance-dependent individuals find it impossible to maintain a controlled use of substances beyond a few months, though some do hold out for as long as a year or two. For therapeutic effectiveness, the clinician may use a controlled drinking contract twice, accepting the person's rationalizations for the failure of the first effort and encouraging the person to try harder with the second effort.

After the failure of the second effort, the therapist is in a much stronger position to say, "I don't think the issue is your willpower or any external factor, but the fact that your central nervous system is addicted. The best choice you can make for yourself is abstinence." Or "Look, you've made a genuine effort, and I think your body is trying to tell you something: It's addicted to this substance and wants more, regardless of what your mind and ego are telling you. I think there is no choice here, for your sake and the sake of your family, but to begin to work on abstinence and accept the fact that you have an addiction." The challenge to the client is built into the process of the intervention; the therapist does not have to be overly confrontational. It also offers a way for the client to save face.

The family is included in this process when the therapist affirms and supports their skepticism and distrust that the substance abuser will succeed in developing control. The therapist frames such skepticism as a normal consequence of the fear and pain that they have already experienced. Encouraging family members to remain skeptical and distrustful is a way of affirming and respecting their fear and their reactions to the suggestion that the substance abuser attempt to abstain from drinking or drugging. The substance-abusing member is told to expect this skepticism and distrust. It is useful to have family members keep a log of the times they suspect drinking or drug use; such a task gives them a way to hold onto their distrust while simultaneously externalizing it, thereby making it easier to tolerate (White & Epston, 1990). They are encouraged to bring the log with them so their entries can be discussed. In the rare situations in which the substance abuser can return to controlled substance use, family members' fears, anxiety, hurt, and anger about the past can become a focus of treatment, as well as how members will handle their emotional interactions when no member is abusing substances.

The therapist needs to help family members, particularly the codependent members, begin a process of emotional separation from enmeshment with (desire to control) and reactiveness to (anger that they cannot control) the substance abuser and to begin work on their own development. The therapist supports the codependent members by letting them know that they have a right to make changes in their own lives, and by suggesting various support and/or educational groups and readings to focus on while the substance abuser works on his or her decision regarding abstinence. This may be the first time family members have worked on creating conscious (i.e., intentional) emotional separation and boundaries within the family.

Family Interventions

In order to get a family member to enter treatment for his or her addiction, the therapist may recommend a process known as a formal "Intervention" (capital "I"), which was developed by Dr. Vernon Johnson (1980, 1986, 1990). The purpose of the Intervention is to break through the substance abuser's denial and confront the person with "the facts" of how his or her use of drugs or alcohol is impairing his or her health and important family and work relationships. This model "brings the bottom up to the drinker rather than having them free-fall to bottom" (V. Johnson, personal communication, August 1978). Family therapists have adapted the Intervention process to align it with the principles of family systems therapy (Speare, 1999; D. Treadway, personal communication, June 1980).

A formal Intervention is a powerful action that unbalances the family from "the strange loops" (Tomm, 1988) of homeostasis that are established in "the wet/dry cycles" of the addiction (Berenson, 1976, 1992). The Johnson Institute Intervention model includes a clearly defined "bottom line," in which the substance abuser will face painful consequences if he or she does not follow the treatment recommendations. Such consequences may include the loss of contact with the family, the loss of the right to live at home, and/or the loss of his or her job. The Intervention process thus intentionally creates the crises that typically will occur over time, while still offering the support of the family (and the employer, if involved in the Intervention) *if* the substance abuser is willing to take the necessary steps toward recovery.

An Intervention requires a great deal of preparation and usually involves a high level of involvement on the part of the therapist to guide those preparations and help family members handle their anxiety as they approach "the day." Family members are coached to develop a script with an opening statement of how they care about the person and how they have seen the alcohol or drug use erode the relationship over time (Jay & Jay, 2000). In the second part a list is presented of specific incidents resulting from the substance abuse, with the date of the incident (or close approximation, e.g., fall of 1999); a description of the incident (e.g., a missed school play or game, an angry interchange about something incidental that became exaggerated); a statement of the emotional experience of the person (e.g., fear, shame, humiliation, disappointment, anger, sadness) in relation to the incident; and, finally, a connection between the incident, the alcohol or drug abuse, and a request that the person take action to become clean and sober.

In the data section on the narrative of incidents, the therapist helps a participant distinguish between single events and repeated ones. For example, if a parent repeatedly fails to show up for school or athletic events because he or she is drinking, the child can state that pattern in a summary statement rather than event by event; however, particularly notable events should be described individually. The important feature of the narrative is to demonstrate that the addiction has been interfering with the relationship for a long time. Finally, there is a closing statement, in which the family member restates what he or she cares for and likes about the person, reiterates how the alcohol or drugs has changed the person and damaged their relationship, then ends with a clear, strong request, again, that the person enter treatment for his or her addiction, get sober, and return to the family as a contributing member. Repetition by family members, emphasizing the seriousness of the situation and the key role the drug or alcohol abuse has played in altering their relationships, is central to the success of an Intervention.

Several preparatory steps are needed in order to create a successful Intervention. The first one is to help the family member who is initiating the therapy to gather the Intervention team (Jay & Jay, 2000). The therapist coaches the individual on how to make phone calls to ask significant people to participate in the Intervention. The second step is to have each individual talk about how the abuse of drugs and alcohol has affected his or her relationship with the chemically dependent person. In the preparation meetings, usually each person's story triggers the memories of other Intervention team members. It is common for suppressed memories of incidents—some painful, some hilarious—to surface. The third step is to work with the intensity of emotions that emerge—anger, humiliation, sadness, and anxiety—to help those who are anxious about confronting the substance abuser to focus their emotion into formulating clear and assertive statements requesting sobriety. If particularly painful memories begin to surface, such as those involving sexual or physical abuse, the therapist may need to see the person individually and create a treatment plan for him or her while continuing to keep the person engaged in the Intervention. The therapist helps the members of the Intervention team identify what they still like about the substance abuser and to separate the behaviors that occur under-the-influence from the individual as a person. The continuum of recovery for the substance abuser and the family is discussed as a vehicle for providing hope for the future.

It is important to have as many people present as possible for an Intervention—immediate and extended family members, family friends, colleagues or fellow employees, and even the employer (Jay & Jay, 2000; Johnson, 1990). Letters from people who cannot be present, including family members, friends, a family doctor or lawyer, can also be useful. Important family members or friends can be present via speakerphone, videotape, or even through computer video streaming.

The establishment of a bottom line is crucial to the success of an Intervention. Helping family members organize themselves to bring "the bottom line up" to the chemically dependent person sets limits and makes everyone feel more empowered. The bottom line has to be serious; it has to have the wholehearted commitment of the Intervention team members behind it. It is only used—and this has to be emphasized—to help the substance abuser take seriously the Intervention and the request to maintain sobriety.

Another important point is how to get the substance abuser to the Intervention location. It is often helpful for family members to state that they are seeking help to learn how to communicate more effectively with the substance abuser. The family members are coached to say that they have a serious problem with their inability to find the right way, the right words, or the right timing, to communicate their fears and concerns, and that they will invite the substance abuser to join them to discuss these issues after they have had a chance to prepare what they are going to say. If there is the possibility that the substance abuser may become violent, suicidal, or run away, then the preparatory meetings have to be kept secret and the Intervention is best done in the home of the family, often in the early morning before the individual has used alcohol or drugs. It is important to include children in the Intervention process, so that they understand that they did not do something wrong that caused the drinking or drugging. Furthermore, children's comments frequently become pivotal in persuading the substance abuser to enter treatment.

It is useful to offer the substance abuser a choice of two treatment facilities. In a situation without easy choices, this tactic gives him or her choices. It is important to emphasize that the substance abuser also can choose to continue to drink or use drugs, but he or she *will* suffer the consequences determined by the family. It is equally emphasized that family members have a right to end their involvement in supporting the substance abuse. This strategy is respectful of the user's "right to" feelings even as it undermines his or her drinking or drug use, paradoxically, by making it an intentional choice. The idea that he or she is making an intentional choice—actually choosing alcohol or drug use over his or her family and friends—has a tendency to intensify the person's embarrassment or shame, which usually increases their motivation to change.

The last issue is to help the family move beyond the Intervention itself. The therapist asks each member to imagine how the family, as a whole, and how each family member individually will be changed by the Intervention and the resulting abstinence. Since people tend to state things generally, such as "better communication," the therapist may need to coach family members to be more specific and detailed, even when they are feeling "drained" by having just completed Intervention preparation. The family also can be encouraged to make a "wish list" of all the things they have been wishing for in the last several years, and to note what actions they are going to take to begin making those things happen. The therapist may have to describe how individuals in other families have had to change during the recovery process, and what the first several years of recovery may look like (drawing on the work of Brown & Lewis, 2000). This process of working together to plan how the family may be changed provides hope and models family planning as an important aspect of recovery (D. Treadway, personal communication, June 1980). It also encourages family members to begin to take responsibility for what they will do for themselves, no matter what the chemically dependent person does.

Treating Indirect Presentations

The indirect presentation of substance abuse problems poses an interesting challenge to the clinician. Rarely can a problem that is presented indirectly be confronted openly during the beginning of therapy. Direct approaches to an indirect presentation of a drug and alcohol problem may reinforce denial, shame, and failure or drive the family away feeling misunderstood, disappointed, and angry. This is the kind of treatment situation that requires what Madanes (1984) and Haley (1987) refer to as "analogic treatment." The presenting problem is understood to be an analogy or metaphor for issues that are not being mentioned.

The therapist proceeds by treating the presenting problem while developing and creating strategies to work with his or her hunches or hypotheses about what is *not* being said. After obtaining sufficient data indicating that alcohol or drug use is interfering with the family's capacity to solve the presenting problem, or when a family member feels safe enough to mention substance abuse, the therapist may be able to bring up the issue indirectly in a story. The story could be about a different family that the therapist felt stumped about, until a member of that family told "an interesting story" about how scared and ashamed everyone was to talk about "some other problems." In working in the frame of embedded metaphors (i.e., a story), the therapist has to look carefully for nonverbal acknowledgments to those passages with which different family members seem to identify (Lankton & Lankton, 1983). It is important not to name the "other" problem but rather to "plant seeds," thus giving permission for family members to bring up other issues, letting them know they will be supported in an exploration of these other issues.

Some families may not walk through any of the doors the therapist opens to discuss the issues of addiction; they may threaten to leave therapy or begin to miss appointments when the therapist addresses the issue gently and indirectly. The therapist will then need to plant a few seeds for the future, so that family members will feel comfortable enough to return to therapy "if anything else comes up." The therapist also can send the family a carefully worded follow-up letter to let everyone know that something important was not addressed. In these communications (they also can be conveyed in a follow-up phone call), the therapist expresses respect for the successful way the family did address certain issues. The therapist also acknowledges that he or she knows there were other things that were not spoken about in the therapy. He or she encourages the family to *not* do anything about those issues until the family or individual members are ready to consider taking action on them. In the treatment of indirectly presented problems, therapy ought to help increase the family's sense of competence by affirming any changes family members make that may motivate them to seek treatment at another time (de Shazer, 1985).

Gender

The therapist needs to be sensitive to issues of gender. It is easy to be unconsciously empathic to one gender in ways that alienate the opposite gender (McGoldrick, Anderson, & Walsh, 1989), or to show bias to same-sex persons who demonstrate a specific role behavior. There is no formula for how to manage this issue; one simply has to pay attention, ask questions, observe what is going on, and listen to how people describe their gender- and social-role functioning when talking about themselves. As Bepko and Krestan (1985) have pointed out, the substance-abusing family is usually rigid in terms of gender role expectations of its members. The therapist can comment on such rigidity, framing things in ways that encourage the development of gender role flexibility for each partner.

Gender differences also may play a role in recovery. Whereas men may consider the development of addictions to be a natural part of participating in male culture, women are often more remorseful and more likely to be aware of the damaging impact of their behavior on their relationships (Straussner & Zelvin, 1997). They will generally have done more secret drinking or drugging and used more combinations of tranquilizers than men, which will leave them in a more depressed state for a longer period during the early recovery. Substance-abusing women often experience a lower sense of self-esteem and a greater sense of shame than men and may need more support to reestablish themselves in the family (L. Sanford, personal communication, March 2004).

Support Systems

It is helpful to have family members attend specialized treatment groups that focus on substance abuse while in family therapy. It is also helpful to have children attend appropriate groups (Hawley & Brown, 1981). In early recovery, the focus of family therapy may be limited to getting people to self-help meetings and working on improving communications skills. During this phase, family sessions, which may take place every 2–6 weeks in conjunction with attendance at support groups, are focused on specific behavioral steps each person needs to take to help the family remain substance free and rebuild trust. The longer the history of addiction and codependency, the greater need to emphasize the stabilization stage (O'Farrell, 1993). The family needs to be informed that complex interactive issues, conflicts, and old hurts will be explored or worked on later in therapy. The therapist can say, "Many families find this phase difficult because they want to clear everything up immediately, especially old hurts and anger, but they have to wait to just get used to one another clean and sober."

When family members are not willing to attend self-help groups or other specialized treatment programs, the therapist must be careful not to push them too hard to do so. It is advisable to take a supportive but skeptical position, stating that the work may be much harder without the help and support of others. The therapist may need to redefine the treatment goals into smaller steps to create the possibility of a positive outcome. One solution to one small problem will help the family build trust in the therapy process and contribute to members' trust in themselves and willingness to consider other suggestions made by the therapist.

Helping Children

Finding ways to include children of substance-abusing parents in treatment can be a challenge (Moe, 1998). Parents often deny that their behaviors have had any impact on their children. To overcome this resistance, therapists can tell parents that it is a routine part of the clinic's or the therapist's treatment procedures to include children in family treatment (Andreozzi, 1996; Zilbach, 1986). If the presenting problem is a child's behavior, it is useful to work with the parents to help them create a solution to it. The therapist also can look for opportunities to praise the parents for effective parenting, thus alleviating some of their fear and shame and rebonding the family in a way that is constructive and empowering. The therapist should refer a parent to a parenting education or support program when appropriate.

The therapist also can include children in a way that empowers them and helps the family: by enrolling them as "co-therapists" or "consultants" who can "help" the therapist understand which one of the parents will be more likely to implement a change the family has discussed. This reversal of hierarchy (Madanes, 1981) conforms to the way parents are already reversing the hierarchy by placing their children in parental roles. This procedure can be effective by adding some humor and consciousness to the process, detoxifying the shame the parents feel in using their children in those ways, building trust, and beginning to realign the hierarchy in an appropriate structure. This approach can be used only when it is clear that no emotional or physical retribution will be directed at the children once the family is out of the office.

Addressing Physical and Sexual Abuse

Issues of physical and sexual abuse, whether child or adult, have to be addressed directly. Children's safety is of the utmost importance. In reporting the family to the child protection authorities, a therapist may have to take a "bad cop–good cop" position, making the state regulations the bad cop and the clinician the good cop who "hates to do this." The clinician must emphasize to the authorities that the family is seeking help, which is a positive step, and, of course, the family must be encouraged to stay in treatment. This is especially important for spouses who feel shame if they have failed to protect their children. In cases of domestic violence, the therapist has to help the family members feel safe—for example, by involving other family members whose presence may reduce or prevent the violence. Furthermore, the therapist should help children and spouses begin treatment in appropriate programs and therapy groups that address issues of violence and abuse. The therapist may recommend separate residence for some family members while continuing family therapy and working on such issues as safety, boundaries, apologies, and forgiveness. The person who has been doing the physical and/or sexual abuse may have to be separated from the family for his or her safety as well as the safety of the family. The clinician has to help the family stop the violence, work with the trauma, and work through what the violence has meant in the family. This may take a great deal of collaborative work and may involve regular contact with other therapists. It may require careful treatment planning for the family as a whole to work through the trauma, and for the member(s) who were abused to forgive the abuser(s) (Dolan, 1991; Haley & Madanes, 1986; Herman, 1997; Madanes, 1990; Miller & Guidry, 2001).

Addressing Distrust within the Family

Clinicians can include the existing distrust as a part of therapy by describing it as a normal aspect of the beginning phases of recovery. The therapist might state: "You ought not to expect to trust one another too much or too soon. It is natural for people not to trust one another after they have been through a painful time, the way you have been. What is really going to matter here is the way you begin to treat one another in this family." Using the concept of congruency, the therapist teaches the family that trust is built not only with words but also with actions.

A useful intervention is to assign "distrust days" that are marked on a calendar, and to ask members to keep anger and hurt journals. "Distrust days" can be every second, third, or fourth day. The therapist tells the family to work seriously at distrusting one another on such days, while working on trust the other days. Members are directed to examine carefully which they like better. All family members are given permission, indeed encouraged, to swear under their breath, to think all sorts of angry, hurt, sad, and distrustful thoughts, and to do a complete review of the past on the distrust days. Such an approach acknowledges what will happen anyway (this is one kind of paradoxical intervention) but brings it under therapeutic control and, more often than not, gives an edge of playfulness to a process that would otherwise be covert and quite painful. It also validates family members' experiences of hurt and anger, increases self-esteem, and decreases shame and guilt by making negative feelings acceptable. The therapist may have to say something seemingly absurd, such as "Look, you and I both know you're feeling all this distrust anyway, so I want you to practice it and get good at it; I don't believe anybody should do anything in a halfhearted way." Sometimes this approach undermines the family members' distrust of one another and bonds them together against the intrusive "outsider" with these strange ideas. Rather than being "fooled" by this pseudo-closeness of the family and their "rejection" of the "outsider," the therapist points to the closeness as progress and builds on it by having the whole family, or dyads, do something together. Such activities can include going to the movies or sports events, shopping, taking a walk or a hike, doing projects around the house, and so forth—thus building on and maintaining the closeness between sessions.

Addressing Communication Issues

Substance-abusing families invariably need help in developing communication skills. The therapist may need to create experiential exercises that help family members understand the behaviors of effective communication, such as speaking in "I" terms. They may need to learn the difference between report and command communication, learn how to change questions that are hidden statements into statements of "I want," "I need," or "I would appreciate it if . . . " For example, the therapist can direct the family to talk with one another for 15 minutes each, or every other, night. During a family communication session, members are expected to report on their day without saying anything confrontative to the other person. They are to speak only about their experience of the day. The therapist has to help the family feel comfortable with the difference between *report* communication, which is often unfamiliar to them, and the more familiar experience of either *command* communication or cold, stony silence. A couple communication training group can be effective in helping the adults learn these skills; then they can role model them for their children and enhance their capacity as parents to establish trust and cooperative, clear communications (McIntyre & Hawley, 1998; O'Farrell, 1993).

Generally family members use "you" terms to project many of their thoughts and feelings onto other family members. Learning to speak directly in "I" terms and in nonmanipulative direct request statements, instead of ones that are veiled as questions, can be awkward for some individuals who grew up in a family in which members spoke to one another indirectly. People from cultural heritages in which speaking in "I" terms is considered impolite may be told that such ways of speaking help the other person, who will then know they are speaking about themselves and not suspect them of being self-centered. For people who are bitter and use "you" phrasing to attack, the therapist can explain that by thinking about "you" all the time, they are projecting all their power to determine their own experience onto the other person, which leads to even greater feelings of disappointment, fear, and frustration.

Conflict Management

Most chemically dependent families do not know how to negotiate their needs or communicate their disappointment or anger without ending up in "a fight." Often the basic rules of conflict management have to be explained and practiced during a therapy session (Bach & Wyclen, 1968; Fisher & Ury, 1991; McIntyre & Hawley, 1998; Stone, Patton, & Heen, 1999). Family members need to learn how to say what they are feeling without raising their voices in anger, and how to think about what they are wanting and needing. They usually have to learn to express and describe the needs that they want to have met in specific, behavioral terms: What behavior or attitude are they wanting to get from another family member during their interactions? It is important that the description be specific and needs-based, not moralistic or vague.

Most family members in early recovery fail to reassure one another that they are willing to try to work things out; the absence of such reassurance provokes feelings of abandonment, fear, failure, and shame. From the viewpoint of the family's experience, anger and conflict are often associated with a "wet," intoxicated state, because in the past, the substance abuser expressed angry, conflicted feelings only when high or drunk. During treatment, discussion of conflictive situations may evoke painful memories (Brown & Lewis, 1999). In worst-case scenarios, the angry feelings can provoke an emotional state in substance abusers known as a "dry drunk"—a state in which they feel intoxicated or are as emotionally negative as when they are drunk or drugged, even though they have no substance in their systems. These issues can be anticipated in the treatment planning by utilizing relapse prevention planning (Daley, 1989; Gorski,

1997; Marlatt & Gordon, 1985; Gray & Gibson, Chapter 7, this volume) so that each family member will have specific guidelines for how to behave if such situations begin to occur.

Working on New Behaviors

The therapist has to follow up with family members about how they did in practicing new behaviors they agreed to try out between sessions. An effective frame for such discussion is to tell family members that they are expected to do only "a little right" and to be sure to make a few mistakes. This instruction can help alleviate some of the self-consciousness family members may experience in trying out new behaviors. Since promises to change have usually been made and repeatedly broken in the past, it is helpful to encourage the family to have low expectations and to take things in small steps. In conjunction with the distrust and conflict management work of early recovery, the therapist can encourage family members to observe one another's mistakes but not to say anything. They are to use their desire to criticize other family members as inspiration "to do their own behavior all that much better." Or, using a journal, they can write down all their criticisms and bring them to therapy, where the therapist will read them later, saying to the family member: "I'll keep these till the end of therapy. Then we'll go over what has and hasn't changed, and what concerns are still true for you. They may even be a good reference to see how far things have come." Such an approach introduces hope by suggesting that there will be a future in which these issues are no longer a problem; it also offers family members a safe place to contain and "leave" the criticism and anger. In addition, it uses feelings of competition and distrust to solve two problems simultaneously: It "captures" the capacity for disappointment, anger, and criticism, and it alleviates the shame attached to experiencing the competition and the desire to criticize by describing it and turning it into a more focused attention to self-process and self-development. Letter writing—describing hopes, fears, expectations, needs, and wants in a reflective way that allows other family members to read and consider them reflectively—is another effective way to slow down process, to encourage reflective consciousness and better boundaries, and to give people more chances to respond in nonreactive ways.

During recovery, there are many new beliefs and behaviors to learn and developmental tasks to accomplish (Brown & Lewis, 1999; Clemmons, 1997; Horberg & Schlesinger, 1992; Ketcham & Asbury, 2000). Both the recovering person and the family members may feed overwhelmed. It is useful to describe the possibilities of recovery to the family, the phases of recovery, and the attitudes and tasks they may want to become interested in learning. The therapist can integrate the stories they are hearing in AA and Al-Anon with the ideas of family therapy, inviting family members to "plan, not project," as they say in the 12-step traditions, what they imagine lies ahead in the next month, the next season, or the next year. This becomes a form of relapse prevention planning by helping members anticipate change and the future. The therapist can invite families to *plan* their future, rather than having the future "happen" to them. The therapist functions as a coach, a planner, an "inviter," and an educator.

The therapist may wish to create experiential exercises that involve directed practice of new behaviors, role playing, letterwriting, and storytelling/metaphor work (Combs & Freedman, 1990; Diamond, 2000; Lankton & Lankton, 1986, 1989; Lovern, 1991). Because family members frequently have no internal references or role models for the suggested behaviors, the therapist may need to be directive (Haley, 1987; Madanes, 1981, 1984), giving specific and detailed instructions for the development of behaviors, cognitive frameworks (beliefs), and affective experiences that will aid family members in accomplishing particular "homework" exercises. The role play in the office helps family members anchor each suggested behavior with an image. For example, instead of having a father and a daughter snarl at each other when Dad arrives home, the therapist may ask the dad and the daughter to teach each other how they want to be spoken to, including voice tone, facial expression, and degree of physical closeness (boundaries). The therapist usually has to comment on the self-consciousness people feel about acting out what they want and help them relax with it. Once again, the therapist prescribes the distrust, predicting its presence and diffusing its impact. Indirectly, the therapist also nurtures, or reparents, the parents by instructing them in how to display a friendly and supportive manner that may be dramatically different from the disrespectful, authoritarian, and even abusive ("Just do it!") way *their* parents treated them. Storytelling is also effective because it allows the therapist to instruct family members in a nonthreatening way (Combs & Freedman, 1990; Lankton & Lankton, 1989). The therapist describes how other families made similar changes, or even made other changes, they were not expecting to make.

During each session, it is important to (1) include everyone who attends, (2) review how they are doing, (3) determine what they think about what is going on, and (4) find a way to connect each person's experience to the experience of the family as a whole. The therapist role models the process of inclusion and fairness, which are usually new values and behaviors. Family members should be supported to do no more than they feel ready to do, and they usually have to be directed in how to set boundaries and limits by asserting "I've had enough" or "No, I won't do that." Addiction could be called the "disease of too-high expectations"; helping people understand their limits helps them understand new ways to manage disappointment, which is the emotional by-product of expectations that are too high or too numerous. The therapist has to help family members learn how to lower and moderate their expectations.

Affirmation, appreciation, apology, and forgiveness are new behaviors and attitudes for a substance-abusing family and will take much practice, because family members will have accumulated much cynicism and bitterness by the time they have come in for therapy. It is important to discuss, in a friendly way, how family members will forget, for example, to demonstrate affection and appreciation after they have worked on learning appropriately affectionate and tender behaviors. This forgetting validates family members' worst fear—that the affection will disappear—and makes that fear more acceptable by encouraging them to expect mistakes. With a sense of humor and empathy, it is useful to reiterate how the men will forget, how the women will be lying in wait for the men to forget, and how the children are already convinced that both parents will fail to "get it right."

Providing an ample supply of affirming, noncondescending praise of every effort to change is important. Given the exaggerated, defensive, and false pride of many substance abusers and substance-abusing families, it is useful to remind people not to take one another for granted. Individuals may need to be coached to apologize when they make mistakes, and to learn to say "thank you" for the positive steps any family members take toward change. It is valuable to prepare a family or a couple for the self-conscious intention and practice these new behaviors require. Analogies to how we learned to walk or ride a bike, back in the days when we were not so self-conscious, are sometimes helpful. Such preparation helps to lower anxiety about self-consciousness and feelings of embarrassment and increases members' tolerance for the effort and resiliency that are required in order to make important changes.

One final—and crucial—new behavior to work on in early recovery is relapse prevention planning for the recovering chemically dependent person and the spouse or partner. Relapse prevention planning involves identifying all the possible events and activities that could trigger the desire to use drugs or drink alcohol (Black, 2000; Daley, 1989; Gorski, 1997; Marlatt & Gordon, 1985). Although there is little literature on relapse prevention planning for family members, the literature written for the recovering alcohol- or drug-addicted person can be applied in principle to the whole family. Each person in the family can contribute ideas about what may trigger substance abuse for the recovering member and trigger increased anxiety and fear for the family members. It is important to assess possible tensions or conflicts around important family events, such as weddings, births, graduations, deaths, or anticipated deaths, and the "unfinished emotional business" among members of different generations (e.g., hurts, resentments, grudges) that may be triggered at those events. The therapist can help family members understand the pain of past events and actively prepare them for upcoming events by identifying the specific attitudes and behaviors that have to be changed to successfully handle these situations. Relapse prevention planning helps the family develop awareness about possibly stressful events and create plans of action to handle those events, an important protocol for all areas of their life for many years to come.

Completing the Contract

The termination of family therapy can be accomplished simply and gracefully when the therapist and the family agree that the work they contracted to do has been completed. If the therapist has reviewed successes and praised the family's accomplishments throughout the therapy, there is little need to do more than reiterate some of the praise and affirmation as part of the goodbye. Some families like to create a ritual as a formal way of symbolizing the end of the work; a review of everything that was and was not accomplished and a formal, solemn goodbye handshake may be part of it. Some families just like to say a quick "Thank you and goodbye." The termination generally should be consistent with the family's social conduct in the therapy.

It is useful to let family members know that if they want to come back, they can. Or, as is done in the Milwaukee Brief Therapy Project (de Shazer, 1990), if they do call back, the therapist can review with them what they might be forgetting to do so that they can remember to do it and stay out of therapy (Berg & Miller, 1992; de Shazer, 1990). This approach often adds a touch of humor and supports the family in remembering that they are now empowered to help themselves. Another way to terminate with families that have had difficulty in learning new behaviors is to suggest playfully, but seriously, that they go home and plan the many ways that they can forget their new behaviors and attitudes. This paradoxical intervention, with its pretending, playful qualities, also can be done in a closing session to block the denial of remembering their commitments to each other.

Another useful way to terminate is to have the clients go home and do a "remember when" or "remember how bad it was" exercise, either writing it down or tape-recording it. Family members are directed to be sure that they become as sad as they can, "and to be sure [they] go over every painful memory to make sure [they] have forgiven each other in proper proportion to the pain [they] experienced." This exercise is particularly useful with families that experienced violence, abuse, and severe shaming behaviors. It may help clear out vestiges of shame and grief, completes the grieving process, creates a boundary with the past, and directs the family toward the future as part of the process of completing therapy. It is usually best for the therapist to have the family practice this in a "near-the-end" session, go home and do it there, then return to describe their experience and complete it in the last session in the safety of her or his office if that is necessary.

CONCLUSION

Families in which alcohol and drug addictions develop become systems that are bound in progressively debilitating processes of poor communication, power struggles, conflict, disorganization, and financial, social, and psychological chaos. These processes profoundly affect each family member and the family as a whole. An effective assessment and differential treatment plan are necessary to undertake this challenging and complex work, and aid in healing the wounds members experienced during the active phases of addiction. The essential components of support for the therapist as he or she helps the family include a willingness to revise and update the assessment to fit new information, a capacity for developing specific experiential exercises that help people learn new attitudes and behaviors, a sense of humor, a willingness to try something different and take creative risks, a willingness to listen carefully to what family members are saying about what is and is not working, a capacity to maintain healthy boundaries, a willingness to apologize for mistakes, a network of reliable colleagues to consult with, and a vision and a faith in the best that is possible in relationships. As Michael Elkin (personal communication, 1991) said, "We are often helped in our own growth by our families as much as we help them in theirs."

ACKNOWLEDGMENTS

The author wishes to thank Shulamith Straussner for her support and consistently good-natured feedback. The spirit of the process only enhanced the work of shaping the complex material of the chapter.

REFERENCES

Andreozzi, L. (1996). *Child-centered family therapy.* New York: Wiley.
Bach, G. R., & Wyclen, P. (1968). *How to fight fair in love and marriage.* New York: Avon.
Bepko, C., & Krestan, J. (1985). *The responsibility trap: A blueprint for treating the alcoholic family.* New York: Free Press.
Berenson, D. (1976). Alcohol and the family system. In P. Guerin (Ed.), *Family therapy: Theory and practice.* New York: Gardner.

Berenson, D. (1992). Interview: Dr. David Berenson, MD. *Family Dynamics of Addiction Quarterly*, 2(1), 1–8.

Berg, I., & Miller, S. (1992) *Working with the problem drinker: A solution focused approach*. New York: Norton.

Black, C. (2000). *A hole in the sidewalk: The recovering person's guide to relapse prevention*. Bainbridge Island, WA: MAC Publishing.

Black, C. (2001). *It'll never happen to me!* (2nd ed.). Bainbridge Island, WA: MAC Publishing.

Brick, J., & Erickson, C. K. (1998). *Drugs, the brain, and behavior: The pharmacology of abuse and dependence*. Binghamton, NY: Haworth Press.

Brown, S. (1985). *Treating the alcoholic*. New York: Wiley

Brown, S. (1988). *Treating adult children of alcoholics*. New York: Wiley.

Brown, S. (Ed.). (1995). *Treating alcoholism*. San Francisco: Jossey-Bass.

Brown, S., & Lewis, V. (1999). *The alcoholic family in recovery: A developmental model*. New York: Guilford Press.

Brown, S., & Lewis, V. (with Liotta, A.). (2000). *The family recovery guide: A map for healthy growth*. Oakland, CA: New Harbinger.

Carter, E., & McGoldrick, M. (Eds.). (1998). *The expanded family life cycle: Individual, family, and social perspectives*. Boston: Allyn & Bacon.

Cermack, T. (1986). *Diagnosing and treating codependence*. Minneapolis, MN: Johnson Institute.

Clemmons, M. C. (1997). *Getting beyond sobriety*. San Francisco: Jossey-Bass.

Combs, G., & Freedman, J. (1990). *Symbol, story, and ceremony: using metaphor in individual and family therapy*. New York: Norton.

Cork, R. M. (1969). *The forgotten children*. Toronto: Addictions Research Foundation.

Daley, D. C. (Ed.). (1989). *Relapse: Conceptual, research, and clinical perspectives*. Binghamton, NY: Haworth Press.

de Shazer, S. (1985). *Keys to solution in brief therapy*. New York: Norton.

de Shazer, S. (1988). *Clues: Investigating solutions in brief therapy*. New York: Norton.

de Shazer, S. (1990, October). *Brief therapy: Constructing solutions*. Seminar presentation at the annual conference of the American Association for Marriage and Family Therapy, Washington, DC.

de Shazer, S. (1994). *Words were originally magic*. New York: Norton.

Diamond, J. (2000). *Narrative means to sober ends: Treating addiction and its aftermath*. New York: Guilford Press.

Dolan, Y. M. (1991). *Resolving sexual abuse: Solution-focused therapy and Ericksonian hypnosis for adult survivors*. New York: Norton.

DuPont, R. L. (1997). *The selfish brain: Learning from addiction*. Washington, DC: American Psychiatric Press.

Elkin, M. (1984). *Families under the influence*. New York: Norton.

Fisher, R., & Ury, W. (1991). *Getting to yes: Negotiating agreement without giving in*. New York: Penguin.

Fossum, M., & Mason, M. (1989). *Facing shame: Families in recovery*. New York: Norton.

Gorski, T. (1997). *Passages through recovery: An action plan for prevention relapse*. Center City, MN: Hazelden Foundation.

Grove, D., & Haley, J. (1993). *Conversations on therapy*. New York: Norton.

Haley, J. (1987). *Problem solving therapy.* San Francisco: Jossey-Bass.

Hawley, N., & Brown, E. (1981). Children of alcoholics: The use of group treatment. *Social Casework, 62*(1), 40–46.

Herman, J. (1997). *Trauma and recovery.* New York: Basic Books.

Hester, R. K., & Miller, W. R. (Eds). (1989). *Handbook of alcoholism treatment approaches.* Elmsford, NY: Pergamon Press.

Horberg, L., & Schlesinger, S. (1992). Developmental tasks in family recovery from addictive disorders. *Family Dynamics of Addiction Quarterly, 2*(2), 46–60.

Jackson, J. (1954). The adjustment of the family to the crisis of alcoholism. *Quarterly Journal of Studies on Alcohol, 15*(4), 562–586.

Jacobs, J., & Wolin, S. J. (1991, March). *Resilient children growing up in alcoholic families.* Paper presented at the National Consensus Symposium on COAs and Codependence, Airlie, VA.

Jay, J., & Jay, D. A. (2000). *Love first: A new approach to intervention for alcoholism and drug addiction.* Center City, MN: Hazelden.

Johnson, V. (1980). *I'll quit tomorrow.* San Francisco: Harper & Row.

Johnson, V. (1986). *Intervention: How to help someone who doesn't want help.* Minneapolis, MN: Johnson Institute.

Johnson, V. (1990). *Everything you need to know about chemical dependence: Vernon Johnson's complete guide for families.* Minneapolis, MN: Johnson Institute.

Kaufman, E. (1985). *Substance abuse and family therapy.* New York: Grune & Stratton.

Ketcham, K., & Asbury, W. (2000). *Beyond the influence: Understanding and defeating alcoholism.* New York: Bantam Books.

Lankton, S. R., & Lankton, C. H. (1983). *The answer within: A clinical framework of Ericksonian hypnotherapy.* New York: Brunner/Mazel.

Lankton, S. R., & Lankton, C. H. (1986). *Enchantment and intervention in family therapy.* New York: Brunner/Mazel.

Lankton, C. H., & Lankton, S. R. (1989). *Tales of enchantment.* New York: Brunner/Mazel.

Lankton, S. R., Lankton, C. H., & Matthews, W. J. (1991). Ericksonian family therapy. In A. S. Gurman & D. P. Kniskern (Eds.), *Handbook of family therapy* (Vol. 2). New York: Brunner/Mazel.

Lovern, J. D. (1991). *Pathways to reality: Erickson-inspired treatment approaches to chemical dependency.* New York: Brunner/Mazel.

Madanes, C. (1981). *Strategic family therapy.* San Francisco: Jossey-Bass.

Madanes, C. (1984). *Behind the one way mirror: Advances in the practice of strategic therapy.* San Francisco: Jossey-Bass.

Madanes, C. (1990). *Sex, love, and violence: Strategies for transformation.* New York: Norton.

Marlatt, G. A., & Gordon, J. R. (Eds.). (1985). *Relapse prevention: Maintenance strategies in the treatment of addictive behaviors.* New York: Guilford Press.

McIntyre, J. (1981–1992). *Assessment approach developed for teaching the family therapy of addictions.* Cambridge, MA: Lesley University.

McIntyre, J., & Hawley, N. M. (1998). *The recovery of love: Treating couples in addiction* [Video]. Boston: NASW.

McGoldrick, M., Anderson, C., & Walsh, F. (1989). *Women in families: A framework for family therapy.* New York: Norton.

Miller, D., & Guidry, L. (2001). *Addictions and trauma recovery: Healing the body, mind, and spirit.* New York: Norton.

Moe, J. (1998). *The children's place: At the heart of recovery.* Tuscon, AZ: Sierra Tuscon Educational Press.

O'Farrell, T. J. (1993). *Treating alcohol problems: Marital and family interventions.* New York: Guilford Press.

O'Hanlon, W. H., & Weiner-Davis, M. (1989). *In search of solutions: A new direction in psychotherapy.* New York: Norton.

Roberts, L. J., & McCrady, B. S. (2003). *Alcohol problems in intimate relationships: Identification and intervention.* Washington, DC: National Institute on Alcohol Abuse and Alcoholism and National Institute on Drug Abuse.

Sanford, C. (2004, March). *The power of shame in addiction treatment.* Paper presented at the Harvard Medical School Symposium on Treating Addictions, Boston.

Seixas, J. S., & Youcha, G. (1985). *Children of alcoholism: A survivor's manual.* New York: Crown.

Stanton, M. D., Todd, T. C., & Associates. (1982). *The family therapy of drug abuse and addiction.* New York: Guilford Press.

Steinglass, P., Bennett, L., Wolin, S., & Reiss, D. (1987). *The alcoholic family.* New York: Basic Books.

Stone, D., Patton, B., & Heen, S. (1999). *Difficult conversations: How to discuss what matters most.* New York: Viking.

Straussner, S. L. A., Weinstein, D. L., & Hernandez, R. (1979). Effects of alcoholism on the family system. *Health and Social Work, 4*(4), 111–127.

Straussner, S. L. A., & Zelvin, E. (1997). *Gender and addictions: Men and women in treatment.* Northvale, NJ: Aronson.

Subby, R., & Friel, J. (1982). *Co-dependence.* Deerfield Beach, FL: Health Communications.

Tomm, K. (1988) Interventive interviewing: Part III. Intending to ask lineal, circular, strategic, or reflexive questions? *Family Process, 27*(1), 1–15.

Treadway, D. (1989). *Before it's too late: Working with substance abuse in the family.* New York: Norton.

Wegscheider-Cruse, S. (1989). *Another chance: Hope and health for the alcoholic family.* Palo Alto, CA: Science and Behavior Books.

White, M., & Epston, D. (1990). *Narrative means to therapeutic ends.* New York: Norton.

Zilbach, J. J. (1986). *Young children in family therapy.* New York: Brunner/Mazel.

CHAPTER 12

Treating the Partners of Substance Abusers

Elizabeth Zelvin

The spouses and partners of alcohol and drug abusers constitute an almost forgotten population in the treatment of alcohol and other drug (AOD) dependence. Traditionally, wives of men with alcoholic problems, in particular, were considered to have a preexisting pathology that led them to select an alcoholic partner and continue to derive secondary gains from his drinking. From the formation of Al-Anon in 1951 to the emergence of the concept of codependency in Minnesota in the early 1970s, attention was focused on the partner of the chemically dependent person as someone adversely affected by alcoholism or other addiction and in need of help. Before long, however, the term *codependent* was co-opted by the fast-growing movement of "adult children of alcoholics" and became synonymous with "adult child," whereas the spouse or partner became a less important figure in the burgeoning chemical dependency literature of the 1980s. A recent literature search yielded only a handful of new articles in 2002 and 2003 on spouses or partners of people with alcoholic or other kinds of substance problems in the United States, many of them focused specifically on domestic violence.

Although the necessity of arresting the enabling behavior of the spouse or partner is a given in addiction treatment, somehow the special plight of the wife, husband, or lover of the alcohol- or drug-abusing person as an individual with his or her own pain, concerns, and treatment needs has not elicited much interest in either the professional community or the recovery movement. This chapter discusses how the partner of the alcohol or other drug abuser is affected and addresses the treatment needs of this important but neglected population.

HOW THE PARTNER IS AFFECTED

Beliefs about how the spouse or partner is affected by chemical dependency have changed over the past few decades. Today we can make a distinction between *enabling*, the protective and controlling behaviors that inadvertently encourage the person to continue abusing substances, and *codependency*, a condition affecting the whole personality and all relationships that arises, in part, from living with a chemically dependent individual. This distinction can help partners detach from the pathological aspects of their relationships (Zelvin, 2002) and move toward recovery.

Myths

The traditional myth about the wives of alcoholic men was that they needed their husbands to go on drinking in order to meet their own neurotic needs. Many, including the wives themselves, believed that the men's drinking was all their fault. The alcoholic person's projection of blame onto his "controlling" partner and her acceptance of that blame was, and is, a key element in the denial system of the alcoholic or addicted relationship. Societal reinforcement of this assumption is evident in the traditional socialization of women to be loyal, accepting, and not overly assertive. Women, as those who carry the gifts and burdens of the relational aspects of culture (Miller, 1986), have traditionally been held responsible for the social and emotional deficiencies of men, especially their husbands and sons. (Husbands of alcoholic women were hardly supposed to exist, thanks to the myth that there were few alcoholic women.) Less obvious, perhaps, was the myth that the wives of alcoholic men were (1) saints who martyred themselves to their husbands' addiction; (2) did not lose their identity, self-esteem, or ability to function because of it; and (3) were able to adapt without much difficulty when their husbands got sober. This view is nowhere more evident than in the "Big Book" of Alcoholics Anonymous (Alcoholics Anonymous, 2001), first written almost 70 years ago, in which the earliest recovering alcoholic men recounted how they had disappointed and shamed their families and wives, who are depicted as long-suffering, flawless, and compassionate. It is well known that Lois W., the wife of the founder of Alcoholics Anonymous (AA), worked for years in a department store to support the fledgling fellowship, coming home to cook for a houseful of drunken "prospects" her husband had taken in, none of whom ever seemed to get sober (Alcoholics Anonymous, 1957)—a prime example of what we would now call enabling by both Lois and Bill W.

The wives of drug addicts seem not to have been mythologized in the same way, perhaps because professional attention focused mainly on the drug addict himself (and addicts were assumed to be male). The notion of the partners of AOD abusers as primary patients who could be helped professionally for their own sake was a product of the Minnesota model of chemical dependency, which was itself based on the 12-step self-help model of AA and Al-Anon (see Spiegel & Fewell, Chapter 6, this volume). This model suggested that AOD dependence, whether to alcohol, heroin, cocaine, or prescription pills, is a disease process requiring spiritual as well as physical and behavioral recovery—a view that is not shared by all substance abuse theoreticians and purveyors of treatment.

The still-evolving myth about partners of substance abusers as codependent contradicts the original mythology in some ways and paradoxically restates it in others. The notion of the spouse's preexisting neurosis was rejected by the family disease model, which acknowledged that living with an alcohol- or drug-addicted person caused significant damage to the partner's emotional, mental, physical, and social well-being. The family disease model also rejected the sainthood myth and acknowledged that a recovery process was necessary for the partner, even if the drinking stopped or the addict left. However, the codependency theorists of the 1980s attributed this condition to the dysfunctional family of origin, seeing the choice of an alcoholic or addicted partner as a reenactment of the preexisting family dysfunction. Only one of these theorists, Schaef (1986), gave due weight to the role of society in producing the addictive relational process and perpetuating codependency, pointing out that "the Ideal American Marriage [has] exactly the same elements as . . . an addictive relationship. . . . Neither partner can function without the other. The lives of the married couple are totally intertwined" (p. 35). Moreover, as pointed out by Zelvin (1988), "novels, theater, movies, and television support a view of the mutually dependent relationship characteristic of alcoholism as not dysfunctional but rather 'romantic' and desirable. . . . Alcoholism itself and its attendant codependency are often viewed in literature and the media as grand and tragic rather than pathological and treatable" (p. 101).

It is well documented that adult children of alcoholic persons, particularly women, tend to marry alcoholic people (Olmsted, Crowell, & Waters, 2003). However, Zelvin (1988) and Schutt (1985) both observed that not every codependent spouse comes from a dysfunctional family. The latter stated: "Some women come from functional families that were relatively happy and stress-free. Yet, if they too fall in love with an alcoholic, they are at risk for developing the dysfunctional behavior that characterizes codependent wives" (p. 9). She added that, given treatment, spouses with such a background may recover more rapidly than other codependents. It is noteworthy that Wegscheider-Cruse (1985) and Woititz (1983), advocating for the concepts of the dysfunctional family system and the adult child of alcoholic parents, became media stars, while Schutt, who was writing about wives at the same time and for the same publisher, did not. The myth that virtually all codependents come from dysfunctional families was reinforced by the powerful adult children of alcoholics (ACOA) movement. This myth still needs to be challenged in the interests of differential diagnosis, prognosis, and treatment of codependency and coaddiction, and also because society must, to some extent, be held accountable for this phenomenon (Zelvin, 1997).

As the myth of spousal sainthood was challenged by the myth of spousal neurosis, the myth of an almost universal codependency has been challenged by myths that, on the one hand, codependency does not exist, and that, on the other hand, it is a stigmatizing label that pathologizes and blames the victim of gender-based psychological or economic oppression (Miller, 1994). The ongoing debate about codependency has moved so far beyond its origins that it fails to focus on the significant others of chemically dependent persons as the key example of such victims.

Enabling

The term *enabling* is used to describe the ways the nonaddicted partner inadvertently perpetuates the drug or alcohol use. Partners of chemically dependent people have been stigmatized by the label of *enabler*. It is more accurate to talk about enabling as the partner's maladaptive behavior in relation to the loved one's addiction—and, by extension, to other dysfunctional family behaviors. For example, it is considered enabling for the partner to take over financial and organizational management of the family if the addict's role normally includes these duties. Such protective behaviors reinforce the AOD-dependent's denial by removing the consequences of his or her chemical abuse. Berating or reproaching the substance abuser also may be enabling. Scolding and accusations arouse the AOD user's remorse, guilt, and shame, and these uncomfortable feelings become an excuse to use chemicals. The user also deflects guilt by projecting blame onto the blaming partner. It is enabling to rescue an addicted person from the consequences of his or her addiction in any way; however, these consequences may appear terrifying to the person who loves the addict. For example, it is hard to refuse money to a loved one who claims that a drug dealer has threatened to break his legs if he does not pay his debts. It is also enabling to attempt to control the addicted person's behavior—for example, to pour liquor down the sink, measure the level in the bottle, or extract promises about whether or how much he or she will drink on a particular occasion. Such behaviors arouse defiance and opposition in the substance abuser, allow the abuser to project responsibility for the consequences onto the enabler, and reinforce the erroneous belief that the uncontrollable—the drug or alcohol dependence—can be controlled.

The Impact of Denial

If enabling is how the spouse or lover attempts to deal with the drinking or drugging, and codependency, at its most pathological, is considered a primary disorder that may result from social and developmental factors as well as the addictive relationship, then how the partner is *affected* by living with someone who is chemically dependent falls between these two extremes. It is all too easy to slip from acknowledging *enabling* as the partner's contribution to the systemic dysfunction to using it as a blaming label that, in effect, makes the nonaddicted partner responsible for the continuing chemical abuse. Without wanting to encourage the spouse to play the passive role of victim, we must remember that he or she is indeed a victim of the bizarre, irrational, and socially unacceptable behavior that can result from substance abuse. It must not be forgotten that the major symptom of chemical dependency is denial. Alcoholic or addicted individuals may deny (1) that they are drinking or using at all, (2) that they have problems at all, (3) that the chemicals have anything to do with the problems, or (4) that they are responsible for the problems. Nonaddicted partners also may (1) deny that the drinking or drugging is going on, (2) minimize its extent, (3) deny their problems as well as the addicted person's, (4) remain oblivious to the relationship between the substance abuse and their problems, or (5) deny that their own behavior has anything to do with the friction in the relationship. Both may deny the label *alcoholic* or *addict,* saying that the alcoholic person "just has a little drinking problem" or "likes his schnapps," that the addict uses cocaine or marijuana "recreationally," or that the daily Xanax or Percocet pill was prescribed by a doctor and is for the abuser's "nerves" or "pain."

As a result of all this denial, the partner gradually develops an unnaturally high tolerance for bizarre, irrational, and unacceptable behavior. Worse, he or she feels confused, fearful, guilty, angry, anxious, depressed, and often even "crazy." As Woititz put it: "You don't know what to believe or what to expect . . . your sense of what is real becomes distorted" (1979, p. 41). Woititz lists the end products of the disease progression for the partner as lethargy, hopelessness, self-pity, and despair. In order to hide the pain, shame, and despair, as well as to minimize the impact of the bizarre behavior on others, the partners isolate themselves. Potential sources of support and help, such as family, friends, and professionals, are cut off. Some marriages are characterized by rage, violence, and mutual recriminations; others bolster the mutual dependence with an image of the couple as "two against the world." Rothberg, looking at the couple from a systems perspective, points out: "People in an alcoholic dyad feel powerless . . . to control each other and are involved in a useless, exacerbating, roller-coaster-like attempt to achieve power and/or control" (1986, p. 73).

Sometimes partners turn to chemicals themselves in order to feel closer to the substance abusers, attempt to control them, or to sedate their own feelings. One wife pours wine from her husband's glass into her own at dinner parties to keep his intake down. Another, distressed by her husband's belligerence when drunk, encourages him to smoke marijuana because it "makes him more cheerful." She smokes along with him nightly, "keeping him company" and sedating her anxiety and terror about her out-of-control marriage and unmanageable life. Neither of these women is necessarily chemically dependent. Their substance abuse may cease when their husbands achieve sobriety. On the other hand, even high-functioning women are at increased risk of alcohol use disorders and illicit substance use when they are married to alcoholic men (Schuckit, Smith, Eng, & Kunovac, 2002) Further exploration of their drinking or drug use patterns and of the level of risk indicated by their own family history would be needed to diagnose or rule out chemical dependence.

Both denial and enabling allow some spouses to appear to be very much in control of their lives. They perform their own and their partners' tasks, have many opinions and much advice for others, and may express a great deal of confidence in their own coping abilities. These traits have caused them to be labeled *overresponsible* (Krestan & Bepko, 1990). They are convinced that they need no help and that no one can be trusted to take care of things as well as they can. In fact, they trust no one, and they are rigidly controlling in order to defend against their belief that if they let go one iota for one second, their whole world will fall apart. This constant need for universal control causes their lives to "become unmanageable," as they will learn to say in Al-Anon. The smallest tasks may feel overwhelming because they are invested with so much magical importance. Says one recovering partner: "It got so getting a parking space was as much of a major crisis as getting married."

Codependency

Codependency is the controversial but popular term—castigated by some, overused by others—for an exaggerated dependence upon a loved object or, by extension, external sources of fulfillment. It is characterized by inadequate or lost identity, neglect of self, and low self-esteem. As previously suggested, it can result from growing up in a dysfunctional family, a relationship with an active alcoholic or addicted person, and/or the socialization to expect external sources of fulfillment and the derivation of identity and self-esteem entirely from a primary love relationship. Incorporating the relational model of women's development into our understanding of codependency (Zelvin, 1999), we can see codependency in women as a series of maladaptive attempts to connect that result "from women's . . . socialization to connect at any price, regardless of the absence of mutuality" (p. 17). It is important to note that forming relationships, even deriving part of one's identity and self-esteem from these connections, is normal, healthy, and desirable. It is, however, the formation of destructive or one-sided relationships that is undesirable or even pathological.

Since the term *codependency* is used so broadly, the concept must be considered along a continuum from the most severe (e.g., someone who clings to a physically and emotionally abusive relationship in spite of being offered viable alternatives) to the mildest (e.g., the highly functional adult child who apologizes when someone steps on his or her foot). Codependent individuals are "people-pleasers" who have an acute need for approval, are terrified of abandonment, fear risk taking, and are unable to express anger. They also may be controlling, rigid, perfectionistic, and overresponsible. They are typically nurturing, whereas it might be said that addicted individuals are typically egocentric. (This may be the best way to distinguish which disorder is primary or needs more attention in treatment when dealing with someone who is both.) Codependent people tend to rescue others at the expense of their own needs. Obversely, they tend to control as a way of distracting attention from their own needs and deficiencies. Codependent people feel as if they are always right, and on the other hand, that they are always wrong. They care deeply what others think, often have difficulty identifying what they want or like, and in relationships tend to be attracted by neediness, unavailability, or a recklessness that complements their own fear of risk. These three attributes are often found in alcoholic or drug-addicted persons. One recovering codependent person ruefully remembers that it seemed perfectly reasonable to explain her attraction to her alcoholic partner by saying, "I'm moved by his problems." Extreme codependent people are often described as "addicted to addicts" or "addicted to relationships." They are obsessed with the beloved object and often believe that their survival, or their partner's, depends on maintaining the relationship. In recovery they must learn to maintain boundaries; identify and express needs; make healthy relationship choices, which they often perceive as "dull" or "boring"; deal with solitude as well as intimacy; and find resources for fulfillment and happiness within themselves as well as in their connections with others.

Although the affected partner enables and denies only in relation to an addicted individual, codependency is a personal trait of the individual him- or herself. It pervades every relationship and attitude toward life and is easily portable from relationship to relationship and from situation to situation. Pathological codependency does not disappear when the codependent person leaves the substance abuser or dysfunctional family. Nor does it disappear when the addicted person recovers. A spouse or partner may stop the enabling behavior and remain codependent. In a recovering relationship, a couple may work hard to reduce their codependent behaviors with each other but find that such behaviors recur in their family of origin, at work, and in their social relationships. Finally, most alcoholic and drug-addicted people themselves are also codependent. Often from dysfunctional families, frequently choosing other addicted people as friends and lovers, and usually surrounded by other addicted people even in recovery, they do not shed these maladaptive traits when they give up alcohol or drugs nor even as they work on their sobriety. Furthermore, recovering substance abusers live in a society that enables codependency by touting the fusion of two egos into a single entity as the ideal of love. In the popular culture's vision of romantic love, personal boundaries dissolve, and the lovers never need to express individual needs or seek support elsewhere. Recovery from codependency requires distinguishing between excessive dependence that entails a loss of self and healthy intimacy. Recovering codependent people must become empowered to form what the relational theorists call mutual and growth-enhancing relationships (Zelvin, 1999).

TREATING THE AFFECTED PARTNER

The conditions of treating the partner of an AOD-dependent individual may vary according to whether the chemically dependent partner is in treatment or is still abusing alcohol or other drugs. Treatment tasks range from stopping the enabling behavior to resolving core codependency issues. Addictions and other pathology also may be present, unacknowledged and untreated, in the partner. A variety of treatment and self-help modalities need to be integrated for effective treatment.

Service Provider Support and Resistance

On an institutional level, the individual clinician's work to engage the partner must be supported by institutionalization of outreach procedures to families and extensive counselor training in understanding family dynamics. Advocacy with administration and funding sources also must take place, especially since treatment of the family may not be considered cost effective. In this age of managed care, "collateral" visits may compete with an already inadequate number of treatment sessions allocated for the substance-abusing partner him- or herself.

Many clinicians, whether recovering AOD abusers themselves or trained to work with an identified patient rather than systemically, resist making real efforts to engage the significant other. If the clinician feels it would violate the patient's confidentiality, his or her boundaries, or the therapeutic relationship to reach out to the partner, then the partner will remain untreated, subject to his or her continued suffering, and liable to sabotage the substance abuser's recovery by continued enabling and codependent behavior. Furthermore, the responsibility for engaging the significant other sometimes falls between the cracks among the intake worker, primary therapist, and family worker, depending upon the structure of the treatment program.

When the AOD-Dependent Partner Is in Treatment

Substance abuse treatment professionals have found that even when an institutionalized commitment to treating families and significant others exists, it is often very difficult to engage the partner of an addicted client in treatment. The response of one wife—"How can I help?"—when told her husband was alcoholic, is unfortunately rare. The wife's offer allowed an alert therapist to respond, "You can go to Al-Anon," thereby quickly engaging the wife in her own recovery. More often, the spouse's response is either to deny the problem altogether or to refuse to participate in treatment on the grounds that it is not his or her problem, but the addicted person's. Denial can be extreme. One wife, for example, after compliantly sitting through a family education series and a review of the facts of her husband's three driving-while-intoxicated (DWI) convictions with high blood alcohol levels, still believed that her husband drank only an infrequent "one or two beers" and that alcohol had caused no problems in their lives. Ironically, spouses who have remained committed to their marriages through many years of embarrassment, neglect, and abuse often choose the moment when the substance abuser finally enters treatment to declare that they have had enough. Some leave, while others cite all the times in the past that they have "helped," to no avail, to justify their refusal to cooperate with family treatment planning.

Partners differ widely in their feelings toward the substance abuser at the moment he or she enters treatment. Some are codependently bonded with the addicted partner and obsessed with his or her treatment and recovery, as they are with every other aspect of his or her drinking or drugging. Others are furious at the AOD abuser. The approach taken to engage partners must be carefully tailored to the individuals. If they claim they will do anything to get their partner sober, they must be told that the most helpful step they can take is to seek recovery for themselves. If they resent and blame the AOD-dependent partner, they may be told that they deserve support and understanding of their own difficult position and that this may be found in self-help and treatment for significant others. For example:

> Deborah had been married for 3 years when her husband, Michael, was mandated to chemical dependency treatment by his company's employee-assistance program. He attended an inpatient rehab program, and she attended weekly family sessions with Michael and his therapist and a group for patients' spouses and partners. At the end of Michael's stay at rehab, Deborah was invited to join an aftercare

group for significant others at the agency's outpatient facility. She did this and attended regularly for more than a year. Initially reluctant to attend Al-Anon, which was strongly recommended by the agency, she began going more frequently after she completed aftercare; 2 years later, she was a regular and enthusiastic member of the fellowship, which she saw as an ongoing support for her own recovery from codependency.

For every case like the one above, there are several like the following:

Peter entered therapy with an alcoholism specialist after several years of sporadic AA attendance without ever achieving more than 90 days of sobriety. His wife, Bonnie, refused several invitations to attend a session, but finally came once. The therapist attempted to engage her by joining with her, and Bonnie reported afterward that she liked the therapist. Peter remained sober for several months, until the therapist's vacation. While she was away, he relapsed. When he came to his first scheduled session on her return, he admitted that he had been drinking; he considered the therapy a failure and refused to return to treatment. He reported that he had concealed his relapse from his wife. Several weeks later, Bonnie called the therapist and requested an appointment. She stated that her husband was drinking and that she wanted help for herself. She also inquired about planned intervention, indicating that several concerned family members and friends were willing to participate. The therapist referred Bonnie to an intervention specialist and also began seeing her weekly. Before an intervention could be made, Peter recommitted himself to AA and became sober again. For several weeks Bonnie continued to attend treatment but had difficulty finding anything to talk about, as things were "going fine"; she eventually dropped out of treatment.

As reflected in the above case, it is common for partners whose own family backgrounds are dysfunctional and those with long histories of codependent relationships to be out of touch with their feelings. Unless a crisis is in progress, they feel that they themselves have no problems and therefore need no help.

When the AOD-Dependent Partner Is Actively Using Substances

When substance abusers are still abusing AOD, their partners typically seek treatment not for themselves but for their addicted partner. They want to know how to make them get into treatment, what they should do to make them stop, or whether they should leave the relationship. Again, the first task is engagement of the partner as the primary client by joining with either his or her anger or concern for the dependent person. While refocusing codependent clients on their own pain and dysfunction, it is appropriate to tell them that changes in their behavior *may* bring about improvement in the partner.

> Harvey, a registered nurse who worked in a large hospital, came in seeking help for his wife, who had a long history of abusing prescription pills and alcohol. He was offered individual treatment and encouraged to attend Al-Anon. After his first meeting, he reported that he disliked Al-Anon because the people there seemed "selfish" and talked only about their own concerns and not about their alcoholic loved one. His therapist explained that these people, like Harvey, were all in Al-Anon because of their love for someone, and that "putting the focus on themselves" instead of being preoccupied with their loved one's behavior was their "medicine," as it was his. The therapist also suggested changes in Harvey's enabling behavior, which included behaving in a controlling way, extracting promises, excessive caretaking, and participating in violent arguments. Harvey immediately began making these changes. Three weeks later, his wife entered treatment.

It is equally important to make it clear that an outcome of sobriety for the partner cannot be guaranteed.

> Pamela came into treatment because she was concerned about the effect of her husband's cocaine and marijuana use on her three young children. She was an impeccable housekeeper and devoted mother who had "no time" for herself because she "had to" perform an infinite number of tasks. She also had fits of anger when she fought with her husband and verbally abused her children.
>
> At the beginning of treatment, her plan was an immediate "geographic" cure, in which she would move to another state and find a job while living with a friend. However, it became clear that she might easily agree to include her husband in the plan, even though its purpose was to get away from him. Early in treatment, she had a pseudohallucinatory episode in which she "saw herself" murdering her husband in a variety of ways. Frightened by this image, she became increasingly committed to her work in therapy. In 8 months of treatment, Pamela learned to express her anger verbally in more appropriate ways; became a regular participant in both Nar-Anon and Al-Anon; found a full-time job and began building financial independence; developed constructive ways of relating to her children and began educating them about addiction as a disease; relinquished many household tasks and allowed them to remain undone if other family members shirked their responsibilities; stopped remaining awake all night when her husband was out getting high, then demanding where he had been upon his return; ceased attending family parties at which all her husband's relatives were drunk or smoking pot; refused to get in the car with him if he insisted on driving while high; and allowed

herself regular outings in which she practiced doing what she liked and enjoying her own company. At the same time, her husband's substance abuse increased, affecting his performance as a building superintendent. When he impulsively quit his job, thereby losing their apartment, which came with it, Pamela was able to find an apartment for herself and the children and leave the marriage.

Treatment Tasks

When the partner of an alcoholic or addicted person is willing to be engaged in treatment, the first task is to change his or her enabling behavior. Untreated partners can enable as destructively in early recovery as in the active situation by trying to control the AOD-dependent person's treatment and AA attendance, by continuing to monopolize decision making in the family, by giving or withholding money, by continuing to express mistrust and contempt, and in a host of other ways. Monitoring the client's engagement in self-help programs—Al-Anon, Nar-Anon, Co-Anon, Families Anonymous, or Codependents Anonymous—and processing resistance to these programs is also a crucial early and ongoing counseling task.

If the codependent partner comes from a dysfunctional family of origin, exploration of this history may begin fairly early, at first gently with psychoeducational information and gradually in more depth. In cases where the dysfunctional family is an actively destructive element in the client's current life, this issue must be addressed more quickly. In other cases, the psychic damage the client has sustained as a child may far outweigh the stresses of the current relationship. Here, too, it would be dangerous to delay addressing the family issues. Many clients, however, are in denial about the impact of their early life on their current relationships and choices. Only after more than a year of treatment was Pamela, for example, beginning to understand that her early loss of an alcoholic father and the codependency of her rigid, controlling mother had affected her.

If the primary problem is dysfunction in the current relationship with an AOD abuser, work on this relationship, especially enabling behavior, will take precedence for a while over core codependency issues. The goal, however, is to lead the client toward a recognition of codependency as a problem of self, irrespective of the chemically dependent relationship. The client eventually may recognize codependency issues in all his or her past and present relationships and way of interacting with the world. Acceptance of the need for treatment and ongoing self-help will follow, whether or not the client remains with the substance abuser and whether or not the addicted partner achieves sobriety. And, of course, working on taking responsibility for one's feelings, not rescuing or controlling the addicted person, and not obsessing about him or her to the point of self-neglect all constitute a start on recovery from codependency. The relational perspective suggests that healthier pattern of connection and the development of a more autonomous sense of self are also primary goals of codependency treatment.

Treatment Modalities

Inpatient treatment for the partners of substance abusers is limited, especially in the age of managed care. At best, family participation brings the significant others together to focus on their codependency issues and also begins to rebuild the relationship by fostering communication between chemically dependent individuals and their partners. Family involvement may be limited to a few sessions of psychoeducation and discharge planning. Traditionally, telling the partner to go to Al-Anon and other self-help groups has been expected to compensate for the deficiencies in family treatment; in reality, getting to Al-Anon and using it effectively, for some clients, is a process that benefits greatly from informed professional help. There is little inpatient care for those whose partners are active substance abusers, although there are a few excellent programs for codependents and adult children that focus on healing the wounds of early family dysfunction. And even these resources are becoming less and less available. Managed care has led to cutbacks in some of the most innovative programs or put them beyond the reach of all but the affluent.

Outpatient programs for significant others usually use psychoeducation and group therapy as their primary modalities. Individual, couple, and family therapy also may be offered. There is evidence that conjoint treatment benefits the partners of alcoholic patients (Kuenzler & Beutler, 2003). It is important to ensure that family education is primarily focused on codependency and the impact of AOD dependence on significant others, rather than on the substance use and problems of the user. Although partners need to be informed about the disease and what to expect, typically they are all too eager to learn about the addicted person's problem while continuing to ignore their own. It is essential that treating staff guard against reinforcing the codependent pathology by putting the alcoholic or addicted person and his or her sobriety in the center of the frame when working with significant others. Similarly, group and individual therapists may find that they must constantly refocus discussion as it drifts inevitably toward the substance abuser's behavior and progress.

The Role of Self-Help Programs

The 12-step programs—Al-Anon and its more recent sister fellowships such as Codependents Anonymous (CODA)—are essential adjuncts to effective treatment that should be used, if at all possible. The combination of cognitive-behavioral change and spiritual comfort that these programs provide cuts the therapist's work in half and makes progress in the codependent's recovery more rapid, more effective, and more lasting. Unfortunately, many clinicians share the codependent's resistance to self-help; they may believe the client's claim that Al-Anon is "just a gripe group" or "not for people who are not religious." The remedy is for treating professionals to be well informed about these programs and about the character of specific meetings in their area. Many addiction professionals are themselves untreated codependents and adult children of alcoholic or other dysfunctional families who may bring this hidden pathology to the workplace and the therapeutic relationship. On the other hand, an increasing number of workers in the field are addressing their own issues and using the concepts of "putting the focus on yourself" and "detachment with love" not only to help their clients but also to eliminate codependency from their helping and professional relationships.

Obstacles to Treatment

In addition to client resistance, the absence or inadequacy of treatment services, and professional lack of understanding or commitment to the addicted person's partner's needs, a major obstacle to treatment is the difficulty many clinicians have in empathizing with the angry and controlling spouse. Such behaviors frequently arouse negative countertransference reactions in clinicians. One social worker, herself recovering from codependency, commented: "I went into the field specifically to advocate for this population, but sometimes I feel so frustrated working with these clients that I want to bang their heads against the wall." Partners of substance abusers are typically angry, self-righteous, impatient, hostile to the therapist, rigid, controlling, critical of their partners, and convinced that they have no need to seek help or to change anything about themselves. They also are convinced that they are sensitive, perceptive, self-aware, good at intimate relationships, and more than tolerant of their partner's shortcomings, although they may feel intolerably victimized by him or her. It is very hard for them to see, for example, that giving up the victim role means not only that they "won't stand for his [her] doing that to me anymore" but also accepting that the way they feel is not the product of what the chemically dependent partner "did *to*" them but is their own responsibility. It is equally hard for them to give up the controlling, critical, "right" stance because it is their defense against self-blame and terror. The clinician must keep firmly in mind that the controlling behavior is not a willful obnoxiousness but an unconscious defense against pain and fear, a symptom that is as far beyond the codependent person's control as bingeing is beyond the alcoholic person's. In exchange for relinquishing their control, these codependents must be offered support and the opportunity to improve their self-esteem.

ADDICTIONS AND OTHER PATHOLOGIES
OF THE SPOUSE OR PARTNER

Frequently one partner's greater alcohol or drug consumption masks an alcohol or drug problem in the other.

> Ted and Gina, who were engaged to be married, came in together with the presenting problem of Ted's heroin addiction. He had been clean for 2 months on his own at the time of the first session. He wanted individual therapy and refused to consider inpatient care. Gina claimed that she was willing to help in any way she could, including paying for the treatment. On questioning them, the therapist discovered that Gina had a history of 2 years of heroin addiction as a teenager, which she had ended on her own; that her father was an alcoholic; and that both she and Ted were heavy daily drinkers. Both Ted and Gina had had a couple of drinks right before the session.

There is no distinction between the identified substance abuser and the codependent partner when it comes to the precept that therapy cannot be done in the presence of chemicals. Before any work could be done, both Ted and Gina had to be educated about the disease process of chemical dependency, and they had to agreed to contract to abstain from all mood-altering chemicals, including alcohol, while in treatment. Attendance at AA and NA was strongly recommended to support their abstinence and provide alcohol and drug education.

Because anxiety and depression are symptoms of codependency, especially in the acute and chronic stages of a chemically dependent relationship, Valium or other benzodiazepines and sugar are frequently the codependent's "drugs of choice." In assessing the coaddicted partner, the worker must routinely ask searching questions about the use of prescribed mood-altering medications and eating patterns. It must be remembered that serious problems with eating are not necessarily confined to the extreme disorders of bulimia, anorexia, or obesity. There is a great deal of denial, both societal and individual, associated with pathological relationships with food and body image. In non-substance-abuse treatment settings, such as mental health clinics, clients presenting with depression or anxiety should be routinely asked about their own and their partner's drinking and other chemical use as well as about their dieting and eating patterns.

Every kind of health, mental health, and social service setting has clients who love a substance abuser and, in many cases, are not aware that this circumstance is closely related to their problems. Because denial is the hallmark symptom of codependency, the worker is frequently the one who must initiate the topic, then explore, assess, gently confront, educate, and support the client while helping him or her move from ego-syntonic to ego-dystonic behaviors to reduce enabling and codependency. This change, in turn, has a positive impact on the affective symptoms.

Depression and anxiety may persist, in some cases, for a significant period even though the client is abstaining from chemicals and other mood-altering substances; refraining from other compulsive behaviors, such as shopping, gambling, or compulsive sex; attending self-help groups and treatment regularly; and detaching emotionally from the addicted person, to the best of his or her ability. In such cases, an additional diagnosis may be made and alternatives should be explored. These may include psychiatric consultation and possible use of psychotropic medications; inpatient codependency treatment; and more focused spiritual or stress-relieving work, such as biofeedback, meditation, physical exercise, or therapeutic body work.

THE RECOVERING RELATIONSHIP

Although treatment for partners of substance abusers has been retarded by managed care, various interventions have been tried and studied, especially in the area of enlisting the spouse to help the alcohol- or drug-abusing partner to achieve and maintain recovery, as in alcohol-related behavioral couple therapy (ABCT; McCrady, Hayaki, Epstein, & Hirsch, 2002). There is still considerable controversy as to whether the couple, as an entity, as well as the recovering individuals, should be treated, especially in early sobriety. In what they call the developmental process of recovery, Brown and Lewis (1999) contend that "the couple can be 'on hold' during the early period and . . . the growth that takes place for each individual will give them a new foundation on which to build a healthy couple relationship later" (p. 20). During the lengthy early recovery phase, they state: "Couples will lead parallel lives until there is a stronger sense of oneself and separateness from the other" (p. 222). At Hazelden, one of the bastions of the Minnesota model, this philosophy is stated in even stronger terms: "It is felt that family members can learn from alcoholics and drug addicts with whom they are not emotionally tied. . . . The Hazelden Family Program is *not* a conjoint experience participated in by the chemically dependent person and his or her family" (Laundergan & Williams, 1993, p.146). In contrast, Wetchler, McCollum, Nelson, Trepper, and Lewis (1993), describing a systemic couple therapy model, maintain that "to ignore the relational context of alcohol abuse is to not offer our clients as powerful a treatment as they deserve" (p. 237). In O'Farrell's (1993) behavioral marital therapy couple group for alcoholic persons and their spouses, the stated goals are to alleviate marital distress and learn better relationship skills, such as improved communication and negotiation. Yet even then, the net effect is to maintain the spouse's subordinate role in the alcoholic drama. Traditional gender assumptions may play a part in treatment models. For example, the wife may contract to monitor the alcoholic husband's daily Antabuse consumption, rather than focusing on her own needs. In a discussion of substance-abusing women, *couple* may be defined broadly: "Partners may be married or unmarried, of the same or different sexes, living together or separated, as long as they define themselves as having a committed, emotional bond with one another" (Wetchler et al., 1993, p. 237). In contrast, the studies of the relationships of male alcoholics tend to be limited to conventional marriages.

Brown and Lewis (1999) suggest a way to support the needs of the couple in recovery while continuing to strengthen both partners individually.

> The adults . . . can now come back together to focus on the "we" of the couple while not losing the hard-won "I." . . . [They] can now build a new healthy couple relationship based on the separateness, the individuality, and individual responsibility each has claimed and developed over the years of recovery. (pp. 253–254)

Many treatment programs for substance-abusing clients are still staffed largely with recovering alcohol and other drug abusers who, however professionalized, have little training or inclination to work with partners and other family members, either individually or conjointly. In some programs, special family workers, usually social workers, deal only with significant others. Substance abusers are told in treatment as well as in AA or NA to "put the relationship on the shelf." At the same time, the codependent partner who tries to talk about his or her marriage in Al-Anon or a codependency group may be told to "put the focus on yourself." The pitfall in this approach is that a relationship that has been wracked by chemical dependency has problems that are not solved by sobriety or codependency treatment, just as codependency issues are not resolved by work on sobriety alone. The recovering person who is trying to deal with the day-to-day difficulties of an established relationship, while being told by therapist, sponsor, and recovering friends to ignore it, is bound to feel unsupported, bewildered, and angry.

Certainly, in some cases, the disease has caused such a rift that the best way to avoid conflict is to direct the partners to their separate recoveries. Equally, if the marriage is in such acute crisis that sobriety is threatened, marital conflict must be addressed immediately. For example, some intervention must be made to deal with violence that does not stop with abstinence. In some cases, however, the counselor and other helpers may be overlooking or minimizing an underlying factor of genuine love between the partners or even dismissing it contemptuously as a manifestation of pathology. The clinician who, in contrast, learns to recognize and acknowledge this love when it exists has a powerful treatment tool. Codependency is often confused with love; however, the love that remains when the excessive dependency of the active situation is removed can be framed as a strength. It is then possible to rebuild the relationship while supporting the individual recovery and autonomy of both partners. In general, a strengths-based relational approach to recovery can be highly effective in empowering the recovering partners.

If the relationship is not addressed, dysfunctional patterns continue even as individual recoveries progress, and the partners may become increasingly alienated from each other. Quarrels about money, differing sexual needs, and pressure from families of origin, eliciting familiar but unconstructive responses, may remain unchanged with sobriety. There also may be acute competition over whose recovery is more important or who is working the program better. Couples in individual recovery only may see each other's program as threatening, feel hostile toward it (a very counterproductive attitude if the codependent person has a hidden addiction problem or the alcoholic person has codependency issues that must be addressed later on), and escalate hostility by accusing each other of "taking my inventory."

An acknowledgment that the couple is an entity that needs and deserves its own recovery is more productive in cases that have at least a hint of a positive prognosis, however buried under resentment and disappointment it may be. In deciding whether a recovering couple can be treated successfully, that spark of love can be used as a diagnostic tool and the basis for a strengths-based approach to change. The therapist must support the recovery of both partners and refrain from allying with one and scapegoating the other.

Working with recovering couples can be both challenging and rewarding. Treatment areas include issues of trust, communication, accepting differences, sexuality, money, and families. These seem to be universal, whether the addict is male or female, or indeed if both partners are addicted, whether the couple is married or in a committed relationship, and whether partners are gay or straight. The therapist has the opportunity to be very concrete and prescriptive in helping partners learn to communicate directly, express feelings, and speak from an "I" perspective instead of accusing, criticizing, and blaming.

A remarkable and little-known resource available in some areas is the 12-step program called Chapter 9. Based on AA and Al-Anon but not affiliated with either, Chapter 9 provides an opportunity for couples to pursue their recovery together, in the company of others addressing the same issues. Like other 12-step programs, it provides a model of recovery and potentiates behavioral and attitudinal change.

CONCLUSION

In recent years, an emphasis on family treatment as essential to the recovery process has waxed and waned as funding streams have dried up and abstinence-based systems and disease models have been challenged by new models that incorporate an expectation that significant others put aside their own needs to participate actively in the addicted person's process of controlling or moderating substance use. Meanwhile, the specific needs of the spouses and partners of alcohol and other drug abusers are still being inadequately addressed. The partner may be viewed simultaneously as enabler, affected partner, and codependent. As enabler, the partner contributes to the chemical abuse by rescuing and controlling behaviors. As affected partner, he or she is adversely affected by the disease, experiencing pain, confusion, anger, fear, guilt, anxiety, and depression. Codependent pathology is independent of any single relationship. It may come from a dysfunctional family of origin, the chemically dependent relationship, existing social norms, or from all of these. In women especially, it may represent a distortion of the healthy need to connect. It is characterized by low self-esteem, an exaggerated dependence on outside objects for identity and fulfillment, neglect of one's own needs, rescue and control of others, approval seeking, perfectionism, fear of risk, and denial of feelings.

The partner of the AOD-dependent individual must be treated as a primary client who needs and deserves help for his or her own sake. Pathological codependency must be transformed into empowerment through healthy connections in combination with increased autonomy. The partner can be treated whether or not the substance abuser seeks help. A variety of modalities is available. Obstacles to treatment include client resistance, professional denial and ignorance, therapists' unresolved codependency issues, a lack of institutional support for codependency or family treatment, and the unattractive presenting personality of the untreated coaddict, whose symptoms may include rigidity, self-righteousness, and control. Self-help programs, such as Al-Anon and Chapter 9, are an invaluable adjunct to treatment.

REFERENCES

Alcoholics Anonymous. (1957). *Alcoholics Anonymous comes of age.* New York: Alcoholics Anonymous World Services.

Alcoholics Anonymous. (2001). *Alcoholics Anonymous* (4th ed.). New York: Alcoholics Anonymous World Services.

Brown, S., & Lewis, V. (1999). *The alcoholic family in recovery: A developmental model.* New York: Guilford Press.

Krestan, J., & Bepko, C. (1990). Codependency: The social reconstruction of female experience. *Smith College Studies in Social Work, 60,* 216–232.

Kuenzler, A., & Buetler, L. E. (2003). Couple alcohol treatment benefits patients' partners. *Journal of Clinical Psychology, 59*(7), 791–806.

Laundergan, J. C., & Williams, T. (1993). The Hazelden residential family program: A combined systems and disease model approach. In T. J. O'Farrell (Ed.), *Treating alcohol problems: Marital and family interventions* (pp. 145–169). New York: Guilford Press.

McCrady, B. S., Hayaki, J., Epstein, E. E., & Hirsch, L. (2002) Testing hypothesized predictors of change in conjoint behavioral alcoholism treatment for men. *Alcoholism: Clinical and Experimental Research, 26*(4), 463–470.

Miller, J. B. (1986). *Toward a new psychology of women* (2nd ed.). Boston: Beacon.

Miller, K. J. (1994). The codependency concept: Does it offer a solution for the spouses of alcoholics? *Journal of Substance Abuse Treatment, 11*(4), 339–345.

O'Farrell, T. J. (1993). A behavioral marital therapy couples group program for alcoholics and their spouses. In T. J. O'Farrell (Ed.), *Treating alcohol problems: Marital and family interventions* (pp. 170–209). New York: Guilford Press.

Olmsted, M. E., Crowell, J. A., & Waters, E. (2003). Assortative mating among adult children of alcoholics and alcoholics. *Family Relations, 52*(1), 64–71.

Rothberg, N. M. (1986). The alcoholic spouse and the dynamics of codependency. *Alcoholism Treatment Quarterly, 3*(1), 73–86.

Schaef, A. W. (1986). *Codependence: Misunderstood—mistreated.* New York: Harper & Row.

Schuckit, M. A., Smith, T. L., Eng, M. Y., & Kunovac, J. (2002). Women who marry men with alcohol-use disorders. *Alcoholism: Clinical and Experimental Research, 26*(9), 1336–1343.

Schutt, M. (1985). *Wives of alcoholics: From codependency to recovery.* Deerfield Beach, FL: Health Communications.

Wegscheider-Cruse, S. (1985). *Choice-making.* Deerfield Beach, FL: Health Communications.

Wetchler, J. L., McCollum, E. E., Nelson, T. S., Trepper, T. S., & Lewis, R. A. (1993). Systemic couples therapy for alcohol-abusing women. In T. J. O'Farrell (Ed.), *Treating alcohol problems: Marital and family interventions* (pp. 236–260). New York: Guilford Press.

Woititz, J. G. (1979). *Marriage on the rocks: Learning to live with yourself and an alcoholic.* New York: Delacorte.

Woititz, J. G. (1983). *Adult children of alcoholics.* Deerfield Beach, FL: Health Communications.

Zelvin, E. (1988). Dependence and denial in coalcoholic women. *Alcoholism Treatment Quarterly, 5*(3/4), 97–115.

Zelvin, E. (1997). Codependency issues of substance abusing women. In S. L. A. Straussner & E. Zelvin (Eds.), *Gender and addictions: Men and women in treatment.* Northvale, NJ: Aronson.

Zelvin, E. (1999). Applying relational theory to treatment of addicted women. *Affilia: Journal of Women in Social Work, 14*(1), 9–23.

Zelvin, E. (2002). Women affected by addictions. In S. L. A. Straussner & S. Brown (Eds.), *The handbook of addiction treatment for women.* San Francisco: Jossey-Bass.

CHAPTER 13

Dynamics and Treatment Issues with Children of Drug and Alcohol Abusers

Roberta Markowitz

It is estimated that there are 26.8 million children of alcoholic parents in the United States (National Association for Children of Alcoholics, 1998), and that one in four children under the age of 18 is exposed to alcohol abuse or dependence in the family (Grant, 2000). In addition, there are hundreds of thousands, maybe millions, of other children whose parents abuse other drugs. Although it is conceptually useful to identify children of alcoholic parents (COAs) or other drug-abusing parents (CODAs) as a population with unique problems, such children do not constitute a monolithic group. Among these children, as among substance-abusing adults, one can find every diagnostic category. Nevertheless, certain commonalities in the behavior of alcoholic and other drug-abusing parents tend to lead to some common pathological outcomes that can seriously diminish the quality of life for their children, even long after these "children" have left the parental home.

This chapter examines the pathogenic circumstances, the dynamics of the resulting impairments, and various treatment issues with this population. Because the research and clinical literature on young and adult children of alcoholic parents is much more comprehensive than that on children of other drug abusers, this chapter, by and large, focuses on COAs.

ETIOLOGY AND DYNAMICS OF
CHILDREN OF ALCOHOLIC PARENTS

In the literature on COAs one frequently sees lists of attributes (e.g., inability to trust, fear of intimacy, external locus of control, and need for control) that are said to characterize this population. These characteristics, however, are certainly not unique to COAs, a fact that has led some to question what substance-abusing families have in common with other types of dysfunctional families that might lead to similar outcomes.

The core commonality in all types of dysfunctional families centers on the existence of some significant degree of impairment in empathy on the part of at least one parent (or primary caretaker). The dynamics of COAs can best be understood as a special case of narcissistic injury suffered at the hands of empathically impaired parents. What makes this a special case is the intermittent presence of behaviors induced by mood-altering substances in parents whose non-drug-involved personalities may be dramatically different from what they appear to be while "under the influence." Children have neither the knowledge nor the experience with which to understand the physiology and behavioral effects of a chemical dependency. In addition to the parents' behavior being directly distorted by the effect of substances, the parents may value their drugs more than their children. As such, the normally powerful parent–child attachment, in which the child is highly valued by the parent, may be supplanted by the parent's attachment to the drug as the chiefly valued object. Because the availability of the substance becomes an all consuming preoccupation for the abuser, the needs and well-being of the child become, by default, a secondary concern at most; indeed, the degree to which the abuser values the child may be dependent on whether the child facilitates or interferes with the parent's use of the substance and related needs. Some spouses may attempt to protect their children from some of the direct consequences of the substance abuse and thereby soften the impact. Many others, however, are as preoccupied with the substance abuser's behavior as the abuser is with the substance; still others simply withdraw or turn to substance abuse themselves, thus becoming similarly unavailable to the child.

Such narcissistic use of the child may or may not be part of a parent's premorbid personality. When sober and drug free during recovery, many parents will express great sorrow and shame in recalling their earlier treatment of their children. However, when substance abuse is present, some degree of empathic impairment is inevitable. This impairment occurs in a number of ways. First, mood-altering drugs affect ego functioning and alter the balance among all the psychic structures. Even in those cases in which abusers behave in a mellow and affectionate way, they are very often preoccupied with their own inner sensations and narcissistic needs and thus are not adequately available to their children. Second, during periods of physical withdrawal or when the drug is not having the desired effect, abusers experience the kind of narcissistic withdrawal that always accompanies illness, making them, again, emotionally unavailable. The added anxiety, depression, tension, and irritability during these periods increases the likelihood that these parents will displace the source of their uncomfortable feelings onto the children, who may then be unfairly blamed and punished. This maltreatment arouses anxiety, confusion, guilt, and anger in the children, who also experience a sense of being "unseen." Third, the occurrence of blackouts, during which the parents do not recall anything that may have been discussed with the children, also can create enormous confusion, fear, and anger, again resulting in the children's feeling of being unseen. Fourth, the substance use often loosens inhibitions and severely impairs parents' social judgment. At such times, the children may become the direct victims of inappropriate and possibly abusive behavior. Even if not directly victimized, if the children see or hear about such behavior, they are likely to experience a sense of helplessness, shame, and humiliation. Finally, nonabusing parents cannot be relied upon for relief, since they are usually overwhelmed and preoccupied with trying to manage the chaos engendered in the family and trying to maintain the illusion of normal functioning. Keeping the "family secret" (i.e., hiding the family shame) makes a mockery of the children's reality-testing abilities, insofar as it demands selective inattention to compelling portions of their reality, both of events and feelings. There is little permission for—indeed, there is often overt discouragement of—the expression of any feelings.

According to Kohut (Kohut & Wolf, 1978), the development of a coherent, well-integrated self requires the presence of responsive–empathic self-objects[1] who can meet the normal mirroring and idealizing needs of the child. As a consequence of minor, *nontraumatic* failures in the responses of mirroring and idealized self-objects, the child begins to develop a mature self by gradually taking over the functions of the self-objects. Archaic mirroring and idealizing needs are transformed into normal self-assertiveness and normal devotion to ideals. Faulty interactions between the child and the self-objects result in a damaged self.

As noted, in a family with alcohol- or other drug-dependent parent(s), one or both are rendered unavailable to meet the child's normal needs for

---

[1]"Self-objects are objects which we experience as part of our self; the expected control over them is, therefore, closer to the concept of control which a grown-up expects to have over his own body and mind than to the concept of control which he expects to have over others. There are two kinds of self-objects: those who respond to and confirm the child's innate sense of vigour, greatness and perfection; and those to whom the child can look up and with whom he can merge as an image of calmness, infallibility and omnipotence. The first type is referred to as the mirroring self-object, the second as the idealized parent imago" (Kohut & Wolf, 1978, p. 414).

mirroring and idealizing. This perspective illuminates the deep sense of shame experienced by many COAs as well as the powerfully felt need to maintain the family secret. The substance abuser may not be able to exercise a normal degree of control—he or she may stumble, vomit, soil him- or herself, or act foolish. Such failures are particularly linked to shame, and to some degree, COAs identify with this shame (Hibbard, 1987). The parent appears degraded in the child's eyes, so that, in addition to the possibility of being directly shamed, the child is shamed, at an even deeper level, because his or her developmental need to identify with an idealized parent is also thwarted.

To understand some of the effects on the child of parental empathic failure, it is helpful to examine what happens in healthy or "good-enough" families.

Jamie has just had one of the most glorious experiences a 9-year-old boy can have: He hit the winning home run in a baseball game. When he arrives home, his mother notices that he is glowing and asks him, in an interested and animated way, what happened at school to make him look so happy. He shares the episode with his mother, relishing the retelling. As he speaks, his mother's eyes are open wide; she is smiling and attentive. When he finishes speaking, she congratulates him enthusiastically, praises him for doing so well, and reflects back to him that she can now see why he looked so delighted when he arrived home.

This exchange has a number of positive effects on Jamie, and he learns a number of things from it. Having his feelings of exhilaration, power, and grandiosity mirrored by his mother validates them, and Jamie is able to sustain the good feelings and internalize them. He receives confirmation that what he was feeling was the correct thing to be feeling under the circumstances, which adds to the integrity of his sense of self and further enhances his self-esteem. He has learned that he can trust an important person to reflect his feelings accurately and that sharing such feelings can multiply the pleasure: There is pleasure in the original experience, in the safety of the retelling, in his mother's reflections of his own pleasure, and in his having pleased her directly. Repeated experiences of this sort help lay the groundwork for healthy intimate relationships.

What happens when such empathic responsiveness is lacking?

Sarah, 10 years old, has been told by a visiting author at school that her story is one of the most charming she has ever read. Sarah is "walking on air," filled with her achievement. On the way home from school, however, some of her excitement is edged out by anxiety because she is not sure in what condition she will find her alcoholic mother when she gets home. On arriving home, she finds her mother up and in the kitchen. Although her mother has not yet begun drinking that day, she is depressed, tense, and irritable because of her craving for alcohol. Sarah's arrival reminds her mother that Sarah had left yesterday's discarded clothing on the floor of her room rather than putting it in the hamper. Sarah attempts to tell her mother about the compliment she received at school. Her mother replies sarcastically that that's great, but if she can put words in such good order on paper, why can't she put her clothing in proper order at home, and proceeds to berate her for being such a "difficult, sloppy child." In her growing anger, her mother starts slamming cabinet doors, pours herself a drink as though to underscore how difficult it is to cope with her daughter, and stomps out of the kitchen. Sarah wonders whether her mother will be able to prepare dinner later.

All the self-enhancing experiences of Jamie's interaction with his mother are absent in this episode. On the contrary, the central experience is one of anxious anticipation followed by shame, anger, and a precipitous drop in self-esteem. Furthermore, Sarah gets the message that she is responsible for her mother's drinking because she is "such a bad girl." Sarah learns that it is not safe to share positive feelings with her mother, because chances are high that they will be shattered; with repeated experiences such as this one, she learns that it is not even safe to allow *herself* to feel such feelings, because they lead to such serious disappointment. She learns to deny her feelings of rejection and abandonment by focusing on a concrete problem.

The experience of the precipitous drop in self-esteem is so very painful that many such children learn to numb their responses to positive experiences: It is felt to be safer to exist in a chronic state of low self-esteem and moderate depression than to take the risk of feeling good about oneself, which is to set oneself up for a fall. Because these children ward off the positive and self-esteem-enhancing feelings that normally accompany compliments or satisfying achievements, there is little to counteract their feeling of being basically bad or flawed. The conviction of being flawed in some very deep, abiding, and fundamental way (which has both conscious and unconscious components) may become an organizing fantasy that can shape much of their lives, expressing itself in excessive feelings of shame. It may be acted out directly (e.g., through social withdrawal) or via a grandiose reaction formation and exhibitionism.

Mr. B., the adult child of an alcoholic father, is a very successful businessman who makes unreasonable demands that everything around him be elegant and perfect. Despite the fact that his wife also works and has primary responsibility for the children, he insists that she change their linens and towels daily. He fights with his colleagues over his periodic demands for special indulgences—such as having a fine bone china tea service for his office. If his wife should bring home a bag of potatoes from the market with a spoiled potato in it, he flies into a rage, becoming verbally abusive and throwing things around. At times, he becomes depressed and has difficulty getting up for work in the morning.

The conviction of being flawed or damaged is typically projected, so that in addition to feeling "I'm lousy," the adolescent or adult COA believes that "You will look at me and see how lousy I am." The sense of exposure is intolerable. Performance situations, even speaking up in a classroom or at a meeting, may give rise to unbearable anxiety or panic attacks. It is not unusual for the resulting feelings of mortification to be dealt with by social withdrawal and isolation, by rages, or by self-medicating use of alcohol or other drugs.

If there is any kind of real bodily defect, even one that is quite minor, the sense of being flawed may be projected onto it. Ms. A., for example, was born with a bump on her head that is visible only to herself and her hairdresser. Yet, in telling her therapist about it at the age of 40, she broke into tears, recalling her belief that no one liked her as she was growing up because of that bump. In the absence of any real external defect, the fantasy of being flawed and/or damaged may remain unconscious and can assume many different forms. Many women, for example, experience themselves as hopelessly stupid or inept or focus on their imperfect body shape, which may lead to an eating disorder or multiple trips to a plastic surgeon. Perfectionism and a desperate need to seek approval develop as a means of warding off any hint of inadequacy or rejection, either of which could trigger the painfully precipitous drop in self-esteem.

ETIOLOGY AND DYNAMICS OF CHILDREN OF ALCOHOLICS OR OTHER DRUG ABUSERS

Much research remains to be done on children of cocaine and heroin abusers. The etiology and psychodynamics appear to be essentially similar to those of COAs, the chief differences flowing largely from the illegality surrounding the use of other drugs. According to Straussner (1994), parents who abuse illicit substances, such as heroin or crack cocaine, are more likely to come from "minority or disenfranchised, low-income groups and/or [be] characterized as having an antisocial personality with poor superego development" (p. 394). The prospect of their children experiencing or witnessing violence, sexual abuse, neglect, and abandonment is high. Whereas the parent's need to seek out drugs can lead to more frequent physical abandonment of CODAs, emotional abandonment is common to both CODAs and COAs. CODAs are more likely to face loss of a parent at an earlier age due to illness, overdose, incarceration, or violence. There is an increased prospect of experiencing homelessness or multiple foster placements, as well as sexually transmitted diseases such as HIV and syphilis. They may observe or be forced into the trading of sex for drugs, as well as participation in other illegal activities. When babies have been exposed to drugs such as cocaine or heroin *in utero*, their addicted mothers, who may have limited ego strengths to begin with, are often quickly overwhelmed by the demands of having to care for a child with neurological and other medical impairments. These mothers may experience the baby as rejecting, suffer an increased sense of worthlessness, and possibly respond by rejecting the child (Levy & Rutter, 1992).

COPING MECHANISMS

Just as a dependent child needs to have certain basic physical needs met in order to survive, so too must certain psychological needs be met: Adequate nurturing and holding, a balanced experience of stimulation and soothing, empathic responsiveness, and reasonable consistency are all necessary for healthy development. When these positive caretaking behaviors are not sufficiently forthcoming, overwhelming anxiety, rage, depression (and, in extreme cases, failure to thrive), and deficits in the sense of self may result. The child generally concludes that he or she is at fault and bad and will seek to have his or her needs met in whatever ways possible. Many authors have pointed out that COAs develop a variety of coping skills to survive in situations where life may be chaotic, unpredictable, frightening, and even dangerous (e.g., Black, 1981; Wegscheider, 1981).

One coping technique that COAs frequently develop is to become overly attuned to parental needs and wishes. In this reversal of roles, children discover that by pleasing or taking care of parents, they can glean at least a facsimile of the nurturing they crave, although their efforts are usually doomed to frustrating failure. Brown (2000) quotes a patient: "I was my mother's confidante from as early as I can remember. I had to listen, sympathize and offer suggestions that would somehow make everything OK. But nothing ever changed. She was the child and I was the ineffective, helpless parent" (p. 168).

In addition to becoming a confidante, comforter, adviser, and supporter of the parents, these children develop a special sensitivity to unconscious signals manifesting the needs of others (Miller, 1981). As with other survival mechanisms that are learned, this one can be very adaptive and provide many secondary gains. Such children are appreciated by friends, in school, or later on the job for their sensitivity, hard work, strongly developed sense of responsibility, desire to please, and need to rescue others (they are represented in large numbers in the helping professions). But these gains come at a high price: the repression of their own wishes, feelings, and needs. These COAs may look very successful on the outside, but they suffer powerful feelings of emptiness and aloneness. Not having access to their own feelings, they have difficulty finding inner sources of satisfaction or tapping creative resources. Such tasks as making career choices or finding a hobby, for example, can be confusing and frustrating. Since inadequate parental empathy causes COAs to feel it is unsafe to act on the basis of their own feelings and needs, they learn to regulate their feelings and actions based on their perception of the feelings and needs of others, leading to boundary confusion and enmeshment. The sense of narcissistic injury is profound.

> Cara, age 7, from a white, working-class family, was referred by her father because of excessive clinging and a "tendency to lie." Her mother had given up custody to the father when Cara was 5 because abuse of crack cocaine had caused her life to become unmanageable. During several of her early years, Cara's father was incarcerated due to illegal drug use. He worked long hours and continued to drink during his limited time with his daughter. Cara was nursed by, and shared a bed with, her mother until age 5. At that time, the mother moved in with a new boyfriend. Cara reported that "the worst day of my life" occurred when her mother left her overnight, evidently to go out in search of drugs. At the time of referral, her parents were engaged in a custody battle. It was clear that both parents had enlisted Cara in telling their sides of the story, and encouraged her to lie to protect them. Even after months of treatment, Cara was not able to form a therapeutic alliance or exhibit a sense of trust. She was uniformly guarded and highly defended. The only time she expressed genuine affect was when, after giving voice to what were clearly her father's words, she expressed the fear that her mother would find out what she had said and would be angry. In play therapy using a dollhouse, people were isolated from one another, each gazing in separate directions. In her play, generally, she was constricted and overly solicitous of the therapist.

Cara needs to yield up her sense of self in order to hold on to her tenuously available parents. As with many of the coping mechanisms that enable children of alcohol- and other drug-abusing parents to survive their difficult and frightening early years, being overly attuned to others—although continuing to yield some rewards—brings with it serious maladaptive consequences later in life. Internal resources of comforting are inadequate, leaving COAs largely dependent on an external source to feel complete. This external focus may help explain the frequency of compulsive behaviors among adult COAs, including eating disorders, substance abuse, gambling, compulsive shopping, and/or addictive relationships. The role reversals, continuing dependence upon external sources for self-regulation, excessive fears about the parents' health and well-being, perfectionism, desperate need for approval, and reaction formation against anger often make it difficult for COAs to separate from parents in reality as well as intrapsychically.

> After years of therapy, Ms. H. was finally able to bring herself to leave her parents at the age of 29 to get married. Both parents were alcoholic, although she was not aware of her mother's alcoholism until, soon after the wedding, her mother developed a life-threatening illness that the doctor declared to have been caused by her drinking. The illness further undercut Ms. H.'s attempts at separation. She became depressed, and even months after the crisis had subsided, Ms. H. continued to feel obligated to spend considerable time with her parents, making biweekly trips to visit them—no easy feat, since they had moved 1,200 miles away! Shortly afterward, Ms. H. became pregnant. Her father, who continued to drink daily, complained bitterly that he could not cope with the limitations his wife's illness had placed on their lifestyle and thought about ending his grief by suicide. Ms. H. believed he would never hurt himself while she was pregnant. She was aware that she had conceived her child as a gift for her father, in order to counter the threatened loss and separation.

Related to the separation issue is the fact that the moods of adult children of alcohol- and other drug-abusing parents are frequently regulated by the feelings of others. When Ms. H. decided to skip one of her biweekly trips, her father called her four times a day because of his own difficulties with separation and infantile dependence. She noticed that she was feeling better than she had in months and realized it was because her father sounded "pretty good" on the phone. She was struck by the degree to which her moods were dependent on her father's state of mind.

According to Cermak and Rosenfeld (1987), COAs, like children who are abused, may suffer from posttraumatic stress disorder. They may develop similar defenses, leading to an extreme need to maintain control. This need for control begins as a coping mechanism that can facilitate survival in a chaotic and unpredictable environment but, because of its rigidity, it has maladaptive consequences. Exerting control often enables COAs to play a role in holding the family together, and this may become a source of realistic pride. But they often cling to the illusion of being in a position to control their substance-abusing parent's behavior. They ascribe the cause of their intermittent abandonment to their own "badness," so that they can continue to view the parent as good (and thereby continue to hope for the caring and connectedness they seek). This misperception perpetuates the illusion and sustains the hope that they can influence the parent's moods and behavior by adjusting their own behavior.

Ms. H. reported receiving nightly spankings up until the age of 10. Although she reported that these spankings were not severe, she recalled that, when intoxicated, her father was quite volatile and explosive and that he would throw and break things, including tearing the heads off her dolls. She reported these episodes with inappropriate affect—smiling, almost laughing—and attempted to minimize their horror by pointing out how guilty her father would later feel. She added that she distinctly remembered deliberately doing naughty things in order to provoke these spankings, as though to say, "You see, it really was my fault, after all, not his."

In a frightening and out-of-control world, Ms. H. had found the one area in which she could experience herself as exerting control. In her reports of these spankings (which were clearly sexualized, thus adding to her guilt), Ms. H. attempted to deny her own anxiety, minimize her father's culpability, and ascribe the cause to her own "badness": If only she were better behaved, her father would have had no cause to hit her. In writing about his work with a severely abused population, Shengold (1989) finds a similar dynamic:

> When one parent can tyrannize, the need for a loving and rescuing authority is so intense that the child must break with the registration of what he or she has suffered, and establish within the mind (delusionally) the existence of a loving parent who will care and who really must be right. . . . (In the adult, there may be a good deal of intellectual awareness of what the parent is like, but the delusion of goodness continues underneath and surfaces when needed.) The child takes on the guilt for the abuse, turning inward the murderous feeling that is evoked by the traumata. . . . The child denies what has happened, sometimes but not always with orders from the tormentor. The parent is right and good; the child must be wrong and bad. (pp. 73–74)

Shengold (1989) explains that the child's need to "break with the registration of what he or she has suffered" results in a kind of compartmentalizing of contradictory images—images that are never permitted to coalesce. This kind of "vertical splitting" transcends diagnostic categories[2] and has powerful implications for the understanding and treatment of this population. Healing can begin to take place only when the client can responsibly own his or her full ambivalence and can truly accept that which is fervently wished for—to have had a good and loving parent—never existed and can never be recreated. Golden and Hill (1991) point out the par-

---

[2]For an excellent discussion of the contributions of the object relations school and Kohut and the self psychologists to this topic, see Wood (1987).

adox in the task of those who need to mourn that which was never enjoyed, as many ACOAs do:

> Childhood may have been endured, may be remembered, or may be denied, but it has not been mourned, because mourning requires letting go. These patients cannot yet let go of the desire for good and loving parents. The recognition that what has been lost in childhood has been lost forever revives the threat of childhood despair which appears to be every bit as devastating now as it was then. (p. 24)

Faced with the chronic overstimulation and emotional deprivation that are typical in chemically dependent families, some children cope through a constellation of acting-out behaviors. They may turn to running away from home, abusing substances, promiscuity, suicidal ideation and behavior, bullying or belligerency with peers, uncooperativeness at school, and antisocial or criminal activities. These behaviors may represent, among other things, direct discharge of overwhelming affect, a seeking of attention and limit setting, identification with the aggressor, reaction formation against feared helplessness, and the turning of passivity into activity. Difficulty dealing with anger is typical. Inability to discharge anger in appropriate ways at appropriate times leads to the building of a well of anger that can be touched off by even small triggers. The resulting overreaction is frightening and leads to more determined efforts to further suppress anger. One client aptly described her experience of her own anger: "It feels like a hard core inside me—like kryptonite—it's toxic and it weakens me."

Dissatisfaction and failure in interpersonal relationships are extremely common complaints among adult children of substance-abusing parents. Fear of intimacy and lack of trust are frequently cited as contributing to the interpersonal difficulties. Equally a problem is *blind trust*. If a child has experienced rejection, abandonment, or abuse, the powerful need for love and attachment will prevent the normal unraveling of the archaic idealization of the parent. This idealization is transferred onto potential love objects during adolescence and adulthood, so that inadequacies and failures in these partners, which may be evident to outside observers, go unperceived by the adult children of substance abusers (ACOSA).

It is common for ACOSAs to find partners who are themselves alcohol or drug abusers, or who are emotionally unavailable for other reasons. Sometimes these attachments seem to blaze into existence precipitously. ACOSAs may report "love at first sight," but these connections are often based on dependency and neediness rather than a relationship of adult mutuality. Sensing the partner's neediness, the ACOSA feels temporarily safe from rejection—a rejection he or she has come to fear but also to expect as normal and inevitable. The partner does inevitably withdraw, based on his or her own fears or conflicts, but the ACOSA, who was blind to the danger signs, assumes the guilt for this rejection and responds with feelings of bad-ness, a painful drop in self-esteem, depression, and such symptoms as diffi-culty eating and sleeping or gastrointestinal problems (Norwood, 1985). These painful interactions represent repetitions of the early parent–child relationship.

As in the childhood experience, the ACOSA sees no relief from the painful affects other than by reuniting with the partner. This scenario may be played out again and again, despite repeated abandonments or even abuse. In addition to denial and an inability to give up this idealization, part of the "blindness" to the character of the partner may be due to the ACOSA's perception of his or her childhood as normal, since there may have been little else with which to compare it. A further motivation for the repetition may be a longing to achieve mastery—the hope that this time it will work out all right, that the trauma can be avoided. Most compelling of all, the need to escape from a pervasive and desperate sense of emptiness almost ensures that the ACOSA will seek to reunite with the very partner who has precipitated the immediate distress. Without outside help, the ACOSA may remain endlessly trapped in a vicious circle with the disap-pointing yet yearned—for partner—or series of such partners.

Recent research on attachment theory has shown a higher rate of vari-ous forms of insecure attachment among COAs compared to children from nonalcoholic families (el-Guebaly, West, Maticka-Tyndale, & Pool, 1993; Jaeger, Hahn, & Weinraub, 2000). This work shows promise in helping to conceptualize the etiology and later expression of the interpersonal diffi-culties of many ACOAs. It may help explain the extraordinary persistence of many ACOAs in remaining in dysfunctional and abusive relationships, as well as, for some, a powerful attachment to compulsive, eating disor-dered, or self-mutilating behaviors. Farber (2000) extensively and inci-sively discusses the relationship between problems in attachment and self-harm.

TREATMENT

Because parental substance abuse leads (at the very least) to impaired pa-rental empathy and therefore narcissistic injury to the children, the first question that arises is whether all COAs require some form of intervention or treatment. There has not been sufficient research to allow us to identify clearly which COAs would be most at risk, and we need to understand more about those factors that seem to mitigate the negative influences of parental pathology. There are certain "resilient" individuals who appear to function successfully despite an apparently traumatizing upbringing (Wolin & Wolin, 1993). Nevertheless, there are two types of intervention that all COSAs should have access to: The first is simply the information that growing up in a chemically dependent home creates an at-risk situation; the second is some basic education about alcoholism and other chemical dependencies. Making such information available alerts the children to specific potential difficulties (this is especially important given our understanding that there is a genetic component to certain types of alcoholism), and it opens the door to individuals to seek help by reducing the shame that is so commonly part of the baggage carried by COAs. Self-help movements such as Al-Anon, ACOA, and codependency groups that have burgeoned since the 1980s are playing an enormously important role in meeting this latter need. In addition, since exposure to alcohol or other drug use during pregnancy can have devastating consequences on the developing fetus (Werner, Joffe, & Graham, 1999), the wide availability of such information may contribute to more responsible decision making on the part of those anticipating parenthood.

COAs are known to be at risk for developing alcoholism or other substance use disorders (Johnson & Leff, 1999). Research also shows a high rate of attention-deficit/hyperactivity disorder (ADHD) among COAs—and, conversely, a high rate of alcoholism among parents of children with ADHD children (Wilens, Spencer, & Biederman, 2000). Substance use disorders and ADHD are both characterized by frequent comorbidity with anxiety, mood, and conduct disorders. ADHD, especially ADHD that is comorbid with conduct disorder or bipolar disorder, is associated with an earlier age of onset, greater severity, and slower recovery from substance use disorders (Wilens et al., 2000). These interrelationships make it imperative that clinicians working with children of alcohol- and other drug-abusing parents be able to recognize, assess, and treat or refer for treatment a broad array of psychiatric difficulties, including ADHD.

Because stimulant drugs are generally the first line of treatment for ADHD, clinicians as well as parents may be extremely concerned about the potential for abusing these prescription drugs or moving on to other drugs of abuse. It is worth noting that a controlled study (Biederman, Wilens, Mick, Spencer, & Faraone, 1999) showed an 85% reduction in risk for substance use disorders for boys with ADHD receiving pharmacotherapy, compared to youth with ADHD who were left untreated.

WORKING WITH YOUNG CHILDREN
OF SUBSTANCE ABUSERS

Children or adolescents living in a substance-abusing family often benefit from participation in a group, which can reduce their isolation, provide peer support, and prepare them for involvement in self-help groups for adolescent children, such as Alateen or Narateen. Clinicians can use all the usual techniques for creating an atmosphere of trust—a critical aspect of beginning treatment—and then enhance this process by demonstrating an understanding of common characteristics of parents who abuse alcohol and other drugs, children's feelings about them, and consequent behaviors. Substance abuse education is an important component of treatment. Concrete suggestions for coping can be provided—for example, steps the child might be able to take to avoid getting into a car with an intoxicated parent. It is important to provide the message that the child is not alone, is not responsible for the parent's drinking or drugging, and cannot control the parent's substance use. Preventive intervention programs, in addition to providing information and education, social support, and skill building in coping strategies and social competence, can be an outlet for the safe expression of feeling and a setting in which to engage in healthy alternative activities (Price & Emshoff, 1997).

Treatment for children and adolescents can help them overcome denial of the parents' difficulties and allow for ventilation of anger. The child needs to know that it is normal to feel angry under certain circumstances; he or she may need help in understanding the distinction between wishes and fantasies, on the one hand, and action, on the other: To wish one's parents dead need not give rise to the kind of guilt one would feel if one were to act on that wish. Clinicians need to be sensitive to the child's ambivalence, however. A child might be feeling unjustly treated and murderously angry, but, at the same time, be very worried about, and fearful of losing, the abusing parent. Conscious fears may include the fear of arrest, accident, illness, and/or death of the parent. Unconsciously, realistic dependence and need for parental protection make loss of the parent's love a terrifying prospect. This terror frequently gives rise to powerful rescue fantasies, which are often unconscious or derivative. They may be displaced onto friends, pets, and so on, It is important for the therapist to assist the child in accepting his or her ambivalence and to point out the unrealistic nature of the wish to rescue the parent.

Children of substance-abusing parents are frequently treated inconsistently and given confusing and conflicting messages, making it difficult for them to trust their own judgment. Therapists can help by providing validation for the child's feelings and perceptions and feedback on what is normal.

TREATING ADULT CHILDREN OF ALCOHOLIC PARENTS

When ACOAs do present themselves for treatment, certain types of issues commonly arise despite the fact that, as mentioned earlier, ACOAs are represented in the full range of diagnostic categories. These issues include proneness to experiencing guilt and shame, fear of anger, an inadequate or damaged sense of self, use of denial, and possibly substance abuse or other forms of compulsive behavior.

Since ACOAs are at increased risk for all types of substance abuse as well as eating disorders and other types of compulsive behaviors, it is important that careful assessments be made of all of these areas and appropriate interventions planned. Not infrequently, ACOAs exhibit the early stages of alcohol or drug abuse, having learned to turn to chemicals as a form of self-medication for painful affects. In these cases relatively minimal intervention—in the form of alcohol and drug education and advice—is often all that is required to help them give up their use of chemicals, because it has not yet become a long-term, chronic problem with its typically entrenched defenses of rationalization and denial.

Low self-esteem and proneness to excessive shame sometimes present obstacles in the beginning of treatment. ACOAs may perceive their very need for treatment as corroboration of their deeply held conviction of being flawed or damaged in some way. This conviction may interfere with their ability to form a therapeutic alliance, because they fear, and fully expect, that if they open themselves up, they will be rejected by a therapist who will see and judge all their flaws. This problem needs to be addressed early on by interventions, offered in an empathic and accepting way, that clarify and illuminate the nature of this anxiety. The clinician also needs to help clients transform excessive shame or guilt from ego-syntonic to ego-alien experiences: The client needs help in redefining the problem from "I am so bad and stupid" to "I am too *quick to feel* bad and stupid." Furthermore, defenses against shame need to be interpreted so that more adaptive behaviors can take their place. By allowing clients to share shameful feelings about the self in a therapeutic environment that is accepting and understanding, the clinician can help clients experience themselves as worthwhile, valuable human beings (Potter-Efron, 1987).

Damage to self-esteem is a specific problem endured by ACOAs; damage to one's very sense of self is a more global difficulty for many ACOAs. Questions such as "What kinds of things do you enjoy?" or "Do you have any hobbies?" are sometimes initially met with surprise and resistance for several reasons: (1) ACOAs have cultivated the art of repressing their own feelings, wishes, and needs; (2) they may be convinced they could not possibly be good at anything; and (3) sharing positive feelings may be felt to be too dangerous because, in their experience, it has often been followed by a precipitous drop in self-esteem. When such clients are able to overcome their own resistance to examining their feelings, surprising examples of interests, hobbies, or desires long suppressed may be voiced. Simply being asked the questions provides permission for them to own their own feelings.

Boundary confusion resulting from damage to the sense of self is frequently an ongoing treatment issue that may manifest in a variety of ways, such as preoccupation with, and a tendency to overreact to, the behavior, thoughts, and feelings of others, including those of the clinician, to the exclusion of the ACOA's own needs. This pattern may become a form of resistance in the treatment when, for example, the client uses it to avoid focusing on him- or herself. The clinician should be careful not to disclose personal information in an effort to keep the boundaries clear and to maximize the client's understanding of this difficulty. The client needs to be enabled to progressively relinquish efforts at regulating his or her feelings through enmeshment with others and to work toward establishing a sufficiently coherent, differentiated, and well-integrated sense of self that can tolerate differences and separation.

> Early in her treatment, Ms. H. complained that her husband made critical remarks about her brother and parents and expressed the wish that "he should be nicer to them." In response to the therapist's request for clarification, she admitted that his comments were warranted, then exclaimed in considerable dismay, "But my parents have been the biggest influence in my life! I *am* my parents; my parents are me! Am I supposed to change at this point in my life and become like my husband?"

Ms. H. experienced her husband's criticism of her relatives as criticism of herself. It was hard for her to imagine that she did not need to replicate her parents *or* her husband—that she could be herself!

Helping ACOAs deal with anger and repressed rage is usually a pivotal issue in treatment. They dread the anger of others, which brings with it the threat of rejection, abandonment, or attack; and they dread their own anger, because it threatens the destruction of the loved object. When the love or attachment of parent or partner seems somewhat secure, ACOAs may engage in provocative behavior as a way of testing their full expectation of rejection. At other times anger may be suppressed or expressed in very ineffectual or self-defeating ways. All of these fears about, and modes of dealing with, anger may be acted out within the context of the therapy as well as in the client's life, in general. For example, the client may not show up for an appointment if he or she is feeling angry at the therapist. If the clinician is able to demonstrate to the client how he or she is handling such feelings, the client may experience considerable relief and, with support, find more adaptive ways of dealing with anger.

COUNTERTRANSFERENCE ISSUES

Certain difficulties of ACOAs, when acted out in relation to the therapist, may contribute to countertransference reactions. For example, it is painful for many ACOAs to acknowledge their dependency wishes. Their expectation is that their needs will never be met, and it is therefore difficult to trust the clinician's implicit offers of help, however much that help may be desired. They may powerfully defend against any display of vulnerability, holding the clinician at arm's length. Therapists who do not understand the dynamics underlying this behavior may feel thwarted and frustrated. Another example involves the many ways in which anger may be acted out. For instance, anger at childhood deprivations may contribute to a sense of entitlement that may be expressed in therapy as dissatisfaction with, or denigration of, helpers, in general, or the therapist, in particular. Again, not understanding these dynamics could cause the clinician to feel personally attacked or inadequate. As in any treatment, if the client is arousing uncomfortable feelings within the clinician, it is vital that the therapist not allow him- or herself to act out those feelings (e.g., by expressing impatience or acting rejecting toward the client). Rather, the clinician must take the time to examine his or her feelings, try to understand the source as it is rooted in the client's conflicts, and demonstrate to the client how he or she is acting out conflicts in a maladaptive manner.

Sensitive treatment by a clinician who demonstrates empathy, patience, and a wish to understand, in a setting that provides consistency and clear boundaries, can make it safe for clients to rediscover a hope of finding relationships of genuine mutuality with truly available partners. They can accomplish this goal by acknowledging their deprivation, working through their sense of shame, and transforming their despair into the kind of mourning that allows them to let go of the illusions of empathic, caring parents (and thereby working through the compulsive need to reenact the childhood trauma). The self that has been injured, frightened, and hidden away can thus emerge as an authentic self, capable of autonomy and a full range of feelings.

CONCLUSION

Given the large numbers of young and adult children of alcohol- and other substance-abusing parents, and given the degree of pain they suffer in childhood and the continuing painful consequences experienced by many of them in adulthood, it is critical for clinicians to be aware of the dynamics common to this population. Appropriate treatment can help clients to overcome excessive shame, guilt, boundary confusion, disabling need for control and approval, and the tendency to repeat their traumatic early experiences. The narcissistic injury and damage to the sense of self, sustained as a result of impaired parental empathy, can begin to be worked through with the help of informed, empathic clinicians.

REFERENCES

Biederman, J., Wilens, T., Mick, E., Spencer, T., & Faraone, S. V. (1999). Pharmacotherapy of attention deficit/hyperactivity disorder reduces risk for substance use disorder. *Pediatrics, 104*(2), e20.

Black, C. (1981). *It will never happen to me.* New York: Ballantine.

Brown, S. (2000). Adult children of alcoholics: An expanded framework for assessment and diagnosis. In S. Abbott (Ed.), *Children of alcoholics: Selected readings* (Vol. 2, pp. 161–188). Rockville, MD: National Association for Children of Alcoholics.

Cermak, T. L., & Beckman, W. (1995). Offspring of alcoholics and other addicts. In R. Coombs & D. Ziedonis (Eds.), *Handbook on drug abuse prevention* (pp. 361–377). Boston: Allyn & Bacon.

Cermak, T. L., & Rosenfeld, A. (1987). Therapeutic considerations with adult children of alcoholics. *Advances in Alcohol and Substance Abuse, 6*(4), 17–32.

el-Guebaly, N., West, M., Maticka-Tyndale, E., & Pool. M. (1993). Attachment among adult children of alcoholics. *Addiction, 88*(10), 1405–1411.

Farber, S. (2000). *When the body is the target: Self-harm, pain, and traumatic attachments.* Northvale, NJ: Aronson.

Golden, G., & Hill, M. (1991). A token of loving: From melancholia to mourning. *Clinical Social Work Journal, 19*(1), 23–33.

Grant, B. F. (2000). Estimates of U.S. children exposed to alcohol use and dependence in the family. *American Journal of Public Health, 90*(1), 112–115.

Hibbard, S. (1987). The diagnosis and treatment of adult children of alcoholics as a specialized therapeutic population. *Psychotherapy, 24*(4), 779–785.

Jaeger, E., Hahn, N. B., & Weinraub, M. (2000). Attachment in adult daughters of alcoholic fathers. *Addiction, 95*(2), 267–276.

Johnson, J., & Leff, M. (1999). Children of substance abusers: Overview of research findings. *Pediatrics, 103*(5 Suppl.), 1085–1099.

Kohut, H., & Wolf, E. S. (1978). The disorders of the self and their treatment: An outline. *International Journal of Psycho-Analysis, 59*, 413–425.

Levy, S., & Rutter, E. (1992). *Children of drug abusers.* New York: Lexington Books.

Miller, A. (1981). *The drama of the gifted child.* New York: Basic Books.

National Association for Children of Alcoholics. (1998). *Children of alcoholics: Important facts.* Rockville, MD: National Clearinghouse for Alcohol- and Drug Information.

Norwood, R. (1985). *Women who love too much.* New York: Simon & Schuster.

O'Connor, M. J., Sigman, M., & Brill, N. (1987). Disorganization of attachment in relation to maternal alcohol consumption. *Journal of Consulting and Clinical Psychology, 55*(6), 831–836.

Price, A., & Emshoff, J. (1997). Breaking the cycle of addiction. *Alcohol Health and Research World, 21*(3), 241–246.

Potter—Efron, R. (1987). Shame and guilt: Definitions, processes and treatment issues with AODA clients. *Alcoholism Treatment Quarterly, 4*(2), 7–24.

Shengold, L. (1989). *Soul murder.* New Haven, CT: Yale University Press.

Sher, K. J. (1991). *Children of alcoholics: A critical appraisal of theory and research.* Chicago: University of Chicago Press.

Straussner, S. L. A. (1994). The impact of alcohol and other drug abuse on the American family. *Drug and Alcohol Review, 13,* 93–399.

Wegscheider, S. (1981). *Another chance: Hope and health for the alcoholic family.* Palo Alto, CA: Science and Behavior Books.

Werner, M., Joffe, A., & Graham, A. (1999). Screening, early identification, and office-based intervention with children and youth living in substance-abusing families. *Pediatrics, 103*(5 Suppl.) 1099–1112.

Wilens, T. E., Spencer, T. J., & Biederman, J. (2000). Attention-deficit/hyperactivity disorder with substance use disorders. In T. E. Brown (Ed.), *Attention deficit disorders and comorbidities in children, adolescents and adults* (pp. 319–339). Washington, DC: American Psychiatric Association Press.

Wolin, S., & Wolin, S. (1993). *The resilient self: How survivors of troubled families rise above adversity.* New York: Villard Books.

Wood, B. (1987). *Children of alcoholism: The struggle for self and intimacy in adult life.* New York: New York University Press.

PART V

Special Issues and Special Populations

Part V has seven chapters that focus on the special issues of working with clients of different ages and with different groups of substance-abusing individuals frequently encountered in a variety of social work settings.

In Chapter 14 the author discusses assessment and treatment of adolescent substance abusers, whereas the author of the next chapter considers individuals at the other end of the age spectrum: older adults. As the material in these two chapters points out, each of these age groups calls for assessment approaches that differ from those used in working with adult populations, and each has its own unique treatment needs.

The aim of the next chapter, 16, is to focus on assessment and intervention with substance-abusing women. Here the author provides data on the latest research on alcohol- and drug-abusing women, including differences not only between women and men but also among women themselves. A common Axis II diagnosis among substance-abusing women is that of borderline personality disorder. This topic is addressed in Chapter 17. After describing the main characteristics, causes, and treatment of borderline disorders, the author considers the main issues that arise when working with substance abusers who also have a borderline disturbance, and identifies the major treatment foci and techniques of use with this difficult group of patients.

The treatment of the gay, lesbian, and bisexual substance abuser is the topic of Chapter 18. The purpose of this chapter is to identify and highlight assessment and treatment issues that may arise when homosexuality is a part of a recovering client's life.

The authors caution clinicians to be cognizant of the wide range of homosexual experiences and to avoid simplistically labeling their clients. In Chapter 19 the author examines the prevalence, etiology, and treatment of substance abuse among homeless individuals. The role of the social worker and the application of innovative approaches for helping this multiple-problem population are highlighted.

Part V ends with a chapter that addresses the numerous physical, psychological, and social issues affecting individuals who acquired HIV/AIDS as a result of intravenous drug use. Here the authors delineate the multiple tasks that confront social workers and other professionals concerned with providing services to this emotionally challenging client group.

Working with substance-abusing clients is not an easy task, but as each of these chapters in Part V points out, it is a challenge that can be successfully addressed with specific knowledge, skills, realistic expectations, and awareness of one's own countertranference reactions.

CHAPTER 14

Assessment and Treatment of Adolescent Substance Abusers

Audrey Freshman

Adolescent substance abuse occurs within a social context of family, school, and community; amid a sociocultural climate that promotes "better living through chemistry." The very society that condemns the use of alcohol and other drugs by young people, and which suffers the consequences of such use through accidents, suicides, criminality, teenage rape, and numerous other problems, spends billions of dollars annually to promote the use of "legal" chemicals such as alcohol, nicotine, caffeine, and prescription medication. Ironically, much of these advertising dollars have been aimed directly at the youth market. Yet the adolescent who becomes addicted is vilified.

The purpose of this chapter is to review current patterns of alcohol and drug abuse among adolescents in the United States, and to identify contemporary approaches to prevention, assessment, and treatment interventions. A systemic approach to conceptualizing this issue is necessary, because adolescent substance abuse can be addressed only within the context of multiple parent/school/community partnerships. Furthermore, the ambiguity around teenage substance use as a "rite of passage" needs clarification at a time when young people are being raised by a "village of elders"—elders who themselves grew up within the drug culture.

CURRENT TRENDS IN ADOLESCENT
ALCOHOL AND OTHER DRUG USE AND ABUSE

Patterns of use and abuse of all substances, ranging from alcohol to other illicit drugs, tend to fluctuate according to ever-shifting trends among adolescents. For example, the popularity of a particular substance (mediated by
such variables as drug trafficking, marketing, and public awareness) can remarkably decrease the use of one substance, such as crack/cocaine, or significantly increase the use of another, such as ecstasy, in any given time. As new
drugs enter the marketplace, a "grace period" exists in which the word of
mouth benefits are quickly touted, whereas the negative consequences are revealed at a slower pace (Johnston, O'Malley, & Bachman, 2003). Thus the
fads may change, but the drug epidemic is kept alive via the introduction of
new drugs and/or the rediscovery of some of the older ones.

Gateway Drugs: Alcohol, Nicotine, and Marijuana

Alcohol, nicotine, and marijuana have come to be viewed as "gateway
drugs," so called for the path that most substance users pass enroute to the
use and abuse of other illicit substances. As a result, these drugs have been
the targets of most prevention efforts. During the 1990s, the onset age of
alcohol, nicotine, and marijuana usage steadily decreased. The 1998 Back
to School Teen Survey (National Center on Addiction and Substance
Abuse, 1999) noted that it is precisely as the 12- or 13-year-old child transitions to middle school that the exposure to illegal drugs increases, while
parental involvement decreases. According to the survey, between ages 12–
15, the proportion of adolescents that smoked cigarettes within the preceding month rose from 2 to 15%, those who reported having been drunk in
the last month increased from 2% to 21%, and the percentage of those
who smoked marijuana jumped from 1 to 34% (National Center on Addiction and Substance Abuse, 1999).

Nationwide trends in licit and illicit drug use among teens are ascer-
tained primarily from data collected by the University of Michigan's Institute
for Social Research. This study, titled "Monitoring the Future Survey"
(MTF) and funded by the National Institute on Drug Abuse (NIDA), was
started in 1975 and continues to be conducted annually with a representative
sample of 8th, 10th, and 12th-grade students throughout the United States.
Overall, the results of the 2003 survey of 43,700 students in 394 schools
showed a slight decrease in the use of alcohol, nicotine, and marijuana.

Although young people have experienced alcohol problems throughout the course of U.S. history, alcohol use is frequently seen as a modern-
day problem (Feigelman & Feigelman, 1993). Currently, alcohol use
remains extremely common, with nearly 78% of students claiming to have
tried it (beyond a few sips) by the end of high school and 62% of 12th

graders having reported being drunk at least once (Johnston et al., 2003). Alcohol is the drug that is most widely used and abused by teens, and the substance most closely associated with such severe consequences as car accidents, teen pregnancy, suicide, and violence (National Center on Addiction and Substance Abuse, 1997). Although teens do not drink as often as adults, their quantity of use in one sitting far exceeds that of their elders. Peer disapproval is lowest for alcohol consumption in comparison to other drugs, and beer remains the most popular form of alcohol consumed, followed by wine coolers (Johnston et al., 2003).

This same MTF 2003 survey found that nicotine use, having risen steadily in all three grades until 1996, has begun to decrease among teens. Reasons for this decrease are attributed to the increase in perceived risk due to adverse publicity, increased cost, and factors related to the aftermath of the tobacco settlement. Nonetheless, there is still reason for considerable concern. In 2002, more than half of U.S. teens reported having tried cigarettes, and by 12th grade, one-quarter were regular users (Johnston et al., 2003).

Marijuana remains the most popular *illicit drug* used in 2002, and, in fact, for the past 27 years of the study. Its use peaked in 1979, dropped until the mid-1990s and continues to remain popular due to its perception of limited risk and ready availability. During 2002, the prevalence rates for marijuana use were 19.2%, 38.7%, and 47.8% for 8th, 10th, and 12th graders, respectively (Johnston et al., 2003).

Of greater importance, especially for prevention efforts, is the cascading effect of these gateway substances in setting the stage for the use of more dangerous drugs. Nicotine was found to be particularly important in the subsequent use of alcohol and marijuana (Duncan, Duncan, & Hops, 1998): Teens who smoke are five and a half times more likely to use marijuana, six times more likely to get drunk at least once a month, and three times more likely to try another illegal drug (National Center on Addiction and Substance Abuse, 1998). Furthermore, statistical analysis of data gathered from 10, 900 9th to 12th graders found that 12–17-year-olds who had used the three gateway drugs (i.e., cigarettes, alcohol, and marijuana) within the past month were almost 17 times more likely to use another drug, such as cocaine or heroin (National Center on Addiction and Substance Abuse, 1997). Conversely, a 50% reduction in the number of teens who smoke cigarettes can cut marijuana use by as much as 16–28%, according to an American Legacy Foundation report (National Center on Addiction and Substance Abuse, 2003).

Other Illicit Drugs

According to the results of the MTF 2002 survey, the prevalence rates for most other illicit drugs of abuse reached peak levels during the mid-1990s and have since leveled off and remained fairly constant. In particular, the investigators found that the use of inhalants peaked in 1995, hallucinogens (including LSD and PCP) in 1996, and amphetamines in 1996–1997. The use of amphetamines and crystal methamphetamine, having increased in the beginning of the last decade, are once again declining among 8th, 10th, and 12th graders. After steadily increasing throughout the 1990s, the use of cocaine showed a large drop in 1999 among 8th and 10th graders, followed by a decrease in use for 12th graders in 2000. Its use was 2.3% (8th grade), 4.0% (10th grade) and 5.0% (12th grade) in 2002. Crack use, however, showed a significant increase among 10th graders in 2002.

In contrast, this same survey found an increase in the prevalence rates of certain other drugs of abuse. For example, the use of steroids has risen substantially among 12th-grade boys. Heroin, having resurged in the earlier part of the decade due to the advent of noninjectable forms, restabilized within the past 3 years and has remained steady at about 1% in each respective grade (Johnston et al., 2003). For the first time in 2002, rates were gathered for the use of opiates such as OxyContin (up to 4% of 12th graders) and Vicodin (9.6% of 12th graders). Interestingly, the use/abuse of stimulants such as Ritalin, commonly prescribed for ADD/ADHD, that are reportedly snorted intranasally is not measured by this survey. In interpreting all of these findings it is important to recognize that the more serious the substance abuse problem, the less likely the adolescent will be attending school and participating in these surveys. This reality skews the data to a more functional population survey (Harrison, Fulkerson, & Beebe, 1998).

Club Drugs

The 1990s ushered in the decade of "club drugs," so named for their association with usage at all-night dances known as "raves." These drugs include Rohypnol, GHB, and Ketamine (Special K), which are mainly central nervous system depressants. Colorless, tasteless, and odorless, they are often referred to as "date-rape" drugs because they can easily be slipped into beverages and ingested unknowingly by an unsuspecting victim. In response to growing concern, Congress passed the "Drug-Induced Rape Prevention and Punishment Act of 1996," which increased federal penalties for use of any controlled substance to aid in sexual assault (National Institute on Drug Abuse [NIDA], 2000a).

Another well-known club drug is MDMA, commonly called "Ecstasy," a synthetic, psychoactive drug with hallucinogenic and amphetamine-like properties (NIDA, 2000b). Originally synthesized and patented in Germany in the early 1900s, the drug remained somewhat dormant until the 1970s, when it was used by some psychotherapists who claimed that it enhanced communication in patient sessions; it reemerged in the mid-1980s, and its use continued to rise yearly through 2001. Recently, peer norms against the use of this drug, along with an increased perception of risk and a leveling off of drug availability, have resulted in the drop in ecstasy use in 2002 (Johnston et al., 2003).

PRIMARY AND SECONDARY PREVENTION OF ADOLESCENT SUBSTANCE ABUSE

One of the best strategies for averting substance use disorders is to encourage abstinence or at least delay the age of onset (Grant & Dawson, 1997). An earlier onset of substance use is highly correlated with future addictive disorders and poorer prognosis (Archambault, 1989; DeWit, Adlaf, Offord, & Ogborne, 2000; Grant & Dawson, 1997; Gruber, DiClemente, Anderson, & Lodico, 1996; Sobeck, Abbey, Agius, Clinton, & Harrison, 2000). There is extensive literature focusing on primary prevention efforts aimed at recognizing the risk factors for substance use disorders. However, focusing on risks has not been the only strategy of primary prevention. A newer model, the strengths-based approach, seeks to enhance protective factors and resiliency (Hawkins, Catalano, & Miller, 1992; Werner, 1982) by focusing on social/life skills, self-esteem building, parenting skills training, education, and media programming.

Identifying Risk Factors

The more risk factors a child or adolescent experiences, the more likely it is that he or she will develop substance abuse problems. Consequently, attending to risk factors affords an opportunity for early assessment of potential problems and interventions targeted at augmenting protection and diminishing further use of substances. However, in the absence of clear warning signs, it is difficult for parents, educators, or mental health professionals to distinguish between the adolescent who is using drugs or alcohol in a social, recreational manner from the teen who is at risk for chemical dependency. Bogenschneider (1991) categorizes much of the body of work on risk factors into six domains:

Individual Risk Factors

- Alienation
- Antisocial behavior
- Anxiety or depression
- Early first use of drugs

Family Risk Factors

- Parent or sibling drug/alcohol abuse
- Adapting to divorce or remarriage, or a marked worsening of family relations
- Distant, uninvolved, and inconsistent parenting
- Negative parent–child communication
- Poor parental monitoring
- Unclear family rules, expectations, and rewards

Peer Risk Factors

- Associating with peers who use drugs
- Perceived use of substances by others

School Risk Factors

- Academic failure
- Low commitment to school
- School transitions
- Poor teaching practices

Work Risk Factors

- Long work hours

Community Risk Factors

- Complacent or permissive community law and norms
- Drug availability
- Lack of concerted law enforcement
- Lack of meaningful roles
- Lack of clarity regarding adolescent status
- Low neighborhood attachment and community disorganization
- Low socioeconomic status

In addition to the individual risk factors mentioned above, gender, cultural, and socioeconomic variables also should be understood.

Gender Differences

Despite the overlap between the sexes with respect to the above risk factors, gender differences do exist. For example, the signs of substance abuse for boys—that is, fighting, drunk driving, and truancy—tend to be outer

directed, whereas for girls the risk factors are more inner directed, less de-
tectable, overlooked, and often misdiagnosed (National Center on Addiction and Substance Abuse, 1996). Studies suggest that substance use disorder follows anxiety and depression in girls but occurs in reversed order for
boys; more research is needed (Angold, Costello, & Erkanli, 1999).

Freshman and Leinwand (2001) believe that a gender-sensitive perspective for adolescent females requires the additional inclusion of the following risk factors: (1) distortion in body image and excessive preoccupation with weight issues, (2) lack of close female friendships, (3) history of
sexual abuse, and (4) a high incidence of suicide attempts. Finally, early onset of menses is associated with earlier initial drug use (Center for Substance Abuse Prevention [CSAP], 1996).

Ethnicity and Socioeconomic Status

Research studies have found that cultural influences and ethnic identification may significantly influence drug use (Straussner, 2001). Adolescents
who strongly identify with their communities and cultures are less vulnerable to risk factors for drug use (Zickler, 2000). African American students
have lower rates of drug use than either white or Hispanic adolescents
(Johnston et al., 2003; Kaminer, 1999; Kilpatrick et al., 2000). Hispanic
adolescents have rates of use that fall between the two groups but are
closer to the rates for whites, although they do have higher rates in the
12th grade of using crack, heroin with a needle, and "ice" (methamphetamine; Johnston et al., 2003).

Friedman and Ali (1998) studied 484 adolescent substance abusers for
the interrelationship between ethnicity and socioeconomic status and drug
use. They found that both the severity and degree of substance abuse was
greater for white than African American teens, with the exception of crack
and heroin use. There was significantly less substance abuse if a family was
receiving welfare than for other socioeconomic (SES) levels. There was no
significant difference between lower SES African Americans and higher
SES whites on the amount of money spent to obtain drugs.

Family Risk Factors

The following family risk factors need to be explored when working with
adolescents.

The Role of Parents. Family background and parenting styles are increasingly receiving attention as critical risk factors and targets of intervention for both prevention and treatment. Of greatest importance is the understanding of the genetic predisposition for substance abuse. Children of

alcohol- or drug-addicted parents are at higher risk of substance abuse—a critical point to understand.

In addition to parental substance abuse, parental absence due to death or divorce and family interaction style have been linked to increased risk of substance abuse in children (Denton & Kampfe, 1994). Parental discord, family disruption, parental nondirectiveness, negative communication style, inconsistent discipline, and lack of closeness have all been noted as important factors that place a child at risk (Denton & Kamfe, 1994; Swadi, 1999). In the families of drug-abusing children, fathers were found to be too distant and disengaged, whereas mothers were too involved or enmeshed (Swadi, 1999). Overly demanding as well as excessively moralistic styles of parenting also were correlated to increased risk of chemical dependency (Lawson, Peterson, & Lawson, 1983). In fact, *extremely high* and *very low* levels of parental monitoring are closely related to adolescent substance abuse, regardless of the presence of parental alcoholism (Swadi, 1999).

The Role of Siblings. Having siblings that are drug involved is related to the risk of substance abuse in adolescents. Needle and colleagues (1986) found that having an older drug-involved sibling not only increased the likelihood of substance abuse but resulted in a decreased age of onset for the younger siblings.

Peer Risk Factors

Bradizza, Reifman, and Barnes (1999), in testing why adolescents drink, discovered that social motives (e.g., drinking is fun and enhances socializing) as opposed to coping motives (e.g., drinking handles worries) are prime reasons for alcohol use among mid- and later-age adolescents. There is also substantial evidence to suggest that peer influence has a tremendous impact on substance-abusing behavior, and it has been indicted as the single factor most likely to predict current drug use (Swadi, 1999). Substance abuse can result from direct peer pressure; it is not just a by-product of subgroup conformity (Swadi, 1999). It should also be noted that the more drug involved the child, the more probable it is that he or she will seek out like-minded friends.

Warning Signals

Jayne, age 15, was recently caught at school holding two joints of marijuana. She denied that the drugs were hers, claiming instead that they belonged to her friend. Her parents were immediately called to school and she was temporarily suspended, pending an evaluation. She was brought to the school social worker, whose job is to decide whether or not she is in need of further assessment. Jayne's parents acknowledged her increased moodiness, depression, rebelliousness, and a tendency to isolate herself from family events, but they believed these to be normal behaviors for an adolescent. She has abandoned her old friendships in favor of a new group of peers that "are more fun and like to hangout and go to clubs." Her parents are aware that she has attended unsupervised parties where alcohol is served but recall that they were similarly involved as teens themselves. They do not believe that she is an "alcoholic," as is her paternal grandfather or her uncles who drink daily. Her grades have begun to deteriorate, and her parents have responded by supplying her with tutors. In response to this latest event, the parents contended that the school personnel were scapegoating their daughter and have considered placing her in another school. Mom and Dad concede that they are beginning to argue more frequently over the management of curfew, money, and consequences for Jayne's rambunctious behavior. Following the screening by the school social worker, Jayne was referred to a clinician in a community outpatient substance abuse agency to determine the severity of the drug problem and what, if any, intervention was indicated.

Understanding the risk factors for substance abuse is only the first step: recognizing the presence of warning signs and acting on this recognition by suggesting the need for further diagnostic assessment and intervention are essential. According to Mooney, Eisenberg, and Eisenberg (1992) some of the warning signs for teens include (1) increasing time spent alone in their room, particularly for adolescents who were not previously loners; (2) increased secretiveness; (3) negative changes in attitude toward school, with friends, in hygiene, in dress; (4) changes in peer-group composition; (5) pronounced mood swings; (6) lying, shoplifting, stealing (money from home); (7) abandonment of extracurricular activities (e.g., sports, clubs, religious services); (8) unpredictable, rebellious behavior; (9) curfew breaking; (10) alcohol on breath; (11) discovery of drug paraphernalia; and (12) obvious hangovers, blackouts, drugged behavior.

ASSESSMENT OF ADOLESCENT SUBSTANCE ABUSERS

Assessment of substance use disorders is far more complicated for adolescents than for adults. Some of the warning signs listed above correlate with the normal behavioral changes that characterize the developmental stage of adolescence. The emotional and physical changes associated with this stage are accompanied by the developmental tasks of achieving individuality, separation, and autonomy, and the assumption of increasingly adult privileges and responsibilities. At this time, adolescents continue to acquire the life skills necessary in making decisions to manage impulses, curb sensation-seeking behavior, delay gratification, and avoid harmful risks. The presence of concomitant learning, physical, or emotional disabilities as well as unresolved sexual orientation and gender identity issues can create additional stress. Many of these stressors, in turn, are linked with the psychological and social causes of substance abuse. In turn, substance abuse or dependence exacerbates the behavior problems commonly associated with normal adolescent development and can cause developmental delays. Unfortunately, the very process of separation and individuation can be stunted (Stanton & Todd, 1982) as the substance-abusing adolescent becomes maturationally incapable of meeting the challenges of adulthood.

The disease of addiction tends to overlap with the "dis-ease" of adolescence; both require careful assessment by the clinician. Assessment requires an understanding of normal adolescent development in addition to awareness of the interrelatedness of individual risk factors, family variables, peer relations, school/vocational performance, legal status, physical health, and psychiatric conditions (comorbidity). Above all, assessment of substance use disorders must involve careful examination of the drug history and pattern of use (i.e., onset and types of substances used, frequency, quantity, and progression over time). Any efforts to control usage or evidence of loss of control (e.g., unsuccessful efforts to stop or limit use) must be examined. Information as to how the adolescent acquires or pays for the drugs (e.g., friends, weekly allowance, dealing, job) needs to be obtained, as it can provide insight into the depth of drug involvement.

Differentiating Use, Abuse, and Dependence in Adolescents

Although not without its limitations, familiarity with DSM-IV criteria is essential when assessing "experimental" drug use versus, abuse and dependence.

Experimental Use

Experimental drug use among adolescents has come to be accepted as a normative developmental phase. The 1999 National Survey of American Attitudes on Substance Abuse and Addiction V (National Center on Addiction and Substance Abuse, 1999) revealed that nearly half of all baby-boomer parents believe that their children will try illegal drugs; 58% of these parents, who regularly used marijuana in their own youth, expect their teenager to use drugs.

It can be hard to distinguish adolescent patterns of experimental substance use from abuse. Harrison and colleagues (1998) note that *any* alcohol or drug use by adolescents occurs in relation to their underage status regarding drinking and the illegal nature of illicit drug use. Using this legalistic frame, drug use can *always* be conceptualized as problematic for adolescents. As a result, these authors believe that in terms of diagnostic assessment of adolescents, the term substance *use* should be abandoned entirely in favor of substance *abuse*, in order to reflect the social disapproval of violation of the law. Apart from the question of legality, Kaminer (1999) notes that in reality, modest or even heavy use of substances can be "adolescence limited"; the progression does not necessarily culminate in a poor prognosis of dependence in young adulthood. Nonetheless, Swadi (1999) cautions us to remember that the vast majority of adult addictions do have their genesis in adolescent experimental use.

Abuse and Dependence

Currently, the DSM-IV is utilized to diagnose substance use disorders in adolescents in spite of the fact that it was developed primarily based on observations of adult populations (Harrison et al., 1998). Thus the interrelationship of substance abuse and the developmental tasks of both early- and late-stage adolescence is not exclusively addressed within the criteria.

Likewise, the DSM-IV diagnosis for substance abuse disorder also has been critiqued as not truly reflective of typical adolescent patterns of use and difficult to distinguish from substance dependence. Diagnosed substance dependence is related to the presence of tolerance, physical problems, withdrawal symptoms, and social and occupational consequences that can take years to develop, and may be difficult to apply to adolescents. For example, the criteria of "impaired control" can be problematic when applied to adolescents whose explicit intention is "to get high or smashed" on multiple substances at a time (Harrison et al., 1998). Many adolescents who use illicit substances do engage in simultaneous polydrug taking that involves the use of two or more substances on the same occasion to increase synergistic effect (Collins, Ellickson, & Bell, 1998). Harrison and colleagues (1998) found that the application of the abuse/dependence diagnostic framework was not supported by their study of 74,008 9th- and 12th-grade students and called for the development of an alternative classification system that is more commensurate with actual teen patterns of use.

Similarly, Pollack and Martin (1999) described a group of "diagnostic orphans," adolescents ages 13–19 who have one or two DSM-IV alcohol dependence symptoms that did not meet either of the DSM-IV criteria for alcohol abuse or alcohol dependence, but who nonetheless were considered to have alcohol problems and were attending alcohol treatment programs. These authors also believe that their results demonstrate the limitations of the DSM-IV criteria for alcohol abuse and dependence when applied to adolescents, particularly during the earlier phases of the illness.

Assessment of Comorbidity

Within the past 10 years, it has become more common to rethink the classification of adolescent pathology in terms of comorbid conditions that precede, exacerbate, co-occur or predict future adult dependency (Angold et al., 1999). Zeitlin (1999) notes that "the heterogeneity of young people with comorbidity for psychiatric disorder and substance misuse suggest that some would better be considered as multiproblem children for whom the necessary conditions are vulnerability, lack of family protection and exposure to a source of drugs" (p. 225). Kaminer (1999) reports that the most common disorders associated with substance use in adolescence are conduct disorders (50–80% of the clinical population) and mood disorders (24–50% prevalence of concurrent depressive disorders, and 7–40% prevalence for anxiety). Suicidal ideation and successful teen suicides have been linked to substance use and abuse disorders (Crumley, 1990; Kaminer, 1999). Aggressive and antisocial behavior in early childhood is another major risk factor for future drug use (Swadi, 1999).

Learning disabilities and attention-deficit/hyperactivity disorder (ADHD) also have a high degree of association within the teen substance-abusing population, although further research is necessary to refine our understanding of these overlapping conditions. Learning disabilities affect as much as 20% of the school-age population in the United States (National Center on Addiction and Substance Abuse, 2000). It is speculated that a child with learning disabilities suffers the same risk factors that set the stage for substance abuse; that is, low self-esteem, academic failure, depression, and an excessive desire for social acceptance/peer pressure. Moreover, a child with a learning disability is twice as likely to also have ADHD (National Center on Addiction and Substance Abuse, 2000). Horner and Scheibe (1997) found that teens with ADHD had earlier and even more severe substance use and negative self-image issues; drugs are seen as an effort at self-medication. These investigators noted that as many as half of all teens diagnosed with ADHD self-medicate with drugs and alcohol (Horner & Scheibe, 1997). Angold and colleagues (1999) believe that the association between substance abuse and ADHD may be mediated by the high incidence of conduct disorder in the latter group. In turn, the interrelatedness of substance abuse, conduct disorder, learning disabilities, and ADHD is illustrative of the multiplicity of variables reported in studies of comorbidity. Other disorders more commonly linked with substance abuse in adolescents are posttraumatic stress disorder secondary to physical abuse, sexual abuse, or the witnessing of violence (Giaconia et al., 2000; Kilpatrick et al., 2000; Lipschitz, Grilo, Fehon, McGlashan, & Southwick, 2000), eating disorders (Zeitlen, 1999), and gambling (Kaminer, 1999).

Much effort has been made to delineate the developmental sequencing and timing of comorbid conditions in order to understand etiology, psychopathology, prevention, assessment, and treatment. More research is necessary to refine current assessment methods. Clearly, a detailed history will enable the clinician to develop a more three-dimensional view of the multiproblem adolescent presenting with substance use. Sensitivity to the role of current chemical usage in either creating or exacerbating psychopathology is always indicated. Evaluation must be seen as an ongoing process. Referral for medication should occur at a time when it is reasonably felt that the adolescent is no longer experiencing the toxic effects of drugs but can benefit from assessment of a comorbid condition; this usually occurs following a period of abstinence.

THE ASSESSMENT PROCESS

The assessment process requires a systemic approach to the understanding of the adolescent within multiple interrelated domains. This process can be facilitated by the utilization of assessment and screening tools, drug testing, the obtainment of collateral information, the presence of family members, and the establishment of rapport to help elicit information.

Assessment Tools

A strong argument can be made for the standardization, reliability, and validity of information that is gathered through the use of assessment tools. For an adolescent caught within a myriad of systems, the uniformity provided by consistent use of such tools can enhance a seamless method of service delivery (Meyers, Hagan, et al., 1999). Instruments such as the Adolescent Drug Involvement Scale simply screen for drug involvement, whereas the Problem Oriented Screening Instrument for Teenagers (POSIT) and the Adolescent Problem Severity Index also measure other dimensions of psychosocial functioning. A more complete listing of adolescent assessment and screening tools is provided by SAMHSA (Substance Abuse and Mental Health Services Administration, 1999a).

The Role of the Clinician

Oftentimes the assessment process marks the first contact that the adolescent has with a helping professional. Understandably, issues of trust abound and there is considerable question as to whether or not an adolescent will accurately self-report his or her drug history (i.e., the type, frequency, pattern, and quantity of substance[s] used). Performance on assessment measures can be complicated by inattention, lack of motivation, disinterest, and reading difficulties (Meyers, Hagan, et al., 1999). Moreover, the focus on assessment tests can impede the rapport building that is necessary for more honest communication.

Inevitably, assessment is best served by a mutually respectful and empathically attuned relationship between adolescent and clinician. Miller (2000) suggests that clinicians use motivational enhancement therapy (MET)—reflective listening, reframing, and support for self-efficacy—in offering hope for change. Feedback to the client of assessment findings is used to enlist client motivation. Likewise, the clinician needs to avoid what Miller refers to as the "confrontation/denial trap" (p. 101). This trap occurs when the clinician is placed in a position of asserting the presence of a problem and the need to change, while the client argues against this position. Instead, he believes that clinicians should "roll with" resistance rather than confronting it directly.

Laboratory Testing

Urinalysis is an essential tool to aid in the assessment process. It is particularly effective in corroborating or disputing the adolescent's self-report regarding recent usage (Winters & Stinchfield, 1995) and can facilitate the adolescent's entry into treatment (Tennant, 1994). However, it must be understood that laboratory findings generally only reveal information as to most recent use (marijuana is the exception, because heavy usage can be detected up to 1 month). As a matter of caution, be aware that many retail and Internet products are sold to adolescents to produce adulterated screens. It is important to understand that the findings of one particular screen do not provide a longitudinal view of drug-taking behavior, nor can these findings be used as a diagnostic tool in lieu of a thorough evaluation.

Collateral Information

The clinician should make every effort to acquire archival information, school reports, relevant mental health and hospital records, and data from interfacing systems, such as juvenile/criminal justice, to support the assessment process. Attention must be paid to issues of confidentiality, and proper permission for release of information should be acquired.

The Role of Family Members during the Assessment Process

The referral of an adolescent for substance abuse assessment is generally viewed as a crisis by all those affected within the support system of the teen. The inclusion of parent(s)/guardian(s) from the outset is instrumental in establishing a treatment rapport with all members affected by a teen's usage at a point in time when they are most receptive to intervention. Instead of inhibiting truthfulness, the presence of family often sets the stage for the beginning of an honest exchange about the scope and context of the adolescent's drug use. Strategic structural systems engagement (SSSE) is an intervention designed to address the challenge of effectively engaging families of substance-abusing youth in treatment. The goal is to begin the work of diagnosing, therapeutic joining, and restructuring the family from the very first (pretherapy) contact, thereby facilitating engagement in therapy (Slesnick, Meyers, Meade, & Segelken, 2000; Szapocznik et al., 1988). Even when working with runaway and homeless youth, use of a family-based treatment-engagement strategy was found to be instrumental to enhancing retention rates and mending relational issues prior to total disintegration of family ties (Slesnick et al., 2000).

Parents are often divided and conflicted with regard to the acknowledgment of their child's substance use. Treadway (1989) noted that parents typically split on the debate between firmness/discipline and nurturance/understanding. It is common to find one parent minimizing, "fixing" problems, and being too understanding of the adolescent in the hopes that he or she will outgrow the behavior. At the same time, the other parent takes an overly determined, limit-setting, and punitive approach, viewing the teen's use of substances as "willful" behavior and the co-occurring failure to grow up as "laziness." The net result is that the parents negate each other's position and fail to respond in a consistent and unified fashion. For this reason, every effort should be made to contact all significant parental figures/guardians whenever possible, regardless of marital status, to attend the initial session. This inclusive meeting can enable divorced parents and stepparents to begin to "work on the same page" and be less vulnerable to subtle manipulations of former rivalries that invariably enable addiction to emerge.

> In the case of Jayne, the assessment reveals that she is using marijuana three or four times a week. She began to drink at the age of 13 and smoked marijuana at age 14. Currently she drinks beer on weekends, sometimes as much as 40 ounces at a time, and shows evidence of high tolerance. At the time of intake, she denied use of other substances, but her drug screen was positive for both cannabis and Ecstasy. She is at increased genetic risk by virtue of the fact that her paternal grandfather is alcoholic, as are some of her uncles. Her parents' use of alcohol and marijuana may be problematic. She has evidenced consequences to her usage in the form of increased difficulties at home, in school, and potentially with the law (i.e., getting caught in possession of marijuana). Her peer group has begun to shift, and she is experiencing depression, isolation, and increased rage. Jayne is resistant to counseling. Her parents have expressed their helplessness and questioned the clinician as to the next steps.

TREATMENT OF THE ADOLESCENT
SUBSTANCE ABUSER

Following assessment, the clinician must decide the appropriate type and level of care, treatment goals, and approaches to accomplish these tasks.

Level of Care

Once the need for treatment has been determined and a multidimensional assessment has been completed, the appropriate level of care must be selected. Safety of the adolescent is a prime concern. Nowadays, placement is determined as much by clinical judgment as by managed care considerations. Meyers, Hagan, and colleagues (1999) note that there is no clear empirical evidence upon which to base these decisions and suggest that three factors be utilized: (1) the severity of the alcohol/drug disorder, (2) the psychosocial profile of the adolescent, and (3) matching the services of the placement to the assessed needs of the adolescent.

Types of Settings

Treatment interventions fall along a continuum of intensity that ranges from minimal outpatient contacts (less than 9 hours a week) to intensive outpatient (6–9 hours or more), to day treatment programs (5-day-a-week programs, sometimes referred to as partial hospitalization and may include schooling) to inpatient hospitalization (rehab and detoxification facilities, halfway houses, and group homes) to long-term residential treatment (therapeutic communities, where the stay is up to 1 year or more). Rounds-Bryant, Kristiansen, and Hubbard (1999) conducted a study of 3,832 adolescent substance abuse clients from short-term (ST) inpatient, long-term residential (LT), and outpatient programs (OT). Of the adolescents within the three modalities, OT adolescents had the lowest rates of drug usage and the least prior drug treatment experiences. They were slightly younger, more likely to be attending school, and the least criminally involved. ST clients were more likely to be white females, with greater indicators of psychiatric impairment. The LT treatment modality had a greater number of male clients, the most African American and Hispanic clients, and the highest proportion of clients mandated by the criminal justice system.

According to the 2002 National Survey of Substance Abuse Treatment Services (N-SSATS), an annual survey of facilities providing substance abuse treatment conducted by SAMHSA, the vast majority of services are provided on an outpatient basis.

Use of the Juvenile Justice System

Many teens come to the attention of the juvenile justice system for substance-related issues. In some states, adolescents can be referred to the family courts and placed on probation by the schools and/or families through the use of PINS petitions (persons in need of supervision). This is often a powerful source of leverage in that court-ordered treatment and monitoring can be the most effective approach to getting many adolescents into substance use disorder services (SAMHSA, 1999b). In the case illustration, if Jayne continues to refuse to attend treatment, one of the strategies available to the clinician is to advise her family to file a PINS petition in order to have the court mandate treatment. Of course, this strategy must be carefully evaluated and other forms of leverage exhausted prior to its consideration.

12-Step Meetings

An invaluable source of adjunctive treatment is the adolescent's participation in 12-step meetings. Many treatment settings incorporate a 12-step approach and encourage participation in several ways by (1) providing institutional meetings, (2) using a psychoeducational model that teaches 12-step recovery, (3) providing "first friends," and (4) encouraging attendance, service, and obtaining a sponsor.

There are some issues of concern that relate specifically to the adolescent population. Some adolescents find it hard to overcome the generation gap or relate to the stories of "old-timers," having not faced the same degree of serious life crises (Feigelman & Feigelman, 1993). Ideally, teenagers should be referred to young-persons groups, led by responsible individuals, with a membership that is appropriate for their age, gender, and culture (SAMHSA, 1999b).

From a clinical standpoint, it is difficult to send an adolescent, such as Jayne, to a 12-step meeting that encourages the definition of self as addict/alcoholic within the context of a disease model, when the degree of severity of use does not yet warrant such labeling. Likewise, the exposure to others in recovery from more serious drug involvement often meets with a great deal of parental resistance. Finally, the adolescent must be helped to understand the importance of "men with the men" and "women with the women" in order to safeguard sexual acting-out behavior on the part of the teen or others in recovery.

TREATMENT GOALS

Treatment goals must address both the individual adolescent and the family.

Goals for the Adolescent

Using a transtheoretical model of change, an adolescent (such as Jayne) must be engaged in the process of developing an alternative life view that does not include substance abuse (Prochaska & DiClemente, 1984). A commitment to abstinence is an essential ingredient and should be contracted for the duration of treatment. Clearly, it would be ideal to extend this commitment into the future. However, this is not easily accomplished; instead the adolescent can be encouraged to develop a sober baseline against which he or she can observe both current and future behavioral changes and consequences, should he or she resume drug-taking behavior (Freshman, 1996). The operationalization of this goal, through successive approximation, often becomes the central task of initial treatment before other psychosocial concerns can be more fully addressed. The overriding aim is to help the adolescent interact in the world without chemical alteration, so that he or she stands a better chance of achieving maturational goals.

Goals for the Family

The very act of seeking help is often a turning point for the family in breaking through their own denial and acknowledging that a problem exists. Premature labeling of "addiction" should be avoided, as it can often create panic and flight from treatment. Conversely, it is equally important not to collude with the family denial of a drug problem or to contract around "other issues" with the hopes that the substance abuse will spontaneously diminish.

The family must be joined in an effort to enable them to make changes that will continue to foster abstinent behavior for their adolescent. This is often accomplished through psychoeducational support groups, in which the family can learn from the experiences of others and seek support for decreasing enabling behaviors, using leverage and contingency planning to maintain their child in treatment (e.g., use of PINS petition, access to driver's education/use of car, increased vigilance around money and teen's whereabouts, enforced curfews, etc.). Conversely, increased privileges can be tied to negative drug screens and improved behavior. As in the case of Jayne's family, it is clear that her parents could benefit from such support and should be encouraged to participate, regardless of whether or not Jayne initially resists attending treatment. Eventually, a family-based treatment approach can be used to target the life-cycle stage of separation–individuation, with its impact upon both the teen and the parents.

Finally, the clinician must become allied with the family in negotiating the significant systems that impact upon their problem and can be incorporated as partners to facilitate treatment compliance. Once again, the clinician must not join with the family's resistance to outside systems (e.g., Jayne's family's view of school as "scapegoating" their daughter). Instead the clinician can broker a cooperative relationship with the school to improve performance. Improved performance enhances self-esteem that, in turn, can mediate against continued drug usage.

EFFECTIVE THERAPEUTIC APPROACHES

Although there is certainly ample evidence to suggest that receiving treatment is better than not receiving it, there remains a paucity of well-developed controlled studies examining the effectiveness of different approaches with adolescents (Booth & Kwiatkowski, 1999; Williams & Chang, 2000). In a review of the literature, family therapy and cognitive-behavioral treatment (CBT) have received the most promising attention (Booth & Kwiatkowski, 1999; Williams & Chang, 2000). Kaminer (1999) also found that in addition to periodic drug urinalysis, these two types of therapeutic approaches (family therapy and CBT) can be even more important to client outcome than the treatment setting (i.e., inpatient, residential, or outpatient). These two approaches are highlighted below.

Cognitive-Behavioral Treatment

Cognitive-behavioral therapy is now one of the most commonly used forms of psychological treatment of substance use in adolescents (Crome, 1999). To achieve and maintain abstinence, CBT is directed at the modification of maladaptive coping skills. Problem-solving, self-monitoring, goal-setting, and decision-making skills are some of the strategies that are taught. Negative affect is addressed through anger management, assertiveness training, and relaxation techniques (e.g., biofeedback, meditation, exercise). Converting negative thought processes into positive thoughts and activities also enhances the capacity to resist temptation and prevent relapse in high-risk situations (Crome, 1999). Communication and social skills training are offered to enhance coping with interpersonal interactions (dealing with criticism, initiating social contacts, etc.).

Relapse prevention, which has now become an integral part of most treatment services (Bell, 1990), focuses on identification of high-risk situations that are emotional triggers for use and learning alternative responses. Other programmatic components of treatment can include behavioral contracting and contingency management. This approach utilizes operant conditioning techniques to reinforce abstinent behaviors (SAMHSA, 1997).

Family-Based Treatment

Perhaps even more compelling are the results of outcome studies since the mid-1980s of family-based treatment with substance-abusing adolescents; these results suggest that this approach is even more favorable than individual or peer group counseling, parent education, or skill-building groups (Liddle & Dakof, 1995). Family-based models are better able to (1) engage and retain clients in drug treatment, (2) lower the dropout rate, and (3) lessen drug-use levels at the point of termination and at 1-year follow-up (Liddle & Dakof, 1995). Simply working with the family through unilateral intervention has been proven to be an effective method of engaging resistant clients in treatment (Meyers, Miller, Hill, & Tonigan, 1999).

Currently, family-based treatment is comprised of several different perspectives. Bry (1977) advocates using a behavioral approach based on the twin assumptions that adolescents are seldom self-referred and that parents still potentially control much of their teen's life. As with CBT, this approach utilizes contingency contracting, family management, parenting strategies, and communication training (Liddle & Dakof, 1995).

Strategic and structural family therapies continue to lie at the heart of treatment as classically described by the work of Stanton and Todd in 1982. These approaches tend to view the adolescent as flagging the symptoms of the family. Treatment is focused on restructuring problematic relationships in terms of boundaries, structural hierarchy, and levels of emotional involvement.

Multifamily therapy groups are invaluable in providing a supportive network of peers for both parents and teens addressing the longitudinal issues of recovery and adolescent development. Often these groups become microcosms of extended family systems, in which intergenerational feedback between adolescents and adults can more easily be exchanged amid the presence of others who share similar concerns.

Integrative models represent the most current trend in family-based treatment (Liddle & Dakof, 1995). These approaches rely on an ecosystems model that transcends the family system, per se, to include a multidimensional view of the various subsystems within which the adolescent interacts: school, peer, juvenile justice, and so on. This approach is most consistent with the call for parent/school/community partnerships in addressing adolescent substance abuse.

CONCLUSION

In a society that worships chemical solutions and places an inordinate value upon youth, it is a perverse truth that the adolescent seeking sophistication through the use and abuse of drugs can seriously impede or irrevocably damage the attainment of his or her adult status. In seeking to address prevention efforts, Flay (2000) asks, "How can we expect youth to continue to hold new attitudes or persist with new behaviors if the social environment does not provide positive role models and reinforcement for such changes?" (p. 1).

The primary bastions of prevention efforts are no longer limited to the school but now include the home, the community, and the mass media. As a result of the research on risk, protective factors, and resiliency, much of these efforts at prevention have become multifaceted approaches to each of these targeted domains. Prevention programs currently include a classroom-based curriculum plus intervention components that include schoolwide climate change, parent involvement or training, mass media, and/or community efforts to modify norms (Flay, 2000).

Likewise, it is no longer acceptable to view the treatment of adolescent substance abuse as the sole province of the lone practitioner using an individual counseling approach. Nor is it desirable to treat adolescents with adult models of chemical dependency that falsely label the teen as an "addict" and are insensitive to the developmental needs of this population. Intervention requires a multisystemic model that can offer comprehensive service delivery of varied modalities to address the plurality of assessed issues that form and maintain substance use and abuse in the adolescent. As with prevention, treatment also must include a convergence of school, family, and community in partnership to avert the consequences of substance abuse or dependence and to enhance the achievement of maturational goals.

REFERENCES

Angold, A., Costello, E., & Erkanli, A. (1999). Comorbidity. *Journal of Child Psychology and Psychiatry and Allied Disciplines, 40*(1), 57–87.

Archambault, D. (1989). Adolescence: A physiological, cultural and psychological no-man's land. In G. Lawson & A. Lawson (Eds.), *Alcoholism and substance abuse in special populations* (pp. 223–245). Gaithersburg, MD: Aspen.

Bell, T. (1990). *Preventing adolescent relapse.* Independence, MO: Herald House.

Bogenschneider, K. (1991). Risk factors for alcohol and drug use/abuse and prevention. *Wisconsin Youth Futures Technical Report No. 10* (pp. 1–15). Madison: University of Wisconsin—Extension.

Booth, R. E., & Kwiatkowski, C. F. (1999). Substance abuse treatment for high-risk adolescents. *Current Psychiatry Report, 1*(2), 185–190.

Bradizza, C. M., Reifman, A., & Barnes, G. M. (1999). Social and coping reasons for drinking: Predicting alcohol misuse in adolescents. *Journal of Studies on Alcohol, 60,* 491–499.

Bry, B. H. (1977). Family-based approaches to reducing adolescent substance use: Theories, techniques and findings. *American Journal of Drug and Alcohol Abuse, 4*(4), 467–478.

Center for Substance Abuse Prevention (CSAP). (1996). Facts about early adolescent girls. Alan Guttmacher Institute. Retrieved December 15, 2000, from www.health.org/gpower/media/forpress/hhsstat.htm

Collins, R., Ellickson, P., & Bell, R. (1998). Simultaneous polydrug use among teens: Prevalence and predictors. *Journal of Substance Abuse, 10*(3), 233–253.

Crome, I. B. (1999). Treatment interventions looking towards the millennium. *Drug and Alcohol Dependence, 55*(3), 247–263.

Crumley, F. E. (1990). Substance abuse and adolescent suicide behavior. *Journal of the American Medical Association, 13*(22), 3051–3056.

Denton, R. E., & Kampfe, C. M. (1994). The relationship between family variables and adolescent substance abuse: A literature review. *Adolescence, 29*(114), 475–496.

DeWit, D., Adlaf, E., Offord, D., & Ogborne, A. (2000). Age at first alcohol use: A risk factor for the development of alcohol disorders. *American Journal of Psychiatry, 157,* 745–750.

Duncan, S., Duncan, T., & Hops, H. (1998). Progressions of alcohol, cigarette, and marijuana use in adolescence. *Journal of Behavioral Medicine, 21,* 375–388.

Feigelman, B., & Feigelman, W. (1993). Treating the adolescent substance abuser. In S. L. A. Straussner (Ed.), *Clinical work with substance-abusing clients* (pp. 233–250). New York: Guilford Press.

Flay, B. R. (2000). Approaches to substance abuse prevention utilizing school curriculum plus social environmental change. *Addictive Behaviors, 25*(6), 861–885.

Friedman, A. S., & Ali, A. (1998). The interaction of SES, race/ethnicity and family organization (living arrangements) of adolescents, in relation to severity of drugs and alcohol. *Journal of Child and Adolescent Substance Abuse, 7*(2) 65–74.

Freshman, A. (1996). The chemically dependent "child" script: Will Peter Pan ever grow up? In J. D. Atwood (Ed.), *Family scripts* (pp. 179–210). Washington, DC: Taylor & Francis.

Freshman, A., & Leinwand, C. (2001). The implications of female risk factors for substance abuse prevention in adolescent girls. *Journal of Prevention and Intervention in the Community, 21*(1), 29–51.

Giaconia, R., Reinherz, H., Hauf, A., Paradis, A., Wasserman, M., & Langhammer, D. (2000). Comorbidity of substance use and post-traumatic stress disorders in a community sample of adolescents. *American Journal of Orthopsychiatry, 70*(2), 253–262.

Grant, B. F., & Dawson, D. A. (1997). Age at onset of alcohol use and its association with DSM-IV alcohol abuse and dependence: Results from the National Longitudinal Alcohol Epidemiologic Survey. *Journal of Substance Abuse, 9,* 103–110.

Gruber, E., DiClementi, R. J., Anderson, N. M., & Lodico, M. (1996). Early drinking onset and its association with alcohol use and problem behavior in late adolescence. *Prevention Medicine, 25*(3), 293–300.

Harrison, P., Fulkerson, J., & Beebe, T. (1998). DSM-IV substance use disorder criteria for adolescents: A critical examination based on a statewide school survey. *American Journal of Psychiatry, 155,* 486–492.

Hawkins, J. D., Catalano, R. F., & Miller, J. Y. (1992). Risk and protective factors for alcohol and other drug problems in adolescence and early adulthood: Implications for substance abuse prevention. *Psychological Bulletin, 112*(2), 64–105.

Horner, B. R., & Scheibe, K. E. (1997). Prevalence and implications of attention-deficit hyperactivity disorder among adolescents in treatment for substance misuse. *Journal of American Academy in Child Adolescent Psychiatry, 36*(1), 30–36.

Howard, M. (1992). Adolescent substance abuse: A social learning theory perspective. In G. Lawson & A. Lawson (Eds.), *Adolescent substance abuse* (pp. 29–40). Gaithersburg, MD: Aspen.

Johnson, G. M., Shontz, F. C., & Locke, T. P. (1984). Relationships between adolescent drug use and parental drug behavior. *Adolescence, 19*(74), 295–299.

Johnston, L. D., O'Malley, P. M., & Bachman, J. G. (2003). *Monitoring the future national results on adolescent drug use: Overview of key findings 2002.* University of Michigan Institute for Social Research, National Institute on Drug Abuse, NIH publication No. 03-5374. Retrieved October 23, 2003, from www.monitoringthefuture.org

Kilpatrick, D. G., Acierno, R., Saunders, B., Resnick, H. S., Best, C. L., & Schnurr, P. P. (2000). Risk factors for adolescent substance abuse and dependence: Data from a national sample. *Journal of Consultation in Clinical Psychology, 68*(1), 19–30.

Lawson, G., Peterson, J., & Lawson, A. (1983). *Alcoholism and the family: A guide to treatment and prevention.* Gaithersburg, MD: Aspen.

Liddle, H. A., & Dakof, G. A. (1995). Family-based treatment for adolescent drug use: State of the science. *NIDA Research Monograph, 156,* 218–254.

Lipschitz, D. S., Grilo, C. M., Fehon, D., McGlashan, T. M., & Southwick, S. M. (2000). Gender differences in the associations between posttraumatic stress symptoms and problematic substance use in psychiatric inpatient adolescents. *Journal of Nervous and Mental Disorders, 188*(6), 349–356.

Meyers, K., Hagan, T. A., Zanis, D., Webb, A., Frantz, J., Ring-Kurtz, S., Rutherford, M., & McLellan, T. A. (1999). Critical issues in adolescent substance abuse assessment. *Drug and Alcohol Dependence, 55*(3), 235–246.

Meyers, R. J., Miller, W. R., Hill, D. E., & Tonigan, J. S. (1999). Community Reinforcement and Family Training (CRAFT): Engaging unmotivated drug users into treatment. *Journal of Substance Abuse, 10,* 291–308.

Miller, W. (2000, July). *Motivational enhancement therapy: Approaches to drug abuse counseling.* National Institute on Drug Abuse (NIDA), NIH publication No. 00-4151, Rockville, MD.

Mooney, A., Eisenberg, A., & Eisenberg, H. (1992). *The recovery book.* New York: Workman Publishing.

National Center on Addiction and Substance Abuse (CASA) at Columbia University. (1996). *Substance abuse and the American woman: Prescription drugs.* Retrieved December 3, 2000, from www.casacolumbia.org/pubs/jun96/predrugs.htm.

National Center on Addiction and Substance Abuse (CASA) at Columbia University. (1997). *CASA adolescent commission report: America's children are smoking, drinking, and using drugs at the youngest ages ever.* Retrieved November 19, 2000, from www.casacolumbia.org/newsletter1457//newsletter_show.htm?doc_id=5832

National Center on Addiction and Substance Abuse (CASA) at Columbia University. (1998). *Teens who smoke cigarettes much likelier to try pot.* Retrieved November 19, 2000, from www.casacolumbia.org/newsletter1457/newsletter_show.htm?doc_id=7041

National Center on Addiction and Substance Abuse (CASA) at Columbia University. (1999). *The National Survey of American Attitudes on Substance Abuse V: Teens and their parents.* Retrieved November 19, 2000, from www.casacolumbia.org/publications1456/publications_show.htm?doc_id=17635

National Center on Addiction and Substance Abuse (CASA) at Columbia University. (2000). *Substance abuse and learning disabilities: Peas in a pod or apples and oranges?* Retrieved December 3, 2000, from www.casacolumbia.org/publications1456/publications_show.htm?doc_id=34846

National Center on Addiction and Substance Abuse (CASA) at Columbia University. (2003). *American Legacy Foundation/CASA report: Reducing teen smoking can cut marijuana use significantly.* Retrieved November 11, 2003, from www.casacolumbia.org/absolutenm/templates/PressReleases.asp?articleid=324&zoneid=46

National Institute on Drug Abuse (NIDA). (2000a). June 1999 advance report: Epidemiological trends in drug abuse: A summary of the proceedings of the June 1999 meeting of NIDA's Community Epidemiology Work Group (CEWG). Retrieved November 26, 2000, from 165.112.78.61/Infofax/clubdrugs. html

National Institute on Drug Abuse (NIDA). (2000b). *Epidemiological trends in drug abuse: Advance report of the Community Epidemiology Work Group (CEWG).* Retrieved November 26, 2000, from 165.112.78.61/CEWG/AdvancedRep/6_20ADV/0600adv.html

National Institute on Drug Abuse (NIDA). (2000c). *Statement of the Director: Congressional testimony: U.S. Senate caucus on international narcotics control.* Retrieved November 19, 2000 from www.drugabuse.gov/Testimony/7–25–00Testimony.html

Needle, R., McCubbin, H., Wilson, M., Reineck, R., Lazar, A., & Mederer, H. (1986). Interpersonal influences in adolescent drug use: The role of older siblings, parents and peers. *International Journal of the Addictions, 21,* 739–766.

Pollack, N. K., & Martin, C. S. (1999) Diagnostic orphans: Adolescents with alcohol symptom who do not qualify for DSM-IV abuse or dependence diagnoses. *American Journal of Psychiatry, 156*(6), 897–901.

Prochaska, J., & DiClemente, C. (1984). *The transtheoretical approach: Crossing the traditional boundaries of therapy.* Homewood, IL: Dow Jones/Irwin.

Rounds-Bryant, J., Kristiansen, P., & Hubbard, R. (1999). Drug abuse treatment outcome study of adolescents: A comparison of client characteristics and pretreatment behaviors in three treatment modalities. *American Journal of Drug and Alcohol Abuse, 25*(4), 573–591.

Slesnick, N., Meyers, R. J., Meade, M., & Segelken, D. H. (2000). Bleak and hopeless no more: Engagement of reluctant substance-abusing runaway youth and their families. *Journal of Substance Abuse Treatment, 19*(3), 215–222.

Sobeck, J., Abbey, A., Agius, E., Clinton, M., & Harrison, K. (2000). Predicting early adolescent substance use: Do risk factors differ depending on age of onset? *Journal of Substance Abuse, 11*(1), 89–102.

Stanton, M. D., Todd, T. C., & Associates. (1982). *The family therapy of drug abuse and addiction.* New York: Guilford Press.

Straussner, S. L. A. (Ed.). (2001). *Ethnocultural factors in substance abuse treatment.* New York: Guilford Press.

Substance Abuse and Mental Health Services Administration (SAMHSA) and Center for Substance Abuse Treatment. (1997). *A guide to substance abuse services for primary care physicians: Treatment Improvement Protocol (TIP) series, 24.* USDHHS Publication No. (SMA) 97-3139, SAMHSA, Rockville, MD.

Substance Abuse and Mental Health Services Administration (SAMHSA) and Center for Substance Abuse Treatment. (1999a). *Screening and assessing adolescents for substance use disorders: Treatment Improvement Protocol (TIP) series, 31.* USDHHS Publication No. 99-3282, SAMHSA, Rockville, MD.

Substance Abuse and Mental Health Services Administration and Center for Substance Abuse Treatment (SAMHSA) (1999b). Treatment of adolescents with substance use disorders. *Treatment Improvement Protocol (TIP) series, 32.* USDHHS Publication No. (SMA) 99-3283, SAMHSA, Rockville, MD.

Substance Abuse and Mental Health Services Administration (SAMHSA), National Survey of Substance Abuse Treatment Services (N-SSATS): 2002 Data on Substance Abuse Treatment Facilities. (2002). Rockville, MD: Author. Retrieved April 1, 2004, from www.dasis.samhsa.gov/02nssats/index.htm

Swadi, H. (1999). Individual risk factors for adolescent substance use. *Drug and Alcohol Dependence, 55*(3), 209–224.

Szapocznik, J., Perez-Vida, A., Brickman, A. L., Foote, F. H., Sanisteban, D., Hervis, O., & Kurtines, W. (1988). Engaging adolescent drug abusers and their families in treatment: A strategic structural systems approach. *Journal of Consulting and Clinical Psychology, 56,* 552–557.

Tennant, F. (1994). Urine drug screening of adolescents on request of parents. *Journal of Child and Adolescent Substance Abuse, 3*(3), 75–81.

Treadway, D. (1989). *Before it's too late: Working with substance abuse in the family.* New York: Norton.

Werner, E. (1982). *Vulnerable, but invincible: A longitudinal study of resilient children and youth.* New York: McGraw-Hill.

Williams. R. J., & Chang, S. Y. (2000). A comprehensive and comparative review of adolescent substance abuse treatment outcome. *Clinical Psychology Science and Practice, 7*(2), 138–166.

Winters, K. C., & Stinchfield, R. D. (1995). *Current issues and future needs in the assessment of adolescent drug abuse. Adolescent drug abuse: Clinical assessment and therapeutic interventions.* National Institute of Drug Abuse (NIDA) Research Monograph, *156,* 146–171. Retrieved December 21, 2000, from 165.112.78.61/pdf/monographs/download156.html

Zeitlin, H. (1999). Psychiatric comorbidity with substance misuse in children and teenagers. *Drug and Alcohol Dependence, 55*(3), 225–234.

Zickler, P. (2000, January 3). Ethnic identification and cultural ties may prevent drug use. *NIDA Notes and Research Findings, 14*(3). Retrieved December 17, 2000, from 165.112.78.61/NIDA_Notes/NNVol14N3/Ethnic.html

CHAPTER 15

Substance Abuse Problems among Older Adults

Kathleen J. Farkas

The number of elderly people in our society has increased substantially during this past century and will continue to increase for the next 50 years. People over age 65 are expected to comprise over 15% of the population within the next 15 years (Bureau of the Census, 1995). The sustained rise in the number of elderly people means that clinicians in all health and human services will be facing the challenges of an aging population. Elderly people have always constituted a subpopulation in need of substance abuse treatment, but their use patterns, problems, and treatment needs are often misinterpreted and unmet (American Medical Association Council on Academic Affairs, 1996). Although some of today's older adults may still feel the influence of temperance ideas, more of them have lived their lives in a social climate that tolerated, if not invited, social drinking. Atkinson (1995) looked at the alcohol consumption patterns of today's middle-aged "baby boomers" and argued that the prevalence of alcohol problems among older adults will increase as the "boomers" become elderly. This chapter provides information and tools to help clinicians recognize substance abuse problems in elderly clients and to make treatment decisions appropriate to their needs.

DIVERSITY AMONG OLDER ADULTS

Work with older adults offers clinicians a variety of challenges (Farkas, 1992; Farkas & Kola, 1997). There exists a wide range of ability, health levels, and resources in people over the age of 60. Gerontologists have grouped the elderly into three age groups: young-old (60–74), old-old (75–84), and oldest-old (85+) (Atchley, 1997). The general rule is that with age comes increasing impairment and need for social services, but chronological age is not always a reliable predictor of function.

In comparison to the general population, substance abuse problems are less common among elderly people (Robins & Regier, 1991). Elderly persons often abstain from alcohol or cut down the amount they drink as they age because of health problems, decreased income, and/or decreased social opportunities. However, a portion of the elderly population does experience problems with alcohol (Adams, Barry, & Fleming, 1996; Barry, Oslin, & Blow, 2001; Liberto, Oslin, & Ruskin, 1992; National Institute on Alcohol Abuse and Alcoholism, 1995). The range of prevalence rates of substance abuse problems among older adults is wide. Liberto and colleagues (1992) have shown that the prevalence of alcohol problems in this population ranges from 3 to 25% for "heavy alcohol use," and from 2.2 to 9.6% for "alcohol abuse." The differences in prevalence are most likely due to differences in samples and data collection sites; clinics, hospitals, and nursing homes are more likely to show higher prevalence rates than community-based studies (Grant et al., 1991).

ALCOHOL AND PRESCRIPTION DRUG USE, MISUSE, AND DEPENDENCE AMONG OLDER ADULTS

Most elderly people drink socially and use alcohol as part of cultural and social events. Many elderly people have been social drinkers their entire lives and continue to enjoy alcoholic beverages during late life. Some literature indicates that moderate alcohol consumption (no more than two drinks per day) is related to lower levels of coronary artery disease (Atkinson & Ganzini, 1994). However, this beneficial finding needs further study and must be weighed against other health risks associated with alcohol use among the elderly. The National Institute on Alcohol Abuse and Alcoholism (1995) has issued low-risk drinking guidelines for elderly people: no more than one drink per day; maximum of two drinks on any drinking occasion; lower limits for women.

A small proportion of elderly people misuses alcohol but do so unintentionally, usually because they lack knowledge about alcohol. Examples of unintentional misuse might be an elderly person who has a drink when he or she is taking medication that should not be used with alcohol. Another example is a person who misinterprets the physical effects of alcohol and misses the connection between alcohol use and the resulting problems.

Unintentional misuse is usually discussed in relationship with over-the-counter (OTC) medications, prescription medications, and alcohol.

Older adults purchase a disproportionate share of all OTC drugs and prescription medications (Condon, 1996; Woods & Winger, 1995). Given the numbers of medications taken, both prescription and nonprescription, it is probable that there will be adverse reactions and mistakes in doses and combinations. The most commonly prescribed psychoactive medications for older adults are benzodiazepines, antidepressants, and opiate/opioid analgesics: all medications that interact negatively with alcohol (Barry, Oslin, & Blow, 2001; Blow, 1998). Educational efforts and prevention strategies are well suited to address unintentional use problems. These efforts and strategies can be as indirect as posting information on bulletin boards or setting out flyers in public places. More direct strategies include having pharmacists and physicians discuss the dangers of mixing alcohol and medications with their elderly clients.

There are also those older adults who have substance abuse and substance dependence problems that require treatment. For those who have problems with alcohol and other drugs, the age of onset of the problem is important for diagnosis as well as for treatment planning. Some older adults have been alcohol- and drug-dependent throughout their lives; they have reached old age with a long history of alcohol and other drug problems. For others, the alcohol and other drug problems began in late life; they have a late onset. For yet another group, the pattern of alcohol and other drug problems is intermittent; they experienced problems early in life, resolved those problems during most of their adult years, and then experienced a resurgence of the problems in late life.

ILLICIT DRUG USE AND DEPENDENCE AMONG OLDER ADULTS

Heroin, cocaine, marijuana, and "street" drugs are used by a small proportion of elderly people (Gomberg, 1996). The Sixth Triennial Report to Congress on Drug Abuse and Addiction Research (U.S. Department of Health and Human Services, 1999) indicated that rates of illicit drug use in 1997 showed substantial variation by age. The rates of illicit use were lower with each successive age group. Only 1% of people age 50 reported current illicit drug use. This estimate, however, is conservative, because people who use illicit drugs, regardless of age, are less likely to be included in household or community surveys.

Data from populations receiving treatment for HIV/AIDS, however, show that intravenous drug-using samples include elderly people (Emlet & Farkas, 2001, 2002). Sixteen percent of the over-age-50 HIV/AIDS sample fell into the injection drug-use exposure category, and 7% of the over-65 group were injection drug users. There is also some indication that the numbers of elderly who use illicit drugs will rise as successive cohorts age. In 1986, 8.1% of adults over 50 with HIV/AIDS had been exposed through IV drug use; by 1996, 16.7% of infected adults over 50 fell into this category (Centers for Disease Control and Prevention, 1996).

RISK FACTORS FOR SUBSTANCE
ABUSE AMONG OLDER ADULTS

A variety of social and physical issues of aging puts the elderly at risk for developing substance abuse problems. First, age-related physical changes such as decline in cellular fluids and increase in body fat serve to increase the impact alcohol and other medications have on the older system. Decreased gastrointestinal metabolization of alcohol results in higher blood alcohol levels for longer periods of time. All of these age-related physical changes may serve to increase the intoxicating effects of alcohol in an older person. Without changing his or her drinking pattern, an elderly person may find that he or she feels dizzy or "drunk." Changes in the body's ability to metabolize alcohol as well as slower reaction times in elderly people have been implicated in the increased risk of physical harm associated with falls or accidents among elderly people (Bucholz, Sheline, & Helzer, 1995). These age-related physical changes also apply to the use of both prescription and OTC drugs.

The social changes of late life also may serve as risk factors. Retirement and loss of work roles (Blow, 1998); loss of spouse (Brennan & Moos, 1996; Bucholz et al., 1995), relatives, and other friends, and the subsequent feelings of grief and loneliness can lead to increased alcohol and other drug use. Alcohol and other drugs may provide solace to those who are alone and isolated. By the same token, retirement also may bring more time to socialize with friends and neighbors and less need to curtail one's drinking to the late afternoon or evening hours.

Alcohol has been associated with increased risk of hypertension, cardiac arrhythmia, and myocardial infarction (American Medical Association, 1996). These are common conditions in elderly populations; the use of alcohol can exacerbate these existing health problems. Chronic health conditions and sleep problems also may increase the use of alcohol and other drugs. Alcohol is a central nervous system depressant and is used by many elderly to self-medicate for sleep disturbances. Insomnia has been identified as a potential factor in the development or relapse of alcohol problems among elderly adults (Liberto & Oslin, 1997). Chronic pain from arthritis and other conditions may present yet another risk factor for substance abuse problems in this population; alcohol and other drugs may be used alone or in combination to self-medicate and manage chronic pain.

ASSESSMENT AND TREATMENT ISSUES

One of the first steps in improving the diagnosis and treatment of alcohol and other drug problems in older adults is for clinicians to examine their attitudes about substance use and abuse by the older adults. Ageism may serve to perpetuate the myth that substance abuse is not a problem for this population. Stigma associated with alcohol and other drug abuse is another factor that may influence attitudes of both clinicians and clients. Elderly women may be especially loathe to admit to substance abuse problems because of the stigma these problems held during their younger years.

Clinicians can easily overlook signs of alcohol and other drug problems in older adults or misdiagnose these problems. In general, the usual indicators of a substance abuse problem may not be evident in an elderly person. For example, an elderly person may not drive, may live alone, and may be retired, thus eliminating three standard areas of assessment: legal problems (driving under the influence), family conflict, and employment problems. Furthermore, the physical problems associated with alcohol and other drug abuse and dependence may be more easily interpreted as a medical condition in an elderly person. Clinicians do not always carefully question older adults about alcohol and other drug use, nor do they use the clients' answers to rule out substance abuse or dependence problems. Often the diagnosis of substance abuse is not considered because it is not expected in an older person.

Building a Therapeutic Relationship for Screening and Assessment

A trusting relationship is the basis of sound clinical work with all phases of substance abuse treatment. Developing a nonjudgmental, supportive stance with an elderly client improves the quality of information a clinician collects and facilitates treatment efforts. Questions about alcohol and other drug use must be explained as standard components of a general health survey. The questions must be asked respectfully and clearly. Many older adults feel ashamed of their use or abuse of alcohol. For these people, disclosure of an alcohol problem may be overwhelming. Successful clinicians convey the facts that alcohol problems among older adults are fairly common, that alcoholism is a disease and not an individual's moral failure, and that many elderly people have entered treatment and done very well in their recovery. Needless to say, the clinician and the client need to have a private place to talk, and the information collected must be confidential.

Screening

The purpose of screening is to separate people who have no alcohol or other drug abuse (AODA) problems from those whose alcohol or drug

(AOD) use warrants a more comprehensive assessment. Because of the complexity of health and social issues in older adults, screening and assessment for substance abuse problems must be considered against the backdrop of multiple physical and mental conditions. Many mental and physical symptoms of AODA, such as loss of memory, loss of balance, and incontinence, mimic some of the common conditions of older adults; therefore, clinicians who are not skilled in AODA screening and assessment may miss the role alcohol or other drugs may play in a person's problems. Clinicians must actively assess and rule out substance abuse with older adults, just as they must do with younger people. The first step in the process is screening: What evidence exists to indicate that additional time and effort should be directed to learning about substance use with this particular client?

An easily administered and interpretable screening tool should be used to discriminate between those who need additional assessment for AODA and those who do not. Screening of the elderly also should include information about the use of prescription and OTC medications. A useful tool that offers a standardized guide for the evaluation of medication noncompliance is the Solano County Senior Medication Education Project Noncompliance Screening Form (Condon, 1996). This 21-question screening form covers a variety of issues that might lead to problems of over- or undermedication in elderly people. It is easily scored, provides baseline information about the types of problems an elderly person might experience with medication, and suggests areas for further investigation.

A variety of tools exist for screening for AODA problems. One of the most popular is the CAGE test (Mayfield, McLeod, & Hall, 1974). CAGE is a mnemonic representing four questions about cutting down on drinking, annoyance in response to criticism of drinking, guilt over drinking, and needing an eyeopener to manage withdrawal symptoms. The CAGE is short, focused, and widely used in treatment and medical communities. However, it is too harsh for some older adults and so may serve to discourage them from talking about their problems.

In talking about alcohol and other drugs with elderly clients, clinicians need to be mindful of language. For many older adults, the terms *drink* and *drinker* may be synonymous with *alcoholic* or *problem drinker*. This may be especially the case for older adults who grew up in abstaining or temperance-minded families or cultures. Similarly, some older adults may be unaware of their alcohol consumption. A case example illustrates this point:

Ms. J., an outreach worker for older adults, made an initial home visit to Mr. T., a 70-year-old man who had severe arthritis and lived alone. Ms. J. and Mr. T. sat at the kitchen table to complete the interview questions. One of the questions was "Do you ever drink alcohol?" Mr. T. responded that he did not drink alcohol. Ms. J. had noticed that the trash can was full of beer cans and that there was a case of beer on the floor. She asked Mr. T. about the beer. "If you don't drink alcohol, who drinks the beer in this house?" Mr. J. was truly puzzled. "Of course, I drink the beer. I just don't drink alcohol—you know, I don't drink whiskey or scotch or any other alcohol."

Specific questions such as "Do you ever have a glass of beer, a glass of wine, or a mixed drink?" produce clearer information than asking about alcohol in general. Often older people will have a drink as part of a celebration but do not think of that as drinking alcohol. A follow-up question to a negative response to the "Do you ever have a glass of beer, etc?" question might be "Might you have a glass of wine or a glass of beer at Christmas or a birthday party?" Cues about occasions are often helpful in triggering a person's recall of his or her use of alcohol.

A screening tool developed specifically for use with older adults is the HEAT (Willenbring & Spring, 1988), another mneumonic that asks open-ended questions and sets a less stigmatizing tone by asking "How do you use alcohol?" This type of question allows a person to talk not only about what he or she drinks, how much and how often, but also about the reasons he or she might use alcohol. How a person uses alcohol is especially important in understanding the cultural practices and health beliefs of the client concerning alcohol. For example:

Mr. V. told his social worker that he did not drink beer, wine, or any other whiskey or mixed drink. However, the worker had often smelled alcohol on his breath. She asked Mr. V. why she might have smelled alcohol when she was around him. He said, "It might be my tonic. Every day I take two shots of whiskey at noon, but that's not drinking, that's medicine."

A third screening tool, the CHARMM (Friedman, Fleming, Roberts, & Hyman, 1996), has the additional strength of setting a timeframe of the past year and asking about the pattern of use, the role of alcohol in a person's life, and the problem of medication–alcohol interactions. These screening tools are helpful only if they are used as part of a larger protocol that allows clinicians to follow up with people who screen positive for alcohol problems.

A longer tool is the Michigan Alcoholism Screening Test—Geriatric Version (MAST-G; Blow et al., 1992). The MAST-G, based on the format of the widely used Michigan Alcohol Screening Test (MAST; Seltzer, 1971; Seltzer, Vinokur, & Van Rooijan, 1975), is a 24-item screening instrument developed specifically for older adults. The test focuses less upon external problems with work, legal systems, and relationship, which are more salient for younger populations using alcohol. It also includes questions about possible physical symptoms; for example, "After drinking have you ever noticed an increase in your heart rate or beating in your chest?" The

MAST-G asks about the use of alcohol to combat loneliness and to aid sleep. A person who responds "yes" to five or more questions out of the 24 is in need of a more thorough assessment for alcohol problems.

Assessment

Assessment is the process by which clinicians explore evidence of substance abuse and interpret that evidence in the form of a diagnosis and treatment plan. The clinician must explore onset patterns, special health and mental health conditions of aging, and the social aspects of later life (Beechem, 2002; Gurnack, Atkinson, & Osgood, 2002). The indicators useful in the diagnosis of substance abuse and substance dependence, as set forth in the fourth edition of the *Diagnostic and Statistical Manual of Mental Disorders* (DSM-IV; American Psychiatric Association, 1994) are not always applicable to elderly people. For example, three of the areas of significant impairment or distress for the diagnosis of substance abuse are (1) failure to fulfill a major role obligation at work, school or home; (2) using substances in situations in which it is physically hazardous; and (3) legal problems. For the elderly person who is socially isolated and does not drive, work, or volunteer, these criteria are not relevant. More appropriate are physical symptoms and health cues for substance abuse. Poor sleeping and eating habits are also significant. Some of the more common medical consequences of alcohol abuse in the elderly are gastrointestinal or other bleeding, psoriasis and signs of immunodeficiency disorders, edema in the lower extremities related to liver impairment, signs of fluid buildup, medication interactions, and electrolyte imbalances (American Medical Association, 1994). However, these medical problems alone are not necessarily indicative of alcohol problems. Cognitive functioning and recall are two other areas that can be affected by alcohol use and abuse. Because older adults with depression or dementia may exhibit the same cognitive and memory deficits as those with alcohol abuse alone, tests such as the Mini Mental State Examination can be helpful in this phase of assessment (Folstein, Folstein, & McHugh, 1975).

Depression is a common diagnosis in the elderly population and can either precede or accompany alcohol use and abuse. The diagnosis and differentiation of depression and dementia are especially important skills for clinicians working with elderly substance abusers. Alcohol and other drug abuse can result in symptoms that mimic depression. Conversely, alcohol and other drugs can exacerbate problems in persons who are suffering from depression, dementia, or both. Careful collaboration with geriatricians and geropsychiatrists can improve the assessments of elderly people who present with decreased cognitive functioning and other symptoms of depression and dementia.

A DSM-IV-based diagnosis of substance dependence requires a person to evidence tolerance and/or withdrawal symptoms. An elderly person may experience alcohol-related problems with low intake because of age-related sensitivity to alcohol that results in higher blood levels. Looking for withdrawal symptoms as a diagnostic indicator may be misleading, because many elderly with late-onset patterns do not develop physiological dependence. The overlap of various medical conditions, both chronic and acute, makes it difficult to interpret withdrawal symptoms in an elderly person. The differential diagnosis of general medical problems and alcohol dependence may require a close working relationship with a physician.

Careful assessment efforts should include family and friends. Family members may be able to provide important pieces of the elder's history regarding medications, alcohol use, and mental health problems. On the other hand, family members may feel embarrassment and shame about the older family member's substance use and try to minimize the problems. Shame and guilt, and thus denial, may be especially problematic if the adult children are struggling with their own substance abuse problems.

Onset Patterns

Researchers and clinicians working with older adults have identified three patterns of onset: early, late, and intermittent (Atkinson, Turner, Kofoed, & Tolson, 1985). The early-onset group includes people who have lived with their substance abuse problems throughout adulthood. These individuals may have histories of multiple treatment attempts and a list of medical and psychiatric problems related to alcohol and other drugs. Their social networks tend to be depleted because of the marital and family difficulties associated with their substance abuse. The early-onset group may include the stereotypic skid row alcoholic homeless person who is elderly, impoverished, and utterly disenfranchised. The prognosis for early-onset clients may be poor because of their long-term denial of the problem, their hopelessness about treatment, limited social support, and their poor emotional skills. These elderly people are also likely to suffer from chronic physical problems, including liver and cardiovascular conditions, and to show some level of cognitive impairment. A harm reduction model that focuses on improved medical care, increased nutrition, and physical safety may be the best approach for the subset of early-onset clients who refuse treatment. More active treatment might include home-based models that focus on medical management of withdrawal symptoms and involvement from 12-step members to increase social support and interaction. Although clinicians may be pessimistic about working with elderly people who have an early-onset pattern, research has shown that relapse rates do not vary with age of onset (Atkinson, Tolson, & Turner, 1990; Schonfeld & Dupree, 1991).

The late-onset group is characterized by a history of drinking or drug use after midlife. People who experience late-life problems may have been social drinkers earlier in life or may even have been abstainers. Because the person presents without a previous history of drinking problems, it is often difficult to diagnose the role of alcohol or other drugs. The physical signs are often misread as medical problems. Late-life substance abuse has been discussed as a reaction to the multiple losses of aging and as a way to cope with problems. Physicians and other health professionals may exacerbate the situation by prescribing additional medications that either interact with alcohol or create an additional addiction problem.

Alcohol and other drug problems that begin in mid or late life often progress rapidly because of the effect of substances on the aging body. The family may not be aware of the person's AOD use and deny any involvement. Another scenario is that the elderly person and his or her family may take extra steps to hide the use of AODs out of fear, guilt, and shame. Even professionals and public officials may see alcohol as a way to soothe the problems elderly people face.

> An inner-city nursing home had opened a new program to provide AODA abuse services to a group of residents. The administration invited a city official to give some opening remarks at the dedication. She stepped to the podium and said, "My granddaddy used to sit on the porch and drink beers all day. It was his last pleasure in life, and I wouldn't want to have seen that taken away from him."

The prognosis for late-onset substance abusers is very good; most have a lifetime of coping skills that do not involve alcohol, and typically they have not been in denial of the problem for decades. Their social support system has not been eroded by years of substance abuse, and they typically do not have chronic physical or mental impairment due to substance abuse. However, late-onset populations are likely to need services to treat depression, grief, and loss issues that may have become worse with alcohol use. Treatment programs geared toward older adults, including inpatient, outpatient or home based, can be successful and should be pursued with both the client and his or her family. Family members also can become a focus of treatment to increase their understanding and awareness so that they can offer informed and useful support. Family members also may need to be evaluated for substance abuse, because any continued abuse by a close relative could put the elderly person at increased risk of relapse.

Intermittent substance abuse is the third onset pattern. In this pattern, the elderly person had an AOD problem earlier in life but was able to recover; then in late life, the problems recurred. This group typically looks similar to the late-onset group and only becomes distinct when asked about lifelong substance use or abuse. Often, a loss in life is associated with the recurrence of the problems, and family members may or may not know about the earlier history. This group is clinically important because the additional shame and guilt that are associated with past substance abuse may compound the shame of the current problems and deter treatment. A competent clinician will incorporate questions about lifelong use into the interview and be sensitive to the effect of earlier problems.

Grief, Loneliness, Isolation, and Pain

One of the core themes in work with older adults is grief. There are many losses associated with late life—social, physical, personal, and psychological. Coping skills that worked in the past may become too difficult to employ or inaccessible to the elderly person. Physical pain from chronic illnesses may pervade daily life, and isolation may compound the distress of that pain. Certainly, the fate of all older adults is not bleak, and late life is not necessarily doomed by ill health and sorrow. However, clinicians must not forget that alcohol and other drugs are powerful in their ability to ease psychic pain and decrease physical distress. In working with elderly clients, it is important to understand the role of AODs. Is alcohol used to enhance sleep? Are OTC drugs taken to ease the pain of arthritis? It is irrelevant that alcohol does not provide long-term relief or that it makes the situation worse in the long term. The clinician must understand the client's reasons for using the substance to be able to introduce the ideas of treatment and to provide some other way of meeting the need the elder person thinks is met by AODs.

Treatment Issues with Elderly People

Regardless of the treatment approach, the core skills needed when working with elderly substance abusers are empathy and the ability to convey support and encouragement. A supportive stance is crucial in encouraging elderly clients to answer screening questions, to consider treatment, or to follow through with aftercare procedures. Taking a nonjudgmental approach toward both substance abuse and the problems of aging are keys to the establishment of a therapeutic working relationship. All of the psychosocial modalities that are used for treatment of substance abuse in younger populations can be adapted to work with the elderly population. Twelve-step groups, cognitive-behavioral therapy, insight therapy, and behavior modification approaches when working can all be useful techniques with elderly substance abusers (Blow, 1998). Useful adaptations include large print and sound amplification to deal with communication deficits, slower pace of treatment, less use of confrontation, and additional opportunity for feedback and evaluation.

Over the past 10 years clinicians have begun to match a person's "stage of change" with treatment procedures to increase the numbers of people who enter treatment and the time they stay in treatment (Miller &

Rollnick, 1991; Prochaska, DiClemente, & Norcross, 1992). An elder person's motivation for active treatment can be assessed through careful questioning and use of the SOCRATES (the Stages of Change Readiness and Treatment Eagerness Scale) tool (Miller & Tonigan, 1996). SOCRATES is a short scale that assesses motivation for change in people with drinking problems. Although it was not developed specifically for use with the elderly population, the questions have face validity for use with this group. A SOCRATES score can be used to determine a client's readiness for change and can assist the clinician and client in determining the most appropriate step. For example, elderly persons who are in a precontemplative phase are not ready for active treatment but might benefit from a "persuasion group," which might meet for an hour a week to discuss AOD use and health issues. Group sessions do not necessarily need to be face to face; they could be conducted via telephone or a computer connection. Telephone and computer-based support groups are especially useful for isolated or housebound elder persons. The tone of the group is nonconfrontational and supportive. The goal of this type of intervention is to increase the elder person's understanding of the risks of continued AOD use and the benefits of seeking treatment or of reducing the amounts currently used. Sometimes older adults do not see any benefit in treatment and are not sure what treatment might mean in terms of changes in their daily lives. The group leader or individual counselor can help the elder person identify areas of his or her life, such as family relationships and health problems, which might be improved if AODs were not used. Persuasion groups are open ended and can be held in health care settings, apartment houses, senior centers, or community meeting rooms. They do not have to be labeled as an AOD treatment meeting. Initially a leader sets the agenda and topics for discussion, but gradually group members can select the topics to reflect their interests and concerns.

Elderly substance abusers who are ready for active treatment can be presented with a series of choices about their care. Do they want to receive treatment at home? Would they prefer treatment from an individual therapist, in a group setting, or a combination approach? Are they interested in a 12-step program or a cognitive-behavioral approach? Does their problem warrant an abstinence-based approach or is harm reduction the goal? Given a menu of options, the older adult and the clinician can tailor the approach best suited for the problem and the circumstances of the individual.

Twelve-step approaches are most common in AOD treatment protocols and include attending meetings, following the 12 steps and 12 traditions, and abstinence from mood-altering drugs. Twelve-step materials such as workbooks and pamphlets are available in large print and can be used as part of individual therapy as well as with groups. Twelve-step meetings can provide inspiration and support, but they can also be intimidating and stigmatizing for elderly people. Age-specific groups, where all members are older, can reduce some of the stigma and isolation elderly people may feel in a mixed-age group.

> Ms. N., 70 years old, talked to her doctor about her drinking. The doctor suggested she try an AA meeting. Ms. N. went willingly to her first AA meeting. She was prepared to accept the term *alcoholic*, even though she did not consider herself to be one.
>
> When she walked in, she noticed that most of the people in the room were in their 20s; she was clearly the oldest person present. However, she was happy that the lead speaker was a young woman. The speaker began to tell the group about her use of alcohol and cocaine. Her story included the facts that she was very promiscuous during her drug use and resorted to prostitution to keep herself in drugs. Ms. N. became more shocked and distressed as the speaker continued. During the comments, when other women in the group said that the speaker's story was similar to their own, Ms. N. feared that the others might think that she had a similar history.
>
> As she left the meeting, Ms. N. resolved that she would never attend another A.A. meeting and would not talk about her problems with alcohol with anyone else.

Before clinicians send elderly clients to 12-step group meetings, they should determine which groups are most appropriate for this age group and the accessibility of the meeting place.

Cognitive-behavioral interventions are well suited for older adults who are cognitively intact. These interventions, which can be used in individual or group formats and can be tailored for both early- and late-onset groups, can be especially useful for late-onset problems in tandem with grief counseling techniques. A cognitive-behavioral approach can help those who have used alcohol to cope with loneliness and grief to identify triggers for loneliness and to substitute other behaviors or attitudes for alcohol use. Friends and family may be involved in these approaches as well.

> Mr. G. had recently lost his wife. She had been ill for several years, and he had taken care of her. After she died, he did not have many ways to fill his time. He was unable to drive and depended on his daughter to grocery shop for him. Once in a while he added a six-pack of beer to the weekly grocery list. Indeed, since his wife's death, Mr. G. had put beer on the list every week. Over the past month, Mr. G. had fallen and become incontinent. His doctor recognized the role alcohol played in these symptoms and asked about it. The social worker and Mr. G. reviewed the triggers for alcohol use and determined that mealtimes and evenings were associated with peak feelings of loneliness. He often drank three or four beers over the course of the evening to combat this loneliness. With Mr. G.'s permission, the social worker

talked with the daughter, who was willing to visit with Mr. G. at meal-times several times a week. The daughter also was willing to view the addition of beer to the grocery list as a signal that Mr. G. was growing lonely and agreed to talk with him about ways to deal with his loneliness before she bought the alcohol for him.

Residential Settings for Treatment

Therapeutic communities have been used in residential treatment, in prisons, and in housing complexes to combat substance abuse. In a therapeutic community all residents are responsible for the good of the group and for meeting behavioral standards. Violations of these standards are dealt with by the group. There has been little written about the assessment and treatment of substance abuse problems in residential settings such as age-segregated apartment buildings, nursing homes, or chronic care hospitals. However, it is reasonable to expect that the principles of therapeutic community could be successfully integrated with in-home individual approaches and used to reach and treat substance-abusing clients in these settings.

CONCLUSION

Substance use patterns of today's middle-aged and young adult cohorts lead epidemiologists to believe that tomorrow's elderly population will have increased substance abuse treatment needs. Since issues of aging and substance abuse are often short-changed in professional training, there may be a particular training gap in the knowledge, values, and skills necessary to treat elderly people who have substance abuse problems. Each practitioner brings his or her own personal and professional experiences in aging and substance abuse treatment (Farkas, 1995). Forward-looking AODA practitioners recognize the need to develop policies and programs to detect and treat elderly people who are either at risk for, or are experiencing, substance abuse problems.

Cross-training models that incorporate information about aging with substance abuse treatment can increase the knowledge of both gerontologists and AODA practitioners. Just as AODA practitioners have educated their professional colleagues about the fact that substance abuse crosses educational, race, and economic lines, they need to increase their efforts to ensure that age does not create a barrier to adequate treatment for elderly people who have substance abuse problems. Dissemination of training materials that emphasize the overlap of the signs and symptoms of health problems, mental disorders, and substance abuse problems in elderly people can sensitize health and human services professionals to the issues of substance abuse in the elderly population. The use of age as a variable in identical case studies can alert professionals to their biases about elderly people and substance abuse issues: Substance abuse problems that are detected in a 27-year-old client may be ignored or misinterpreted in the 72-year-old. Adding a brief screening tool and training workers to make referrals to substance abuse treatment agencies could improve agencies' effectiveness at identifying and addressing the needs of at-risk individuals. Heeding the changes necessary to accommodate the physical and communication needs of older adults can help make AODA services more accessible and effective for these clients.

Researchers need to address questions about age- and cohort-related changes in substance use and abuse patterns. Cohort-related issues require longitudinal studies of people moving from middle age to late life. Will future cohorts of elderly people continue to decrease their use as they age? Will tomorrow's elderly population continue to use alcohol and other drugs at the same rates they did during their middle-aged years? Age-related research is needed to address the role of age in treatment effectiveness. What are the most effective service delivery strategies for AODA treatment of elder people? Which treatment models are most effective and why? AODA and gerontology clinicians and researchers can work collaboratively to develop knowledge that can help not only older adults but substance abusers across the lifespan.

REFERENCES

Adams, W. L., Barry, K. L., & Fleming, J. F. (1996). Screening for problem drinking in older primary care patients. *Journal of the American Medical Association*, 276(24), 1964–1967.

American Medical Association Council on Academic Affairs. (1996). Alcoholism in the elderly. *Journal of the American Medical Association*, 275, 797–801.

American Psychiatric Association. (1994). *Diagnostic and Statistical Manual of Mental Disorders* (4th ed.). Washington, DC: Author.

Atchley, R. C. (1997). *Social forces and aging* (8th ed.). Belmont CA: Wadsworth.

Atkinson, R. M. (1995). Treatment programs for aging alcoholics. In T. Beresford & E. Gomberg (Eds.), *Alcohol and aging* (pp. 186–210). New York: Oxford University Press.

Atkinson, R. M., & Ganzini, L. (1994). Substance abuse. In C. E. Coffey & J. L. Cummings (Eds.), *Textbook of geriatric neuropsychiatry* (pp. 297–321). Washington, DC: American Psychiatric Press.

Atkinson, R. M., Tolson, R. L., & Turner, J. A. (1990). Late versus early onset problems drinking in older men. *Alcoholism: Clinical and Experimental Research*, 14, 574–579.

Atkinson, R. M., Turner, J. A., Kofoed, L. L., & Tolson, R. L. (1985). Early versus late onset alcoholism in older persons: Preliminary findings. *Alcoholism: Clinical and Experimental Research*, 9, 513–515.

Atchley, R. C. (1997). *Social forces and aging* (8th ed.). Belmont CA: Wadsworth.

Barry, K. L. Oslin, D. W., & Blow, F. (2001). *Alcohol problems in older adults: Prevention and management.* New York: Springer.

Beechem, M. (2002). *Elderly alcoholism: Intervention strategies.* Springfield, IL: Charles C. Thomas.

Blow, F. C. (1998). *Substance abuse among older adults: Treatment Improvement Protocol (TIP), series 26.* U.S. Department of Health and Human Services, Publication No. (SMA) 98–3179. Rockville, MD.

Blow, F. C., Brower, K. J., Schulenberg,J. E., Demo-Dananberg, L. M., Young, J. P., & Beresford, T. P. (1992). The Michigan Alcoholism Screening Test—Geriatric Version (MAST-G): A new elderly-specific screening instrument. *Alcoholism: Clinical and Experimental Research, 16,* 372.

Brennan, P. L., & Moos, R. H. (1996). Late-life problem drinking: Personal and environmental risk factors for 4–year functioning outcomes and treatment seeking. *Journal of Substance Abuse, 8,* 167–180.

Bucholz, K. K., Sheline, Y., & Helzer, J. E. (1995). The epidemiology of alcohol use, problems, and dependence in elders: A review. In T. Beresford & E. Gomberg (Eds.), *Alcohol and aging* (pp. 19–41). New York: Oxford University Press.

Bureau of the Census. (1995). *Statistical brief: Sixty-five plus in the United States.* U.S. Department of Commerce, Economics and Statistics Administration, Washington, DC.

Centers for Disease Control and Prevention. (1996). *HIV/AIDA Surveillance Report, 8*(2), Atlanta, GA.

Condon, V. A. (1996). Medication management and the elderly. In C. Emlet, J. Crabtree, V. A. Condon, & L. A. Treml (Eds.), *In-home assessment of older adults: An interdisciplinary approach* (pp. 107–130). Gaithersburg, MD: Aspen.

Emlet, C., & Farkas, K. (2001). A descriptive analysis of older adults with HIV/AIDS in California. *Health and Social Work, 26*(4), 226–234.

Emlet, C., & Farkas, K. (2002). Correlation of service utilization among midlife and older adults with HIV/AIDS: The role of age in the equation. *Journal of Aging and Health, 14*(3), 315–335.

Farkas, K. J. (1992). Alcohol and elderly people. In F. Turner (Ed.), *Mental health and the elderly: A social work perspective* (pp. 328–354). New York: Free Press.

Farkas, K. J. (1995). Training health care and human services personnel in perinatal substance abuse. In R. R. Watson (Ed.), *Drug and Alcohol Abuse Reviews, Vol. 8: Drug and alcohol abuse during pregnancy and childhood* (pp. 13–35). Totowa, NJ: Humana Press.

Farkas, K. J., & Kola, L. A. (1997). Recognizing and treating alcohol abuse and alcohol dependence in elderly men. In J. I. Kosberg & L. W. Kaye (Eds.), *Elderly men: Special problems and professional challenges* (pp. 175–192). New York: Springer.

Folstein, M. F., Folstein, S. E., & McHugh, P. R. (1975). "Mini-mental state": A practical method for grading the cognitive state of patients for the clinician. *Journal of Psychiatric Research, 12,* 189–198.

Friedman, L., Fleming, N. F., Roberts, K. H., & Hyman, S. E. (Eds.). (1996). *Source book of substance abuse and addiction.* Baltimore: Williams & Wilkins.

Gomberg, E. S. L. (1996). Alcohol and Drugs. In *Encyclopedia of gerontology, Vol. 1* (pp. 93–101). New York: Academic Press.

Grant, B. F., Harford, T. C., Chou, P., Pickering, R., Dawson, D. A., Stinson, F. S., & Noble, J. (1991). Prevalence of DSM-III-R alcohol and abuse and dependence: United States, 1988. *Alcohol and Health Research World, 15*, 91–96.

Gurnack, A., Atkinson, R., & Osgood, N. (Eds.). (2002). *Treating alcohol and drug abuse in the elderly.* New York: Springer.

Liberto, J., & Oslin, D. (1997). Early versus late onset of alcoholism in the elderly. In A. M. Gurnack (Ed.), *Older adults' misuse of alcohol, medicines, and other drugs: Research and practice issues* (pp. 113–131). New York: Springer.

Liberto, J. G., Oslin, D. W., & Ruskin, P. E. (1992). Alcoholism in older persons: A review of the literature. *Hospital and Community Psychiatry, 43*(10), 975–984.

Mayfield, S., McLeod, G., & Hall, P. (1974). The CAGE questionnaire: Validation of a new alcoholism screening instrument. *American Journal of Psychiatry, 131*, 1121–1123.

Miller, W. R., & Rollnick, S. (1991). *Motivational interviewing: Preparing people to change addictive behavior.* New York: Guilford Press.

Miller, W. R., & Tonigan, S. J. (1996). Assessing drinkers' motivation for change: The Stages of Change Readiness and Treatment Eagerness Scale (SOCRATES). *Journal of Addictive Behaviors, 10*(2), 81–89.

National Institute on Alcohol Abuse and Alcoholism. (1995). *The physicians' guide to helping patients with alcohol problems.* NIH Publication No. 95-3796, Rockville, MD.

Prochaska, J. O., DiClemente, C. C., & Norcross, J. C. (1992). In search of how people change: Applications to addictive behaviors. *American Psychologist, 47*(9), 1102–1114.

Robins, L. N., & Regier, D. A. (1991). *Psychiatric disorders in America: The Epidemiologic Catchment Area Study.* New York: Free Press.

Schonfeld, L., & Dupree, L. W. (1991). Antecedents of drinking for early- and late-onset elderly alcohol abusers. *Journal of Studies on Alcohol, 52*, 587–592.

Seltzer, M. (1971). The Michigan Alcohol Screening Test: The quest for a new diagnostic instrument. *American Journal of Psychiatry, 127*, 1653–1658.

Seltzer, M., Vinojur, A., & Van Rooijan, L. (1975). A self-administered short Michigan Alcoholism Screening Test (SMAST). *Quarterly Journal of Studies on Alcohol, 36*, 117–126.

U. S. Department of Health and Human Services. (1999). *Drug abuse and addiction research: Sixth triennial report to Congress*, U.S. Department of Health and Human Services, Washington, DC. Available at www.nih.gov/STRCIndex.html

Willenbring, M., & Spring, W. D. (1988). Evaluating alcohol use in elders. *Generations, 12*(4), 27–31.

Woods, J. H., & Winger, G. (1995). Current benzodiazepine issues. *Psychopharmacology, 118*, 107–115.

CHAPTER 16

Assessment and Intervention with Alcohol- and Drug-Abusing Women

Patricia A. Pape

In ancient Rome, an alcoholic woman was considered to be such an affront to society that she could be legally put to death. She could also be put to death for adultery. It was simply assumed that a woman who drank or got drunk was also sexually promiscuous. Even today, women who are alcoholic or drug addicted (or both) are often treated with rejection, disgust, prejudice, apathy, or indifference. The purpose of this chapter is to review the research on substance-abusing women, including differences between women and men and among women themselves. Issues related to assessment and treatment are discussed.

PREVALENCE OF ALCOHOL
AND DRUG ABUSE IN WOMEN

In the best of ways, women in the United States are closing the gap with men: They are corporate officers, law firm partners, physicians, professors, military personnel, and other types of professionals that were not options in the past. At the same time, in the worst of ways, women are closing the gap with men in the extent to which they abuse alcohol, tobacco, legal and illegal drugs, and in the high price they pay for it. According to recent studies, 215 million women smoke, 4.5 million abuse or are addicted to alcohol, 3.5 million misuse prescription drugs, and 3.1 million regularly use illicit drugs (National Center on Addiction and Substance Abuse, 1996).

Although these numbers are lower than the corresponding figures for men, the gender gap is closing. The first major national analysis of alcohol, cigarette, and illicit drug use in a representative sample of women showed dramatic increases over the last three decades in the initial use of alcohol and drugs by girls ages 10–14 (Substance Abuse and Mental Health Services Administration [SAMHSA], 1997). In the early 1960s, girls between the ages of 10 and 14 represented about 7% of new users of alcohol. By the early 1990s that percentage had increased to 31, reflecting an increase of 9.5 times the overall rate of initial drinking by young females over the last 30 years. Moreover, in the early 1960s, only 5% of 10- to 14-year-old girls reported that they had used marijuana; in the early 1990s, the figure had risen to 24%. In addition, during 1961–1965 and 1986–1990, females generally initiated alcohol use at later ages than males. However, by 1991–1995, the gender differences in age-specific rates of alcohol initiation became negligible. It is evident that substance use is an increasingly significant aspect of women's lives, and it is starting earlier and earlier.

Other key findings relating to substance abuse among women include the following points (SAMHSA, 1997):

• Approximately a fifth of pregnant women under the age of 44 had used alcohol in the month preceding the survey, and nearly a third of those who drank reported having three or more drinks on the days they drank.
• Nearly a fifth of pregnant women under the age of 44 smoked cigarettes in the past month, and more than a fourth of those who smoked reported smoking a pack or more a day.
• Among adult women, the highest prevalence of any illicit drug use in the past year was found among those ages 18–34, those who were unemployed, those who had never married, and those who initiated substance use at an early age (15 years or younger).

RISK FACTORS FOR ALCOHOL MISUSE

Factors that may increase women's risk for alcohol abuse or dependence include genetic influences, early initiation of drinking, and violent victimization (National Institute on Alcohol Abuse and Alcoholism [NIAAA], 1999). A large study of twins provides the strongest evidence yet on the development of alcoholism in women (Kendler, Neale, Heath, Kessler, & Eaves, 1994). Heritability of alcoholism liability ranged from 51 to 59%, with the balance of the variance (41–49%) attributed to environmental factors.

Using data collected in a large general population survey, Wilsnack, Vogeltanz, and Klassen (1997) found that women who reported being sexually abused in childhood were more likely than other women to have experienced alcohol-related problems and to have one or more symptoms of alcohol dependence. Physical abuse during adulthood also has been associated with women's alcohol use. One study found that significantly more women undergoing alcoholism treatment experienced severe partner violence compared with other women in the community, although the data do not indicate whether the association was causal (Miller, 1998).

DIFFERENCES BETWEEN WOMEN'S AND MEN'S ALCOHOL CONSUMPTION

Research studies have documented how women's patterns of alcohol use, antecedents, and risk factors differ from those of men. Women experience more severe health and social consequences, face unique issues related to pregnancy, and are more vulnerable to physical abuse and sexual assault. These findings are of vital importance in recognizing and meeting the special needs of women when designing and implementing prevention and treatment services (Covington, 2002; Straussner, 1997).

Women appear to be more vulnerable than men to the many adverse consequences of alcohol use. For example, research suggests that women are more susceptible than men to alcohol-related organ damage and to trauma resulting from traffic crashes and interpersonal violence (NIAAA, 1999). Furthermore, studies also show that when women and men are given equal amounts of absolute alcohol per pound of body weight, women reach higher peak blood alcohol concentrations. This difference is related to the higher percentage of body fat and less body water in women than in men of similar body weight (NIAAA, 1999). Since alcohol is distributed throughout body water, it is less diluted in women. To make matters worse, percent of body fat in women increases every decade, so their tolerance of alcohol diminishes as they age (Roberts, 1999).

Studies also show that the level of sex hormones in the body determines the effect alcohol has on women. For example, women are more easily intoxicated just prior to their menstrual period, and women using birth control pills have an additional complication: Because both alcohol and birth control pills are metabolized in the liver, alcohol remains in the body longer, and these women will have higher blood alcohol levels (Straussner, 1985).

Alcohol dependence has been found to progress more quickly in women; this is called the "telescoping" effect. The progression itself may be different from that of men. Women will develop alcohol-induced liver disease with lower intake and fewer years of drinking than men. They are more likely than men to develop alcohol-induced hepatitis and to die from cirrhosis. Heavy drinking among women correlates with infertility, lack of sexual functioning, inability to reach orgasm, irregular menstrual cycles, and early menopause. Whether these factors precede or result from heavy alcohol use needs to be further addressed (Blume, 1988).

The psychological differences between women and men who abuse alcohol are also well documented. Women experience more depression and anxiety and have lower self-esteem. Women are more apt to start drinking in reaction to a specific stressful event, often a relationship or role loss. In comparison to men, who often drink to be sociable, women tend to drink to escape and self-medicate (Straussner, 1985).

Studies of women in treatment indicate that they are more likely to come from families in which there is a history of alcoholism (National Center on Addiction and Substance Abuse, 1996; NIAAA, 1999). Gomberg (1980) reported more loss and more depression as well as other psychiatric problems in their families. Studies also show that women are more apt than men to attempt suicide, usually by overdosing with legally prescribed pills, and to have primary affective disorders. Women also report more severe problems with amphetamines and tranquilizers and use more legal drugs, most of which are prescribed by male physicians. The use of stimulants, such as cocaine and amphetamines, to lose weight or overcome depression is common among women (O'Connor, Esherick, & Vieten, 2002; Straussner, 1997).

DIFFERENCES AMONG SUBGROUPS
OF SUBSTANCE-ABUSING WOMEN

In addition to differences between male and female substance abusers, there are differences among subgroups within the female population on a number of variables: socioeconomic status, employment status, sexual preference, and age, ethnic, racial, and cultural factors. Summaries of some of these findings are reported by Wilsnack (1990), Straussner (1985, 1997), and O'Connor and colleagues (2002).

In terms of socioeconomic status, rates of drinking (nonabstention) tend to be higher among women who have higher levels of education and income; however, rates of alcohol *problems* and *dependence* are not consistently related to socioeconomic levels (Straussner, 1985; Wilznack, 1990).

Among racial groups, alcohol use is more prevalent among white women, and black women have higher rates of abstention. However, black women are more likely to drink heavily and to use crack cocaine. Hispanic women are more likely to abstain and less likely to drink heavily than either black or white women (NIAAA, 1999). Available data regarding Native American women suggests that they experience higher rates of drinking, leading to higher rates of fetal alcohol syndrome and alcohol-related deaths, including death from liver cirrhosis, than either black or white women (NIAAA, 1999).

Wilsnack (1990) found little evidence to support the once-popular belief that women who fill multiple roles are at especially high risk for alcohol abuse. In fact, women who combine marital and employment roles may have lower rates of alcohol problems than women who lack these roles. "Role deprivation" may increase women's risk for unrestrained or self-medicative use of alcohol and/or other drugs.

EFFECTS OF MARIJUANA, COCAINE, AND HEROIN ON WOMEN

With the exception of marijuana, women are less likely than men to use illicit drugs, such as cocaine and heroin (National Center on Addiction and Substance Abuse, 1996). However, as indicated previously, gender differences in drug use among the younger populations are narrowing.

Use of Marijuana by Women

According to research studies, women who are between 19 and 40 years old are as likely as men to have used marijuana (National Center on Addiction and Substance Abuse, 1996). Marijuana has been the subject of mixed messages dating back to the 1960s social movements. The increased denial related to drug addiction in women, in general, is compounded by the specific denial related to the physical addiction of marijuana. This denial becomes a barrier to women getting treatment for marijuana addiction.

It is estimated that 20% of people who try marijuana become daily users (Chacin, 1996). Even weekly usage may become addictive, due to the build-up of delta-9-tetrahydrocannabinol (THC) in fatty tissue. THC is 200 times more soluble in fat than in blood—which may present unique problems for women, whose baseline fat content is greater than men's. Some of the harmful effects of marijuana include memory impairment, hormonal and gonadal disruption, lung disease, increased risk of schizophrenia, and various forms of cancer. Long-term THC use causes cell abnormalities, alters normal cell division, affects genetic makeup of new cells, and lowers cell immunity (Chacin, 1996).

Marijuana also has far-reaching effects on the reproductive system. Specific effects on females include decreased femininity due to increased amounts of testosterone, infertility due to interruption of the menstrual cycle, and irreversible damage to the supply of eggs from the ovaries. The use of marijuana also may lead to pregnancy complications and fetal effects such as premature births, low birth weights, birth defects, and increased infant mortality rates. Nursing mothers can transfer THC to their babies through their breast milk (Chacin, 1996).

Use of Powder and Crack Cocaine by Women

In both women and men, cocaine use can cause heart attacks, hypertension, strokes, seizures, malnutrition, and infections from intravenous injection sites. Other common consequences of cocaine use are increased risk of AIDS, syphilis, tuberculosis, hepatitis B, and suppressed immune function (National Center on Addiction and Substance Abuse, 1996). A 1996 study by Bowersox showed that women were less sensitive to the effects of cocaine and that hormonal fluctuations play an important role in women's responses to the drug. An increase in certain hormone levels causes women's mucous membranes, including the nasal passages, to secrete more mucous. This additional mucous may act as a barrier to the absorption of cocaine if women snort the drug during the luteal phase of their menstrual cycle. Consequently, women's response to cocaine will differ at different phases of their monthly cycle. Patterns of craving and response to withdrawal also can fluctuate with the menstrual cycle.

Forty percent of all crack addicts are women (National Center on Addiction and Substance Abuse, 1996). Crack cocaine is cheap, it is smoked rather than injected, and it gives a temporary sense of confidence that women report liking. Unfortunately, trading sex for money to buy drugs has become a deadly practice among many crack-addicted women (National Center on Addiction and Substance Abuse, 1996). The crack epidemic also has fueled an explosion in the female prison population. By 1991, a third of female inmates were serving time for a drug offense, compared to a fifth of men. Although men still outnumber women, the number of female inmates is growing faster than the number of men (National Center on Addiction and Substance Abuse, 1996; van Wormer, 2002).

Since the advent of crack cocaine in the mid-1980s, there has been a sharp increase in the number of crack-exposed newborns. Child abuse and neglect reports, mostly related to alcohol and drug abuse, rose 64% from 1985 to 1994. The percentage of children in foster care under age 4 who have been exposed prenatally to drugs more than doubled from 1986 to 1991 (National Center on Addiction and Substance Abuse, 1996).

Use of Heroin by Women

The past decade also has seen an alarming rise in heroin use among women. Heroin is an analgesic, or pain suppressant, whose effects are stronger and reach peak effects much faster than its predecessor, morphine. Heroin produces intense euphoria, reduces anxiety, and is even more addictive than morphine. As tolerance levels increase and more of the drug is needed to achieve the desired effect, one alternative is to switch the route of administration from snorting or smoking to that of intravenous drug use (National Center on Addiction and Substance Abuse, 1996).

There has been an increase in the number of young women who are smoking or sniffing heroin rather than injecting it. This may be the result of the increased purity of the drug, which makes this kind of use feasible, coupled with lower prices due to increased supplies. Another common trend is "cross-lining"—the practice of snorting one line of heroin followed by one line of cocaine (Chatham, Hiller, Rowan-Szal, Joe, & Simpson, 1999).

Research studies by Chatham and colleagues (1999) and Powis, Griffiths, Gossop, and Strang (1996) highlight significant gender differences among heroin users. Heroin-addicted females were younger, less likely to inject the drug, used it for shorter periods of time, and more dependent on it than their male counterparts. Moreover, women tended to use cocaine in addition to heroin, whereas men used alcohol. Women were also more apt to be unemployed, receiving welfare, and have more dependent children than men. Female heroin users were more likely to have a regular sex partner who used heroin and were more likely to have been injected first by their male sexual partner. Whereas males financed their heroin use through criminal acts such as theft and drug dealing, women turned to prostitution. As pointed out by Straussner (1997), "men sell drugs, while women sell themselves" (p. 21).

Women and HIV

The increasing risk of women who are intravenous (IV) drug users for HIV infection warrants special attention (Friedman, 1997). Few of these women reported using condoms during vaginal, oral, or anal sex, and a large proportion do not use new or bleach-cleaned needles, yet share needles with two or more persons, often daily. Many of these women further compromise their immune systems, as well as their judgment, by the use of alcohol. The majority of these women are in their prime childbearing years and many have substantial child-care responsibilities (Friedman, 1997).

Why do these women continue to put themselves at risk by practicing unsafe sex with multiple partners? The answers lie in the issues of sexual abuse, violence, and victimization. Women with such histories tend to have low self-esteem, dissociate frequently, experience phobic reactions, and have difficulty with intimate relationships. A history of painful or victimizing experiences, combined with fear of a currently abusive partner, interfere with a woman's ability to assert herself and to reduce HIV risks. Until she feels empowered to make choices, she is at high risk for victimizing relationships and HIV infection.

IMPACT OF ALCOHOL AND OTHER
DRUGS ON FETAL DEVELOPMENT

The National Institute on Drug Abuse (NIDA) conducted the National Pregnancy and Health Survey during 1992; it was the first national survey of drug use among pregnant women in the United States (Mathias, 1995). The results indicated that 5.5% of the 4 million women who gave birth in 1992 used illegal drugs while they were pregnant. Marijuana and cocaine were the most frequently used illicit drugs.

The survey also found a high incidence of cigarette and alcohol use among pregnant women. There is already evidence that use of these legal substances affect the health of both the fetus and the mother during and after pregnancy. The survey also demonstrated a strong link between cigarette smoking, alcohol use, and the use of illicit drugs in this population. The conclusion drawn is that health care practitioners must monitor *both* licit and illicit drug use during pregnancy.

The survey also examined differences in amount and types of drugs used by several racial and ethnic groups of women. Overall, 11.3% of African American women and 4.5% of Hispanic women used illicit drugs during pregnancy. Pregnant African American women had the highest rates of cocaine use, mainly crack, and pregnant white women had the highest rates of alcohol and cigarette use (Mathias, 1995).

The Centers for Disease Control report that drinking among pregnant women has increased dramatically in recent years: The number who consumed any alcohol increased over 60% from 1992 to 1995, and frequent drinking (seven drinks or more in 1 week, or five on one occasion) among pregnant women grew fourfold (Drug Strategies, 1998).

The impact on children born to women using alcohol and other drugs can be devastating, as the following points demonstrate:

• The rate of infant deaths increases by 50% when mothers smoke during pregnancy. In addition, smoking by mothers doubles the incidence of sudden infant death syndrome (SIDS), results in higher respiratory infections, and leads to lower birth weights—20% of low birth weights in babies are caused by smoking (Drug Strategies, 1998).

• Alcohol is the leading known preventable cause of birth defects and mental retardation. There are more than 7,000 fetal alcohol syndrome (FAS) babies born each year. This most extreme manifestation of alcohol effects includes growth retardation, facial dysmorphology, central nervous system anomalies, and morphologic abnormalities. Less severely affected babies are considered to have fetal alcohol effects (FAE). Incidence of FAE is estimated to be three to four times that of FAS. The cost of caring for infants, children, and surviving adults with FAS exceeds $2 billion annually (Drug Strategies, 1998).

• Complications found among cocaine-using women include premature birth, SIDS, low birth weight, and premature separation of the placenta. Cocaine is considered more dangerous to the unborn baby than any other illicit drug (Chasnoff, 1989).

• Women using marijuana gave birth to babies who were 3 ounces lighter and one-fifth of an inch shorter than babies of nonusing mothers. These babies also had a smaller head circumference, suggesting possible problems with brain development (Moulton & Moulton, 1984).

• Infants exposed to narcotics undergo a characteristic withdrawal sequence called the neonatal abstinence syndrome. These newborns show increased sensitivity to noise, irritability, poor coordination, excessive sneezing and yawning, and uncoordinated sucking and swallowing reflexes. As noted above, for marijuana use, these babies tend to have smaller head circumferences, raising questions about brain growth that could affect mental functioning, such as memory (NIDA, 1992).

Researchers have found that although women have decreased their rates of drug use during pregnancy, they do not totally discontinue drugs (NIDA, 1992). This finding points out how powerful drug addiction can be, given the fact that concern for her unborn baby is usually the ultimate incentive for a woman to abstain from drugs.

ISSUES RELATING TO FAMILIES OF ALCOHOL- AND DRUG-ADDICTED WOMEN

Three major domains affecting the families of alcohol- or drug-addicted women are (1) family-of-origin issues; (2) the effects of the woman's substance abuse on her present family; and (3) the high correlation between alcohol/drug abuse and domestic violence. All three domains need to be addressed during treatment.

Family-of-Origin Issues

Women who develop alcoholism have a higher percentage of alcoholic relatives, especially an alcoholic biological mother, than women who develop other problems. Women with an alcoholic father have higher rates of depression, an inability to make friends as children, somatoform illnesses, eating disorders, greater problems with intimacy, and a high propensity to marry an alcoholic male. In contrast, women with an alcoholic mother have higher rates of chemical dependency (Ackerman, 1987).

Effects of Substance Abuse on a Woman's Family

Several characteristics are commonly seen in substance-abusing women's current family: (1) the women are less likely to be in a long-term relationship than substance-abusing men, because men are much more likely to leave their addicted wives or partners, whereas women stay with their addicted husbands; (2) addicted women are emotionally, and sometimes physically, unavailable to their children, which impacts on their development; and (3) the rules and roles in these dysfunctional families generally perpetuate denial and secret keeping.

Connection between Alcohol/Drug Abuse and Domestic Violence

In 1992, a NIDA-funded epidemiological study of posttraumatic stress disorder (PTSD) and substance abuse demonstrated what most clinicians have been observing: a link between the victimization of female children and women and the subsequent initiation of alcohol and other drug abuse (NIDA Notes, 1992). Parental substance abuse and family violence affects a large number of children. The rate of child abuse or serious neglect is 1500% higher in substance-abusing families than the national average (Illinois Advisory Council on Alcoholism and Other Drug Dependency, 1995). Research indicates that the abuse of the mother may be the single most important risk factor for child maltreatment.

ISSUES OF SUBSTANCE-ABUSING WOMEN IN THE WORKPLACE

Although there have been gains for women in the workplace, including decreases in the wage gap and in occupational segregation, the structure of the workplace is still directed toward the needs of men (Nakken, 2002; Pape, 1999). One of the principal barriers to women's full participation in the paid labor force is the disproportionate responsibility women continue to bear for the well-being of home and family, in addition to their full-time jobs outside the home. These are the "superwomen" who are also vulnerable to substance abuse (Pape, 1988). Whereas multiple roles of family and work do not increase alcohol problems, "superwomen" are those who take on way too much and demand perfection of themselves, resulting in burnout and substance abuse.

Research studies indicate that working women are less likely than men to be identified with alcohol- and other drug-related problems, and that women require different types of outreach strategies in the workplace (Copeland & Hall, 1992; Nakken, 2002). Research on the constructive confrontation model, often used by employee assistance programs (EAPs) to break through denial and motivate men to get treatment for substance abuse, shows that it does not work with women (Reed, 1994). This approach may, in fact, be contraindicated for women, because self-blame and shame, not denial, tend to be their primary dynamics.

BARRIERS TO TREATMENT

Women are still not being identified as substance abusers or as being dependent on drugs or alcohol, nor are they entering treatment, at the same rate as men. This "disgraceful discrepancy" (Pape, 1986) has been documented in much of the research literature. Estimates indicate that at least one of three alcoholic persons in the United States is female, yet only one of 20 of these women is in treatment in a given year. Among other drug abusers, two of five are women, but only one of 50 is in treatment (Reed, 1994). A good place to find and identify alcohol- and drug-dependent women is in the doctor's office. It is common knowledge that women are more apt to visit their primary care physician for health concerns than are men, and these physicians are less likely to diagnose substance abuse and addiction in women than in men (Cyr & Moulton, 1993).

Research on the obstacles and barriers to women seeking treatment consistently identify lack of child care, lack of transportation, and lack of insurance or other financial resources. Additional barriers to treatment utilization and to treatment effectiveness for women fall into two categories: external or systemic barriers, and internal or individual barriers (National Center on Addiction and Substance Abuse, 1996).

Some of the external, systemic barriers include (1) male-oriented identification processes and treatment models, (2) involvement with partners who use substances themselves, (3) greater pressure from family and friends *not* to enter treatment, (4) lack of diagnosis or misdiagnosis by medical professionals, (5) inadequate training and sensitivity of health professionals to women's unique needs, and (6) lack of comprehensive services in a single location. Internal, individual barriers include (1) high levels of shame and guilt due to the internalization of society's stigmatization, (2) fear of leaving or losing children, (3) fear of abuse from, or loss of, a partner, (4) lack of self-esteem, and (5) lack of information about services (National Center on Addiction and Substance Abuse, 1996).

Pregnant drug abusers face unique barriers to treatment, the most formidable of which is the lack of available and appropriate drug abuse treatment services for pregnant women, including the specialized prenatal care and postnatal services that they require.

TREATMENT NEEDS OF WOMEN

Beyond removing barriers to access, successful treatment programs for women must address their special medical, psychological, and social needs. Childhood sexual abuse, eating disorders, domestic violence, depression, anger, shame, anxiety, suicide attempts, PTSD, and lack of parenting skill are only some of the treatment issues that need to be addressed.

Many substance-abusing women need basic medical care, drug-free housing, and education and job skills training. Vocational as well as economic issues and limitations are common, as are educational deficiencies. Some may be illiterate, and many lack basic communication and assertiveness skills. They also may have legal as well as child welfare concerns. Learned helplessness and a sense of powerlessness are pervasive. Lack of education regarding HIV/AIDS and issues of safe sex, especially for injecting drug users and partners of injecting drug users, need to be addressed during treatment. Special medical problems, especially gynecological ones, due to the telescoped development of their disease must be diagnosed and treated. In addition, substance-abusing women need basic information about diet and nutrition. Providing comprehensive services in one location, as well as providing linkages to other needed support services, increases women's attendance at treatment sessions. Finally, women-only therapy groups and self-help groups have shown better outcomes than the traditional treatment approaches (National Center on Addiction and Substance Abuse, 1996).

Women suffer a triple stigma from alcohol and drug addiction: (1) the general stigma of chemical dependency, (2) the double moral standards, wherein women are placed on a "pedestal," with higher moral expectations than those for men, and (3) the continued association of drinking and drug use with sexual promiscuity. Women turn this triple stigma against themselves, internalize it, and create two major issues with which they must deal in the recovery: guilt and shame.

Another special issue for women relates to the centrality of relationships in their lives: as daughters of alcoholic parents, as partners of substance abusers, and as parents. Involving a woman's family in her treatment produces better outcomes. In addition, women need more realistic, individualized aftercare plans that accommodate relationships, as well as recovery, work, or school commitments. For many women, developing fulfilling friendships with other women is an essential ingredient to healing and growth (Byington, 1997).

In general, women tend to evaluate themselves in terms of their deficiencies, to be unaware of their strengths, to blame themselves for all of the problems in their lives, and to have higher levels of guilt and shame than men. Consequently, gender-sensitive assessments must move from a deficit model to a competence model. Such a model focuses on assessing a woman's sense of competence, her vulnerabilities, and the stresses she experiences (Mejta, Lewis, & Engle, 1995).

Issues in the Screening and Assessment of Women

In order to help women with alcohol and other drug problems, we must be able to identify those problems. However, almost all of the well-known screening instruments have been developed for, and validated on, male populations, and are based on male substance abuse thresholds, symptoms, and problems (Lieber, 1993).

Alcohol screening questionnaires may be less valid for women than men for several reasons (Bradley, Boyd-Wickizer, Powell, & Burman, 1998): First, the increased stigma associated with women who drink heavily may cause them to underreport alcohol use and related problems. Second, women are less likely than men to experience the overt social consequences of heavy drinking, such as employment, economic, or legal difficulties, and therefore they may be missed by screening questionnaires that target these experiences. On the other hand, women are much more apt to report internal and personal correlates of alcohol abuse, such as depression, feelings of isolation, anxiety, and conflicts in relationships. These inner-directed symptoms are much less visible. Third, women suffer from adverse consequences of drinking at much lower levels of consumption than men. Therefore, questions related to quantity are much less reliable and sensitive in identifying alcohol abuse or dependence in women (Blume, 1988; Lieber, 1993).

The CAGE, AUDIT, and TWEAK questionnaires are considered optimal instruments for identification of alcohol dependence in women (Bradley et al., 1998). However, it may be necessary to use different cutoff points in women than in men. Recommended cutoff points for women are 2 points or more for the TWEAK; 4 points or more for the AUDIT; and 1 point or more for the CAGE (Bradley et al., 1998).

Screening is only the first step in the assessment of alcohol and other drug problems. If women have positive screening results, they need to be assessed for current substance use, adverse consequences, symptoms of dependence, and motivation to change. An extensive alcohol and drug history must be taken, paying particular attention to the use of prescribed medications and any delayed withdrawal symptoms from sedatives.

It is also important to do a thorough differential diagnosis to determine if there is primary substance use disorder, or if it is secondary or co-existing with another mental disorder. In females, depressive, anxiety, and eating disorders often coexist with alcohol abuse (Straussner, 1997). In addition, a complete family history, particularly noting any mental illness or chemical dependency, going back two or three generations, is important. Information about current living situation and significant relationships is also a crucial part of the assessment, because of the priority women place on relationships and the importance of their roles as wife and mother to their own identity. Finally, because substance-abusing women tend to exhibit more physiological problems than men, a comprehensive physical examination, including a gynecological exam and a pregnancy test, is extremely important.

Intervention

Treatment of Alcohol Abuse

Some of the major issues substance-abusing women bring into treatment include low self-esteem, codependency resulting from their extreme socialization as nurturers of others, and an inability to identify and express their own feelings, especially anger, and needs. For example:

> Susan, a 35-year-old single parent, came in as a self-referral to her company's EAP. Susan had three children, ages 5, 7, and 12, and her 12-year-old daughter was getting into trouble at school. Susan talked about the stress related to her career advancement in the company, attending school to finish her MBA, and trying to parent her three children by herself. She had no extended family, no support system, and no leisure time in her life. Her "reward" for getting through her days was to "relax after the kids are in bed, drinking a couple of brandies and reading a good book before I fall asleep." Often she could not fall asleep, and so a few months ago her doctor had prescribed sleeping pills, to be taken only "occasionally, when she needed them."
>
> When questioned further, the following information was gathered: Susan's father and grandfather both had problems with alcohol; the "couple of brandies" were 4 ounces each, more than she needed to relax, but she had developed a tolerance for alcohol; she occasionally had blackouts; she was now taking at least one, sometimes two, sleeping pills each night in order to sleep (further evidence of tolerance); and finally, she had promised herself the month before that she would stop taking the pills, but had suffered such anxiety and insomnia that she had returned to using them.
>
> The diagnosis for Susan was alcohol dependence (DSM-IV 303.90). Treatment recommendations included an outpatient chemical dependency program where she would receive education about her disease; family therapy to work on the problems involved with single parenting; and a women's sobriety group and attendance at AA meetings. Today, Susan has been abstinent for 2 years, is successfully parenting her three children, still attends AA, and is involved in an ACOA therapy group to address the affects of growing up with an alcoholic father.

Historically, male-modeled programs have focused only on the addiction and on changing the patterns of an individual's alcohol or drug use, without addressing the circumstances surrounding the addiction. In the past decade we have learned the importance of the *context* in women's addiction problems. Women's chemical dependency does not exist in isolation but is an interactive factor with their social, economic, and cultural contexts (Brown, 2002). The acute powerlessness of being chemically dependent compounds with the essential powerlessness of being female in our society—and the results are devastating. By recognizing the interconnectedness of women's lives with those of family members, partners, children, and others in the communities, and by providing gender-sensitive services for women, we can empower these clients to make changes in their lives beyond the mere cessation of drinking or drug use, and to play an integral part in their own healing and reintegration. The model of treatment for women must provide comprehensive services for multiple problems.

Female clients tend to respond well to self-esteem-building counseling strategies. Motivational interviewing (Miller, 1983), an alternative to the traditional confrontational model of interviewing typically used with substance-abusing clients, works well with women (see Hanson & El-Bassel, Chapter 2, this volume, for additional information). Four aspects of motivational interviewing are stressed when working with women (Mejta et al., 1995): First is the *deemphasis on labels*. Rather than focusing on identifying "diagnosis," this approach focuses on the problems the client defines and what solutions might resolve them. Second is *internal attribution*. If women see themselves as powerless and helpless, such beliefs can become self-fulfilling prophecies. Changes that are attributed internally are usually longer-lasting. Women need to see themselves as responsible for changing themselves. Third is *individual responsibility*. The client herself decides what is a problem and what needs to be done about it. She is the "expert" on herself; the clinician is a resource, guide, and support person. The assumption is that the client is a responsible and capable adult. The fourth aspect is *cognitive dissonance*, which is a discrepancy between the client's behavior and her beliefs about herself. This discrepancy is uncomfortable and leads her to attempt to overcome the dissonance. The higher her self-esteem and self-respect, the more apt she is to change.

A sense of self-efficacy arises from a self-made judgment that the person can successfully solve a problem or accomplish a task. People with high feelings of self-efficacy tend to be more successful; substance-abusing women, in general, tend to have a low sense of self-efficacy. Motivational interviewing can be used at intake to (1) encourage women to take responsibility for their own treatment, (2) identify their own ideas about the positive and negative consequences of changing their substance use behaviors, (3) deal openly with doubts and fears about change, and (4) freely choose their treatment goals. During treatment, motivational interviewing can be used to help women identify situations that place them at risk for relapse and practice the countermanding coping strategies to prevent relapse.

In general, strategies that focus on a women's strengths, resources, and behaviors from her past that have helped her to survive difficult circumstances can help her to change her negative beliefs about herself and to increase her feelings of self-worth. Specific strategies that have been identified as working well with female clients include a focus on collaborative relationships, behavioral/self-management training, self-control training, self-esteem training, supportive women's groups, and gender-sensitive family/couple counseling (Lewis, 1995).

A relational model of treatment, based on women's psychological development (Miller, 1986), takes into account the centrality and continuity of relationships throughout women's lives. Forming and enhancing relationships are central to a woman's sense of personhood and critical to her sense of efficacy and effectiveness. The self-in-relation theory shifts the emphasis from a "separate self" to that of a "relational self" as the core self-structure in women and as the basis for growth and development (Byington, 1997; Surrey, 1985).

The relational model of treatment provides an empowerment approach for women. This model view humans as always expanding, growing, and capable of changing. It is a capacity-focused approach wherein the clinician is a facilitator or companion on the journey, rather than the authority or the expert. This model assumes that there are many paths to growth and recovery and that clients have their own best answers within themselves.

A woman's experience with addiction cannot be separated from the realities of sexism in our society. Every dimension—its causes, consequences, subversive hidden quality, and its treatment—is shaped by a woman's subordinate and devalued status that informs the ways of seeing, defining, and dealing with human behaviors (Sandmaier, 1992). In feminist therapy women help women facilitate change in a nonhierarchical, reciprocal, and supportive way (Levine, 1989). Feminist counseling is *not* a technique. It is an approach that works within an explicit feminist framework. Such an approach helps us to reexamine assumptions about the traditional male hierarchical models of power as power *over,* versus the female model of power as empowerment, or power *to.* This vision is particularly relevant to our work with substance-abusing women, because issues of power and powerlessness are always at the core of chemical dependency (see Brown, 2002).

Many women talk about feeling a "spiritual void" or "emptiness." To address this issue, substance-abusing women need to develop a new set of recovery-based beliefs and values and some sort of spiritual view or sense of purpose, meaning, and connectedness with others. Often, attending a self-help group and working the 12 steps of a recovery program such as Alcoholics Anonymous or Narcotics Anonymous provide this deeply needed dimension. In addition, these self-help programs appear to be the best modality for dealing with the shame that is so prevalent among female substance abusers. Many women feel more comfortable at women-only self-help groups, and most communities provide such resources.

Brief family systems therapy, in combination with the addictions model of treatment, is often very important in helping women. A major goal is to get family members to focus on themselves, their feelings, and their needs, and to stop focusing on the chemically dependent woman. Family members may need to receive professional treatment as well as participate in self-help recovery groups such as Al-Anon, Nar-Anon, Alateen, or Adult Children of Alcoholics. It is also important to screen family members for their own addictions and to refer them for help, if appropriate. Family rules, roles, boundaries, communication styles, expression of anger, conflict negotiation, dealing with losses (both during the active abuse and in recovery), and having fun and recreation without the use of substances are all issues that need focused attention.

Treatment needs to address both the cognitive and behavioral aspects of dealing with the real world. Women need to learn to manage people, places, things, and feelings in order to reduce the risk of relapse. They need to identify the relapse cues, both internal and external, that are specific to them. Women also need permission to be assertive and to put their needs first—particularly difficult to do for a woman who is in a relationship with a male substance abuser, which all too often leads her to frequenting places where alcohol and other drugs are available. Often she needs to end this relationship, but doing so takes time and does not usually happen until she has found other, more satisfying, relationships.

Women also need to set career, vocational, or educational goals. Much of the literature points to the importance of setting goals in areas where women feel competent and can experience self-mastery and pride in their accomplishments. Increased feelings of independence, a sense of personal power and security, and a greater willingness to take responsibility for their own lives are the results.

Treatment of Illicit Drug Use

Treatment issues specific to women addicted to opiates must address the legal consequences of their addiction. The Harrison Act of 1914 marked the beginning of the criminalization of the use of narcotics. Consequently, the history of a heroin addiction is one of reduced life options. The heroin-addicted woman often turns to illegal activities to support her habit and enters the world of crime. Such activities are often sex-role related, such as selling sexual favors for money to buy drugs, further locking the woman into a deviant lifestyle.

Methadone maintenance as a treatment for narcotic addiction is a phenomenon with unique dynamics. Rosenbaum and Murphy (1990) identified several phases in the treatment of women using methadone. The initial phases involve the surrender of control as the woman is put on a structured routine that includes mandatory clinic attendance, urinalysis, and counseling. Entering this phase is often accompanied by a sense of relief. In the next stage, of "stabilization," the correct dosage of methadone is attained, and the woman begins a lifelong relationship with this drug. She is viewed as a "success" when she breaks from her deviant lifestyle and reenters conventional adult frameworks. A woman deemed a "failure" continues in the heroin world and uses methadone as a fallback drug. In the final phase, that of "disillusionment," the woman resents the control to which she us subjected in the lifelong need to mandatory report to the methadone clinic and the identity of being a "half-junkie." Being a successful methadone patient, paradoxically, impedes detachment from methadone. The most pervasive obstacle to getting off methadone is fear: of long-term withdrawal symptoms, of emotional vulnerability, and of the lack of structure and social life that clinic attendance provides.

Regardless of the drugs used or the treatment approach, women, in general, have more difficulty returning to the conventional world than do men; they carry a deeper stigma and, as a consequence, find it more difficult to secure and keep jobs as part of their recovery. Middle-class recovering women have more options, although even for them these are generally fewer than for men. And finally, women who user drugs intravenously are at high risk of HIV and AIDS, making them the outreach worker's greatest challenge. Issues concerning sex-roles and stigma make IV-drug-using women the most difficult to reach at-risk population.

Although cocaine-abusing women exhibit symptoms common to all substance-abusing women, the intensity of their compulsion to use makes them prone to particularly high relapse rates. Three major treatment issues—grief, sexuality, and assertion—have a major impact on positive treatment outcomes for this group. Cocaine-addicted women exhibit a more intense bonding with their drug of choice—they are "in love with their drug." The memory of the pain of their addiction is overshadowed by the memory of the pleasure. They are giving up the most intense love affair they have ever known. They need to be educated about the stages of the grieving process to understand that the intensity of many of their emotions is directly related to their grieving over the loss of cocaine.

The unspoken sexual concerns these women bring into treatment can impede their progress. They need to be reassured that their numerous and unusual sexual encounters are the norm for cocaine-abusing women; their guilt, anger, and humiliation must be processed thoroughly. Some of the guilt and shame comes from their embarrassment over having enjoyed some of those experiences and their belief that, were they to share this with others, they would be seen as "sick" and "perverted." Women-only groups provide the safe and respectful atmosphere needed to work on these issues.

Basic assertion training can be a powerful treatment modality that opens up a new world of options, enhances self-esteem and self-respect, and helps these women deal with risky situations.

Betsy, a 24-year-old white woman, was referred by the court system for her heroin addiction. She had been using heroin off and on for 6 years and had finally been arrested for possession of a controlled substance. She had gone through withdrawal while she was in jail and was drug free when she came in for treatment.

In keeping with the competence model and using a feminist counseling approach, the initial assessment and treatment planning focused on the strengths and competencies Betsy could use in her recovery program. She was intelligent, highly motivated, empathic, and nurturing as a mom. Among her vulnerabilities was the tendency to care for others but not herself. Stresses in her life included homelessness, unemployment, singly parenting her 8-year-old son, lack of a sober support system, and dysfunctional relationships with men.

Betsy completed the intensive outpatient program and the 1-year Women's Sobriety Group aftercare program, attended two NA meetings per week, and got an NA sponsor with whom she had weekly contact. Betsy and her sister (also a recovering drug addict) moved back home with their parents and found jobs on different shifts so they could watch each other's children when they were not working. During her treatment she found out she was pregnant, which surprised her because she had assumed her lack of menstrual periods was simply a symptom of her heroin use. The father of the child moved away and did not support her. She was able to get short-term welfare support as well as some financial support from her church.

Betsy learned to identify and express her feelings, especially anger; identify and ask for what she needed; and nurture and care for herself as well as others. She improved her problem-solving, decision-making, and assertiveness skills. Today, 3 years later, she is still drug free, attends NA weekly, has been promoted three times on her job, got her GED, and has plans to go to college to obtain her degree in business administration.

COUNTERTRANSFERENCE ISSUES

First and foremost, we must examine our own denial, which supports and maintains societal denial, and our own tendencies to buy into the myths and stereotypes related to chemically dependent persons, in general, and substance-abusing women, in particular. Many helping professionals were the oldest child, the "family hero," and the caretaker in their chemically dependent family system.

Often as adults they are personally uncomfortable talking about chemical dependency and, in turn, project their feelings onto the client because of their own experiences with parental substance abuse. If they have not acknowledged and worked through their own issues, both in therapy and in a 12-step program, they will surely get in the way of attempts to help clients.

For example, Joe, a social worker whose mother suffered from alcohol and drug abuse during his growing-up years, was always making excuses for, and rescuing, female clients who were substance abusers. He took phone calls any time of the day or night, gave out his home phone number, did not set healthy boundaries, and did not hold his clients accountable for their behavior. Joe was encouraged to go to Al-Anon and also to engage in a therapy group for adult children of alcoholics. As a result of doing this, his changes have had a positive impact on his ability to work in a healthy way with female substance-abusing clients.

CONCLUSION

During the past decade, the abuse of alcohol and other drugs by women has been recognized by many as one of the top health problems in the United States today. Although we have made gains in the assessment and treatment of female substance abusers, we have generally ignored the larger system of which women are a part.

Data indicate that many of the issues specific to female substance abusers are a consequence of the social structure in which they live and the oppression they experience as a result of that structure. We need to modify the social, political, and economic contexts of women's lives. Four ways this can be accomplished are: increasing their opportunities in the workplace; redistributing responsibilities of home and family; eliminating violence against women and children; and eliminating poverty (Pape, 1999). Social workers, because of their unique training and positioning, can participate in mentoring, advocacy, and social activism to enlighten and change beliefs, attitudes, and behaviors toward substance-abusing women. We owe it to ourselves and to our clients to take all of the necessary steps to fulfill the unmet needs of this special population.

REFERENCES

Ackerman, R. J. (1987). A new perspective on adult children of a Alcoholics. *EAP Digest, 7*, 25–29.

Blume, S. B. (1988). *Alcohol/drug dependent women*. Minneapolis, MN: Johnson Institute.

Bowersox, J. A. (1996). Cocaine affects men and women differently, NIDA study shows. *NIDA Notes, 11*(1), 3.

Bradley, K. A., Boyd-Wickizer, J., Powell, S. H., & Burman, M. L. (1998). Alcohol screening questionnaires in women: A critical review. *Journal of the American Medical Association, 280*, 166–171.

Brown, S. (2002). Women and addiction: Expanding theoretical points of view. In S. L. A. Straussner & S. Brown (Eds.), *The handbook of addiction treatment for women: Theory and practice* (pp. 26–50). San Francisco: Jossey-Bass.

Byington, D. B. (1997). Applying relational theory to addiction treatment. In S. L. A. Straussner & E. Zelvin (Eds.), *Gender and addictions: Men and women in treatment* (pp. 31–46). Northvale, NJ: Aronson.

Chacin, S. (1996). Women's marijuana problems: An overview with implications for outreach, intervention, treatment, and research. In B. L. Underhill & D. G. Finnegan (Eds.), *Chemical dependency: Women at risk* (pp. 129–167). New York: Haworth Press.

Chasnoff, I. J. (1989). Drug use and women: Establishing a standard of care. *Annals of the New York Academy of Sciences, 562,* 208–210.

Chatham, L. R., Hiller, M. L., Rowan-Szal, G., Joe, G. W., & Simpson, D. D. (1999). Gender differences at admission and follow-up in a sample of methadone maintenance clients. *Substance Use and Misuse, 34*(8), 1137–1165.

Copeland, J., & Hall, W. (1992). Comparison of women seeking drug and alcohol treatment in a specialist women's program and two traditional mixed-sex treatment services. *British Journal of Addiction, 87*(9), 1293–1302.

Covington, S. S. (2002). Helping women recover: Creating gender-responsive treatment. In S. L. A. Straussner & S. Brown (Eds.), *The handbook of addiction treatment for women: Theory and practice* (pp. 52–72). San Francisco: Jossey-Bass.

Cyr, M. G., & Moulton, A. W. (1993). The physician's role in prevention, detection and treatment of alcohol abuse in women. *Psychiatric Annals, 23*(8), 454–462.

Drabble, L. (1996). Elements of effective services for women in recovery: Implications for clinicians and program supervisors. In B. L. Underhill & D. G. Finnegan (Eds.), *Chemical dependency: Women at risk* (pp. 1–21). New York: Haworth Press.

Drug Strategies. (1998). *Keeping score 1998.* Retrieved May 19, 1999, from www.drugstrategies.org/ks1998/health.html

Female crime victims with stress disorder more likely to abuse drugs. (1992). *NIDA Notes, 7*(5), 12–13.

Friedman, E. G. (1997). The impact of AIDS on the lives of women. In S. L. A. Straussner & E. Zelvin (Eds.), *Gender and addictions: Men and women in treatment* (pp. 197–222). Northvale, NJ: Aronson.

Gomberg, E. S. L. (1980). Risk factors related to alcohol problems among women: Proneness and vulnerability. In *Alcoholism and alcohol abuse among women: Research issues.* Washington, DC: U.S. Government Printing Office.

Illinois Advisory Council on Alcoholism and Other Drug Dependency (1995). *Illinois commitment to restoring healthy families: A strategy for effective alcohol and other drug services for women.* Springfield: State of Illinois Department of Alcoholism and Substance Abuse.

Kendler, K. S., Neale, M. C., Heath, A. C., Kessler, R. C., & Eaves, L. J. (1994). A Twin-family study of alcoholism in women. *American Journal of Psychiatry, 151*(5), 707–715.

Levine, H. (1989). Feminist counseling: A woman-centered approach. In V. Carver & C. Ponee (Eds.), *Women, work, and wellness* (pp. 230–231). Toronto: Alcoholism and Drug Addiction Research Foundation.

Lewis, J. A. (1995). Strategies that work for women substance-abuse clients. In C. L. Mejta, J. A. Lewis, & J. A. Engle (Eds.), *Training the gender-competent substance abuse counselor* (pp. 3.27–3.28). Springfield: Illinois Department of Alcoholism and Substance Abuse.

Lieber, C. S. (1993). Women and alcohol: Gender differences in metabolism and susceptibility. In E. S. L. Gomberg & T. D. Nuremberg (Eds.), *Women and substance abuse* (pp. 1–17). Norwood, NJ: Ablex.

Mathias, R. (1995). NIDA survey provides first national data on drug use during
pregnancy. *NIDA Notes, 10*(1), 6.

Mejta, C. L., Lewis, J. A., & Engle, J. (1995). *Training the gender-competent substance abuse counselor.* Springfield: Illinois Department of Alcoholism and Substance Abuse.

Miller, B. A. (1998). Partner violence experiences and women's drug use: Exploring
the connections. In C. L. Wetherington & A. B. Roman (Eds.), *Drug addiction
research and the health of women* (pp. 407–416). Rockville, MD: National Institute on Drug Abuse.

Miller, J. B. (1986). *Toward a new psychology of women* (2nd ed.). Boston: Beacon
Press.

Miller, W. R. (1983). Motivational interviewing with problem drinkers. *Behavioral
Psychotherapy, 11,* 147–172.

Moulton, C., & Moulton, O. (1984). Biological effects of marijuana. *Drug Abuse
Newsletter, 6.*

Nakken, J. (2002). Addiction and women in the workplace. In S. L. A. Straussner &
S. Brown (Eds). *The handbook of addiction treatment for women: Theory and
practice* (pp. 377–398). San Francisco: Jossey-Bass.

National Center on Addiction and Substance Abuse. (1996). *Substance abuse and the
American woman.* New York: Author.

National Institute on Alcohol Abuse and Alcoholism (NIAAA). (1999). *Alcohol
alert* (No. 46). Rockville, MD: U.S. Department of Health and Human Services.

National Institute on Drug Abuse (NIDA). (1992). *National pregnancy and health
survey-drug use among women delivering livebirths: 1992.* Rockville, MD: National Clearinghouse for Alcohol and Drug Information.

O'Connor, L., Esherick, M., & Vieten, C. (2002). Drug- and alcohol-abusing women.
In S. L. A. Straussner & S. Brown (Eds.), *The handbook of addiction treatment
for women: Theory and practice* (pp. 73–98). San Francisco: Jossey-Bass.

Pape, P. A. (1986). Women and alcohol: The disgraceful discrepancy. *EAP Digest,
6*(6), 49–53.

Pape, P. A. (1988). Superwoman and alcohol: The unrecognized link. *EAP Digest,
8*(3), 25–30.

Pape, P. A. (1997). Shedding light on domestic violence. *Chicago Life, 1*(2), 3.

Pape, P. A. (1999). Women, EAPs, and substance abuse treatment: A decade in review.
EAPA Exchange, 29(15), 18–19.

Powis, B., Griffiths, P., Gossop, M., & Strang, J. (1996). The differences between
male and female drug users: Community samples of heroin and cocaine users
compared. *Substance Use and Misuse, 31*(5), 529–543.

Reed, B. G. (1994). Women and alcohol, tobacco, and other drugs: The need to
broaden the base within EAPs. In M. Lundy & B. Younger (Eds.), *Empowering
women in the workplace: Perspective, innovations, and techniques for helping
professionals* (pp. 179–201). New York: Haworth Press.

Roberts, B. (1999, August 6). The invisible addict: Women and chemical dependency.

Paper presented at the International Doctors in Alcoholics Anonymous (IDAA), Tucson, AZ.

Rosenbaum, M., & Murphy, S. (1990). Opiates. In R. C. Engs (Ed.), *Women: Alcohol and other drugs* (pp. 111–117). Dubuque, IA: Kendall/Hunt.

Sandmaier, M. (1992). *The invisible alcoholics: Women and alcohol* (2nd ed.). Blue Ridge Summitt, PA: Human Services Institute and TAB Books.

Straussner, S. L. A. (1985). Alcoholism in women: Current knowledge and implications for treatment. In D. Cook, S. L. A. Straussner, & C. Fewell (Eds.), *Psychosocial issues in the treatment of alcoholism* (p. 65). New York: Haworth Press.

Straussner, S. L. A. (1997). Gender and substance abuse. In S. L. A. Straussner & E. Zelvin (Eds.), *Gender and addictions: Men and women in treatment* (pp. 3–27). Northvale, NJ: Aronson.

Substance Abuse and Mental Health Services Administration (SAMHSA). (1997). *New national study on substance use among women in the United States Released*. Retrieved July 24, 2001, from www.hhs.gov/news/press/1997pres/970922.html

Surrey, J. (1985). *Self-in-relation: A theory of women's development* (Work in Progress, No. 13). Stone Center, Wellesley College, Wellesley, MA.

van Wormer, K. (2002). Addictions and women in the criminal justice system. In S. L. A. Straussner & S. Brown (Eds.), *The handbook of addiction treatment for women: Theory and practice* (pp. 470–486). San Francisco: Jossey-Bass.

Wilsnack, S. C. (1990). Alcohol abuse and alcoholism: Extent of the problem. In R. C. Engs (Ed.), *Women: Alcohol and other drugs* (pp. 17–30). Washington, DC: Alcohol and Drug Problems Association.

Wilsnack, S. C., Vogeltanz, N. D., & Klassen, A. D. (1997). Childhood sexual abuse and women's substance abuse: National survey findings. *Journal of Studies on Alcohol, 58*(3), 264–271.

CHAPTER 17

Substance Abusers with Borderline Disorders

Eda G. Goldstein

As a result of increasing interest in the differential assessment and treatment of individuals who present with a dual diagnosis (Attia, 1988; Blume, 1989; Brown, Ridgely, Pepper, Levine, & Ryglewicz, 1989; Evans & Sullivan, 2000; Mulinski, 1989; Osher & Kofoed, 1989), attention has turned to a particularly challenging group of clients who show both borderline disorders and chemical dependency. Although studies of the comorbidity of borderline personality disorder and substance abuse reveal variable rates, from a low of 11% to a high of 87%, numerous studies found that it was over 55% (Dulit, Fyer, Haas, Suillivan, & Frances, 1990; Hatzitaskos, Soldatos, Kokkevi, & Stefanis, 1999; Kiesler, Simpkins, & Morton, 1991; Morgenstern, Langenbucher, Labouvie, & Miller, 1997).

There are different explanations for these findings on the high comorbidity of these two disorders, including the views that individuals with borderline disorders are vulnerable to abusing alcohol and drugs because of their developmental deficits; that chemical dependency produces borderline symptomatology; and that both substance abuse and borderline personality disorder are caused by similar developmental factors and circumstances. Although in some instances, chemical dependency may result in what appears to be borderline traits, it is more likely that a substantial number of substance abusers also is borderline (Dirksen & Hendriks, 1991).

Because it usually is more difficult to treat substance abusers who have borderline disorders than those who do not, it is important for those working in the field of chemical dependency to be knowledgeable about the special treatment needs of patients who present with both conditions. After describing the main characteristics, causes, and treatment of borderline disorders generally, this chapter considers the main issues that arise when working with substance abusers who also have a borderline disturbance, and discusses major treatment foci and techniques with this group of patients.

CHARACTERISTICS OF BORDERLINE PERSONALITY DISORDERS

The fourth edition of the *Diagnostic and Statistical Manual of Mental Disorders* (DSM-IV; American Psychiatric Association, 1994) classifies borderline conditions on Axis II as a type of personality disorder if at least five of the following eight characteristics are present: (1) a pattern of unstable and intense interpersonal relationships characterized by extremes of idealization and devaluation; (2) impulsiveness in at least two areas that are potentially self-damaging (e.g., spending, sex, substance use, shoplifting, reckless driving, binge eating); (3) affective instability—that is, marked shifts from baseline mood to depression, irritability, or anxiety, usually lasting a few hours and only rarely more than a few days; (4) inappropriate intense anger or lack of control of anger (e.g., frequent displays of temper, constant anger, recurrent physical fights); (5) recurrent suicidal threats, gestures, or behavior, or self-mutilating behavior; (6) marked and persistent identity disturbance manifested by uncertainty about at least two of the following: self-image, sexual orientation, long-term goals or career choice, type of friends desired, preferred values; (7) chronic feelings of emptiness or boredom; and (8) frantic efforts to avoid real or imagined abandonment.

In addition to DSM-IV's atheoretical approach to the borderline diagnosis, a review of the voluminous literature on borderline disorders from a psychodynamic developmental perspective shows that the following 13 major characteristics are common among individuals with borderline disorders (Goldstein, 1990).

Identity Disturbances

Individuals with borderline disorders are confusing and unpredictable patients. They tend to portray themselves either as "all good" or "all bad," making it difficult to get a three-dimensional sense of who they are. They may repeatedly use others to buttress their frail sense of identity. Abrupt and radical shifts in feelings, attitudes, and behavior may occur within hours, days, or weeks, seemingly without reason.

Splitting and Related Defenses

Splitting, the main defense of individuals with borderline disorders, segregates two conscious, contradictory feeling states, such as love and anger or admiration and disappointment, so that a friend, family member, or therapist, for example, who is viewed as all good suddenly may be seen as all bad. Selected personality traits become associated with goodness or badness, for example, an individual may view assertiveness negatively and compliance favorably, or may acknowledge his or her submissiveness and cooperativeness while denying the existence of independent or rebellious thoughts, feelings, or behavior.

Other related borderline defenses are (1) *denial*, in which there is an inability to acknowledge selected aspects of the self or of others that conflict with the individual's image of self or other; (2) *idealization*, in which there is a tendency to see self or others as totally good in order to ward off frightening impulses; (3) *devaluation*, in which there is a penchant to see self or others as all bad; (4) *omnipotent control*, in which a person with a highly inflated sense of self attempts to control others totally; and (5) *projective identification*, in which a person continues to have an impulse, generally an angry one, which, at the same time, is projected onto another person, who then is feared as an enemy who must be controlled.

Problems in Impulse Control

Individuals with borderline disorders generally are impulsive in one or more areas of their lives. Their impulsiveness may be chronic and seemingly without environmental triggers, or episodic in response to internal or external events, such as blows to self-esteem, loss, or the threat of abandonment. In addition to substance abuse, such impulsiveness often shows itself in eating disorders, self-mutilation, at-risk sexual behavior, manipulative suicidal threats and acts, financial mismanagement or gambling, physical abuse, and violence.

Problems in Anxiety Tolerance

Many individuals with borderline disorders are anxious most of the time or they have recurrent, disabling bouts of diffuse anxiety. They may experience dread when they awaken in the morning or sometimes in the middle of the night; they become disorganized or overwhelmed by increases in stress; they may experience panic reactions intermittently in response to life events, especially separations.

Problems in Affect Regulation

Individuals with borderline disorders often escalate rapidly in their feelings; thus, for example, irritation becomes rage, sadness becomes despair, loneliness becomes aloneness, and disappointment becomes hopelessness. They become overwhelmed by either positive or negative feelings that are too intense. Seemingly happy at one moment, they plunge into a painful depression the next or show intense and inappropriate anger, temper tantrums, or affect storms. When these displays are coupled with impulsiveness, people with borderline disorders can become frightening in their physical violence or self-destructive behavior.

Negative Affects

Often complaining of chronic depression, many people with borderline disorders show persistent feelings of anger, resentment, dissatisfaction, and envy. Sometimes they experience inner emptiness and feel bereft of positive or meaningful connections to others or even to themselves.

Problems in Self-Soothing

Individuals with borderline disorders lack the capacity for self-soothing. They are at the mercy of any upsurge of uncomfortable feelings and have "no money in the bank" to draw upon in moments of stress. They become overwhelmed by feelings of panic, rage, and aloneness. Even minor separations such as leaving a therapy session can generate panic that prompts the client to engage in desperate efforts to maintain the contact. Some individuals immerse themselves in activities of all sorts or engage in addictive or other types of self-destructive behavior in order to escape from their feelings.

Abandonment Fears

Individuals with borderline disorders commonly show fears of abandonment. Some attempt to merge with others in efforts to deny or ward off their aloneness and to reassure themselves that they will never be abandoned. They seek constant proximity to, or contact with, those upon whom they are dependent and want to know their exact whereabouts or minute details of their activities. At the same time, most individuals with borderline disorders have a need–fear dilemma that makes them ward off or withdraw from the positive experiences with others for which they long; their profound ambivalence creates an oscillating cycle of clinging and distancing behavior. When they are not feeling intense loneliness, many individuals with borderline disorders manage their abandonment fears by regulating interpersonal closeness; that is, they engage in many superficial relationships, which allows them to avoid intimacy.

Problems in Self-Esteem Regulation

Individuals with borderline disorders are extremely dependent upon others and upon external sources of approval. Consequently, their self-regard is highly vulnerable and may undergo radical swings depending on the nature of the feedback they receive from others or the degree to which they live up to their own perfectionistic standards. Some individuals show either highly grandiose or devalued conceptions of their abilities and talents and tend to feel either very entitled to special treatment or unworthy of help; sometimes they fluctuate between these extremes. Even seemingly minor disappointments or comments can lead to rage reactions, feelings of worthlessness, shame, humiliation, and fits of self-loathing.

Superego Difficulties

Although some individuals with borderline disorders show an absence of guilt and empathy in their dealings with others and are even capable of ruthless and exploitative acts, many experience remorse, self-contempt, and self-recriminations after they mistreat others. Nevertheless, they find themselves unable to stop the very behavior that they hate.

Intense and Unstable Interpersonal Relationships

Intimacy is a problem because persons with borderline disorders tend to merge with others or regulate closeness so that it is not threatening. Moodiness, possessiveness, insecurity, highly charged interactions, and a sense of victimization by others are common. Fights, accusations, and sudden breaks frequently occur and are usually related to feelings of being rejected or abandoned. Separations are difficult, however, and cause anxiety and severe depression that may lead to desperate and often seemingly manipulative and attention-getting behavior, such as suicidal threats and attempts or other types of acting out.

Reality Testing and Psychotic-Like Features

Individuals with borderline disorders show distorted perceptions of reality that usually are not, however, bizarre; furthermore, their capacity for reality testing is maintained. For example, they may seem convinced that they are psychic, dying of an incurable illness, or being punished for their success, but they become more realistic when more reality-based explanations for their perceptions are presented. Showing problems in their sense of reality, as evidenced by feelings of depersonalization and derealization, people with borderline disorders may experience themselves as outside of their bodies or may feel as if they are walking on a strange planet. Distortions of body image, such as feeling too fat when they are, in fact, slender, are common.

Problems in Self-Cohesion

Some individuals with borderline disorders are vulnerable to psychotic decompensation under stress. They have a profound lack of self-cohesion that leaves them susceptible to transient periods of fragmentation that can be quite disturbing. When in equilibrium, these individuals can maintain a sense of self-cohesion by regulating the degree of intimacy in their relationships. In this manner, they avoid the loss of ego boundaries involved in close interpersonal connections.

CAUSES OF BORDERLINE PERSONALITY DISORDER

There are different perspectives on the causes of borderline disorders: developmental, family systems, biological, and trauma based.

Developmental Failures

Most psychodynamically oriented theorists and clinicians view borderline disorders as stemming from faulty development. A controversy exists regarding whether borderline pathology reflects a type of intrapsychic defensive structure that arises to ward off conflict and that must be modified, usually through a highly confrontative, interpretive, and limit-setting treatment approach (Kernberg, 1975, 1984; Masterson, 1972, 1976; Masterson & Rinsley, 1975); or alternatively, whether it reflects developmental failures that result in deficits or underdeveloped elements in the personality and that require treatment that builds, strengthens, and consolidates internal structure (Adler, 1985; Blanck & Blanck, 1974, 1979; Buie & Adler, 1982; Kohut, 1971, 1977, 1984). Neither the conflict or deficit model, however, sufficiently takes into account the mounting evidence documenting the traumas of sexual abuse and violence in the histories of female individuals with borderline disorders (Herman, Perry, & van der Kolk, 1989; Kroll, 1988; Wheeler & Walton, 1987).

Family Systems Pathology

Family-oriented theorists view the family of origin and current interpersonal interactions as generating and sometimes perpetuating borderline pathology. Borderline characteristics in the family system include primitive defenses such as splitting, denial, idealization, and projective identification; conflicts around autonomy and dependence; enmeshment and overinvolvement; and neglect and rejection (Goldstein, 1981a; Grinker, Werble, & Drye, 1968; Gunderson, Kerr, & Englund, 1980; Shapiro, Shapiro, Zinner, & Berkowitz, 1977; Walsh, 1977). Couple dynamics show collusion, distortion, and vicious cycles of mutual frustration (Schwartzman, 1984; Slipp, 1988; Solomon, 1985; Stewart, Peters, Marsh, & Peters, 1975).

Biological Factors

Some researchers believe that borderline disorders reflect an underlying affective or mood disorder (Akiskal, 1981; Klein, 1977). The evidence for viewing borderline pathology as a form of affective disorder treatable with antidepressants is not conclusive, although it seems clear that some individuals with borderline disorders also may present with depression and may benefit from medication (Kroll, 1988).

Impact of Trauma

Another important contribution to our understanding of individuals who present with borderline features stems from the recognition that dissociated experiences of childhood trauma, usually related to sexual abuse, are at the root of an unusually high percentage of those individuals who are diagnosed as borderline. Some patients argue that they have been misdiagnosed and really are trauma survivors suffering from a complex variety of posttraumatic stress disorder (Corwin, 1996; Gunderson & Chu, 1993; Herman, 1992; Herman et al., 1989; Kroll, 1993).

ASSESSING SUBSTANCE ABUSERS WITH BORDERLINE DISORDERS

Because substance abuse can either mask or intensify many traits that are characteristic of individuals with borderline disorders, the question of whether a "true" borderline disorder exists requires a careful assessment. It is more useful to think of borderline disorders and substance abuse as coexisting in some individuals rather than to try to establish whether one disorder is primary and one is secondary or whether one is causing the other.

Evans and Sullivan (2000) suggest several guidelines for determining, generally, that a substance abuse is accompanied by a psychiatric disorder: (1) when the maladaptive traits or symptoms existed prior to the substance use; (2) when the traits and symptoms are qualitatively different from those usually encountered among most substance abusers; (3) when the individual continues to show difficulties after a period of abstinence (e.g., 4 weeks); (4) when there is a positive family history for mental disorder; (5) when there is a history of multiple treatment failures; and (6) when there is improvement on nonaddictive neuroleptic medications. Unfortunately, in assessing substance abusers with borderline disorders, these decision-making rules are less certain than with other types of psychiatric disorders. Because borderline defenses distort patients' inner experience and perceptions of others and the world, it is difficult to get an accurate history from these individuals. Likewise, because of their identity problems and shifting states, it is hard to get a sense of who the individual really is.

Substance use usually begins very early in individuals with borderline disorders: during, and sometimes even before, adolescence. In some instances the substance use intensifies anxiety, depression, and self-destructive and violent behavior, whereas in other cases, it quells the uncomfortable feelings. Thus, diagnosing such individuals during abstinence or inpatient treatment can be misleading because they appear better when they are in structured settings or are not stressed by life demands, separations, interpersonal closeness, and so forth. Because their chronic storms generally are episodic in nature, and they may show good control in between such episodes, it may take some time before their characteristic difficulties are observed. By this time, they may be discharged and lost to follow-up, unfortunately, because their deeply entrenched ego and self deficits leave them vulnerable to slips and ongoing problems in maintaining abstinence.

It is not clear that substance abusers who have borderline disorders are distinctive from other substance abusers with respect to their family histories. Although many come from overtly dysfunctional families in which there was (and may still be) physical and sexual abuse and substance abuse, others come from families in which there are more subtle, though nevertheless malignant, difficulties.

The best assessment tools are an accurate history of the person's development, personality functioning, and symptoms and systematic observation over time. It usually is necessary to obtain information from multiple sources and to focus particularly on how clients cope during periods in which they are not using drugs as well as on the triggers for, and patterns of, drug use.

THE NEED FOR AN INTEGRATED
TREATMENT APPROACH

Substance abusers with borderline disorders find it difficult to maintain a stable sobriety; or, if they do stay sober, they are likely to resort to other types of dysfunctional behavior. They constitute a large number of those who are designated as treatment failures or who drop out of, or are asked to leave, such services because of their seeming "noncompliance." Despite the success of 12-step programs with many people who have borderline disorders, some have trouble adhering to such programs. Mental health practitioners, often biased toward seeing substance abuse as a form of self-medication for underlying personality difficulties, have tended to neglect treating the substance abuse directly when they see individuals with borderline disorders in psychotherapy. Likewise, programs that do aim at ameliorating the substance abuse often ignore these individuals' personality problems—problems that significantly affect their recovery. Staff in substance abuse facilities are usually focused on the chemical dependence itself and typically lack knowledge about the nature of borderline pathology and the special treatment needs of those who present with this disorder.

Even those individuals with borderline disorders who are engaged in treatment that is specifically geared to their needs have difficulties in developing and maintaining a therapeutic alliance; indeed, they show a stormy treatment course. They arouse strong emotions in therapeutic personnel and challenge usual notions about what is supposed to occur in treatment. They present frequent crises, miss appointments, break off treatment abruptly, mutilate themselves or engage in other destructive behavior, threaten suicide and make actual suicide attempts, do not comply with agency or therapeutic requirements, and request personal information, additional time, or extratherapeutic contact. Consequently, it is common for therapists to feel insecure and as if they were "walking a tightrope" in the treatment.

Staff difficulties in treatment collaboration are frequent in work with substance abusers who have borderline disorders. These difficulties are particularly evident in inpatient and residential settings. In settings that house substance abusers who reflect a range of other psychiatric disorders, including units for patients with dual diagnosis, patients with borderline disorders often are at the center of discord because of their need for, and ability to elicit, special treatment or to provoke conflict. Disputes among staff typically center on how to work with a particular client, who is likely to be viewed by some staff members as dependent and fragile and in need of empathy or special treatment, and by others as hostile and belligerent and requiring firm limits and structure.

Family relationships of individuals with borderline disorders also present problems. Couple interactions are turbulent and conflicted. Parent–child relationships generally are characterized either by rejection or enmeshment.

In working with substance abusers who have borderline disorders, an integrated approach is necessary (Minkoff, 1989). It is generally advisable to treat both the underlying personality disorder and the substance abuse, because it is potentially just as futile to assume that substance abuse will cease with psychotherapy alone as to believe that abstinence will suffice or even be possible in the presence of such profound ego and self deficits. There are differences of opinion, however, as to how to accomplish this complex task. Furthermore, to achieve such an approach the usual dichotomy between the mental health and substance abuse treatment models needs to be bridged (Mulinski, 1989; Ridgely, Goldman, & Willenbring, 1990; Wallen & Weiner, 1989). It is important for clinicians to draw on diverse theoretical formulations and models and to individualize the treatment.

Individual Psychodynamic Psychotherapy

Long-term individual psychodynamically oriented psychotherapy that is based on drive, ego, object relations, and self psychological thinking is an important modality in the treatment of individuals with borderline disorders. Specific approaches differ, however, in whether they emphasize confrontation, interpretation, limit setting, and structure versus empathic understanding and responsiveness, ego building, and corrective experiences (Goldstein, 1990).

In working with patients who have borderline disorders and are also substance abusers, individual psychotherapy should be utilized even in the earliest stages. A crucial focus of the first phase of the treatment is to help these patients develop better ways of dealing with their pressing needs and impulses so that sobriety can be attained and maintained. In later stages of the treatment, more reparative work can be done.

Establishing a Therapeutic Holding Environment

Because individuals with borderline disorders generally are chaotic and impulsive and prone to radical shifts in their feelings, the establishment of a therapeutic environment that helps them to feel safe and to contain their impulses is essential in the beginning stage of treatment. Stability, consistency, clarity about expectations, and limits are important in achieving these goals; however, the treatment framework should be individualized, flexible, and empathic rather than mechanistic. Clients who are angry, provocative, demanding, impulsive, or disorganized can benefit from strict rules to help them maintain control of their behavior, whereas those who are anxious, fearful, depressed, dependent, and volatile may need more access to the therapist or other staff and a more flexible approach. Because lack of object constancy and absence of self-soothing capacity propel these patients into impulsiveness and panic, therapists need to find ways of helping them maintain positive connections with them and managing their intense feeling states between sessions. Some authors (Wells & Glickauf-

Hughes, 1986) have suggested using transitional objects, such as items from the therapist's office that are associated with the therapist, journal keeping, and visualization to achieve these purposes.

Whether or not to expect total abstinence as an immediate goal with patients who have borderline disorders is a controversial question. The answer is clearer when the substance abuse is out of control and having obvious and immediately destructive consequences for the individual or others. In these instances, steps must be taken to enable the client to become free of alcohol or drugs. Although such abstinence may be possible to achieve on an outpatient basis in some instances, in most situations an inpatient phase of treatment is necessary. When the substance abuse is erratic, even though severe, and the client shows more denial, the therapist's timing in placing expectations for sobriety on the client and the use of a stepwise therapeutic process are important in the treatment. The therapist may need to wait until the therapeutic alliance is stronger and he or she has more leverage with the client before making abstinence a clear condition of the treatment.

Waiting does not imply inactivity or that the therapist ignores the client's substance abuse. It is advisable (1) to let the client know that abstinence is a goal; (2) to keep the negative consequences of substance abuse in the forefront of the treatment; (3) to identify the defenses that protect the abuse; (4) to identify the underlying problems in self-soothing, abandonment fears, and so forth, that give rise to the abuse; (5) to acknowledge and explore the gratification obtained from the abuse; (6) to explore fears of, and resistance to, abstinence; and (7) to problem-solve with the client about the ways of controlling the abuse. The therapist must be vigilant about his or her own fears of raising these issues with the client or the erroneous belief that eventually the client will gain control of his or her substance abuse as a matter of course. Unfortunately, therapists can unwittingly become "enablers" too (Levinson & Straussner, 1978). Usually it is necessary to pressure the client to take decisive action at some point, but it may take a long time before this tactic can be effective (Chernus, 1985).

Setting Limits and Creating Structure

Unfortunately, patients' fears of abandonment, problems with closeness, absence of self-soothing mechanisms, and panic and rage reactions—which make them feel more alone and alienated—do not easily permit them to experience being "held" by a worker's consistency, accessibility, empathy, or limits. The client's actual life circumstances also may present stresses that stimulate impulsiveness and that overshadow the therapeutic holding environment, especially at the beginning of treatment. Some individuals may require active and protective interventions, such as the use of hospitalization, day treatment, 12-step programs, or other types of external structure. To the degree that limits and structure are needed, it is important for the therapist to engage these clients in a collaborative problem-solving effort to identify what factors, conditions, or resources will enable them to contain their impulses and self-destructive behavior. Although the use of contracts that spell out consequences is helpful, the therapist working with individuals who have borderline disorders needs to recognize their vulnerability to slips and crises. There should be sufficient flexibility in the treatment structure to help clients through these crises without their being discharged or terminated from treatment.

Confronting versus Empathizing

Some authors have stressed the usefulness of confronting the defenses of patients with borderline pathology (Kernberg, 1975, 1984), and in work with substance abusers generally (Chernus, 1985; Fewell & Bissell, 1978; Wallace, 1978). In contrast, others have emphasized a more empathic approach (Brandchaft & Stolorow, 1984; Levin, 1987). Clinicians in the latter group argue that too great an emphasis on pointing out and controlling maladaptive defenses and behaviors may escalate rather than diffuse aggressive outbursts or other forms of self-destructive behavior, because clients are likely to feel attacked. Those who work with these individuals with these individuals need to see beyond their often angry, provocative, grandiose, and seemingly manipulative behavior to their underlying anxiety, desperation, diminished self-esteem, fears of abandonment, feelings of being unlovable, and hopelessness. A nonjudgmental attitude is essential.

It may be necessary to address self-defeating behavior, but it is generally preferable to do so in ways that show an understanding of these patients' inner states and difficulties in soothing themselves. Empathically relating to the urgent needs that clients experience, exploring their origins in clients' early life, and pointing out negative consequences of behavior that the individuals may have learned in order to survive early neglect, abuse, or other kinds of trauma—all are nonthreatening paths toward addressing self-defeating behaviors. The therapist should employ "experience-near-empathy" (Kohut, 1984; Wolf, 1988) in which he or she tries to feel what it is like to "walk" in the client's "shoes." For example, the therapist might say that the client's need to get immediate relief from his or her emotional pain through the use of a chemical is understandable, particularly since no one in the client's early life ever responded to his or her feelings or offered needed protection. This effort to understand subjective experience is calming and soothing to a disturbed client.

Ego Building

Most of us take for granted certain capacities that individuals with borderline disorders often lack, such as the ability to recognize and verbalize feelings, soothe ourselves, maintain positive connections when alone or frustrated, and empathize with others' motivations and feelings. Deficits in these areas impair individuals' ability to cope effectively; treatment must attempt to help these clients restore, develop, or strengthen their adaptive coping mechanisms or restructure the environment to be more responsive to their particular personality needs and weaknesses (Blanck & Blanck, 1974, 1979; Goldstein, 1995; Weick, Rapp, Sullivan, & Kisthardt, 1989). Although such an approach may initially focus on here-and-now issues and must consider clients' ability to tolerate exploration of their feelings and past traumas, it is inadvisable to attempt to help clients manage their emotional states only through cognitive or behavioral means, or to consistently divert the focus of treatment away from their feelings. Helping substance abusers with borderline disorders get in touch with what is disturbing to them, track the relation between their feelings and their use of substances, and get validation for their needs can have soothing and ego-strengthening effects.

The Therapist's Use of Self

The traditional psychoanalytic view that therapists should remain neutral and frustrating of patients' needs should be reexamined when working with substance abusers who have borderline disorders (Goldstein, 1994). Because these clients are so profoundly arrested in development, this stance may reexpose them to the neglect they experienced early in life. At times, therapists may need to be more real and to selectively meet the client's needs rather than to interpret the client's efforts to get his or her needs met as manipulations. This does not mean that the therapist should always gratify the client's requests, because doing so may (1) put the therapist in the position of enabling, (2) stimulate regressive behavior, or (3) eventually lead to therapist burnout or anger and withdrawal. What is important is providing a type of "optimal responsiveness" (Bacal, 1985) based on what is likely to help the client to function more adaptively. For example, the therapist may indicate his or her availability to clients for brief telephone calls between sessions, clearly specifying when these may occur.

Working with Trauma

Most skilled clinicians are more cautious and recognize that trauma-based treatment is no less complicated or time consuming than other long-term approaches. In addition to the more usual borderline symptomatology that clients who have a trauma history typically present, they are (1) highly distrustful of relationships, (2) use defenses and engage in behaviors that protect their traumatic memories and that have helped them to survive, (3) often cannot tolerate confrontative techniques, (4) tend to become involved in situations in which they experience repeated revictimization, and (5) are not readily able to do the work of the treatment because of their sense of interpersonal threat and their variable ego functioning, which may make it hard for them to tolerate the working through of their traumatic experiences. Some overzealous practitioners have pressed these clients to deal with early trauma, only to find that this approach has a disorganizing effect. Considerable attention must be given to (1) the creation of a holding environment for these clients, (2) validation of their survival skills, helping them avoid situations in which they are revictimized, and (3) the sensitive timing of interventions that can engage clients in the trauma recovery work.

Managing Countertransference

There is general consensus that therapists are especially vulnerable to problematic reactions that can obstruct their work with individuals who have borderline disorders because of the impact of these clients' urgent needs, aggressive behavior, and primitive defenses. There has been a tendency to say that these clients "induce" particular responses in those around them in order to rid themselves of uncomfortable feelings. There is a risk in assuming that inducement is always the case; such a view, after all, tends to hold the client responsible for what the therapist is feeling. Although a client's provocative and even obnoxious behavior may result in a therapist becoming angry, rejecting, or feeling helpless, it is possible that the therapist contributed to the client's behavior by uttering an insensitive or harsh comment. Or, the therapist may feel particularly defensive because of having a hard day. Even if the client is inducing a reaction in the therapist, it is important to explore the reasons for the client's behavior rather than act on one's feelings.

Cognitive-Behavioral Treatment

More recently, cognitive-behavioral approaches that focus on altering the client's dysfunctional ways of thinking and behavior have increased in popularity in the treatment of clients with borderline disorders (Dungee-Anderson, 1992; Heller & Northcut, 1996; Linehan, 1993). These approaches rely heavily on educative and cognitive restructuring techniques, task assignment, modeling, exercises, and problem solving. For example, Heller and Northcut (1996) describe their use of cognitive-behavioral techniques in working with these clients' pattern of affective–cognitive splitting, problems in affect regulation, and faulty attributions. Likewise, Dungee-Anderson (1992) recommends what she calls a self-nurturing approach that teaches the client "to recognize and differentiate both the underdeveloped reality ego and developmentally arrested child components of the split-ego structure by their affective and behavioral characteristics" (p. 295). The mastery of separateness and independence/autonomy are central to the work, although the tasks involved are unique to each client, based on his or her history and developmental issues. The therapist is a teacher and modeler of more positive skills that the client is helped to practice in exercises.

Linehan (1993), who has the most systematic and well-studied approach (but also strict and confrontative), advocates giving relentless attention to modifying the client's most disruptive target behaviors in order to increase and sustain the client's level of motivation and commitment to treatment. Her first-stage target behaviors involve decreasing suicidal, therapy-interfering, and quality-of-life-interfering behaviors and increasing behavioral skills in the areas of core mindfulness, interpersonal effectiveness, emotional regulation, distress tolerance, and self-management. Her second-stage goals are aimed at reducing posttraumatic stress; and her third-stage goals include increasing respect for self and achieving individual goals.

Although cognitive-behavioral approaches make different assumptions about the origins and nature of borderline pathology and utilize a different set of technical interventions than are characteristic of psychodynamic approaches, there is much to be learned from them about breaking problems down into manageable parts and conceptualizing them in ways that are more accessible to the client's ego. The ability to think, process information, problem-solve, and perform other cognitive skills is an important component of ego functioning. Indeed, it could be argued that a client's self-concept or way of viewing others reflects how he or she has learned to think as well as what he or she has experienced.

It is possible, furthermore, to translate psychodynamic concepts into cognitive-behavioral terms in order to make it easier for these clients to grasp and assimilate. For example, we can help clients think about their defense of splitting by talking about how they view themselves or others in black-and-white/all-or-nothing terms. Their problems with self-soothing can be described as not being able to identify their feelings, talk themselves through certain feelings, or find ways of relieving their feelings. Likewise, a psychodynamically oriented clinician may integrate certain aspect of these cognitive-behavioral approaches, such as the use of cognitive restructuring, educative modeling, and task-oriented and problem-solving interventions, into his or her armamentarium without becoming mechanistic.

The Role of Psychotropic Drugs

Although the common view is that psychotropic drugs do not help substance abusers who have borderline disorders and are generally contraindicated because they tend to be abused, there are some positive indications for the use of medication with clients who show depression, panic states, or disorganized thinking (Zweben & Smith, 1989). A rule of thumb is to give antidepressant drugs, such as SSRIs, for a concurrent mood disorder or panic states and small doses of major tranquilizers for pathology that is close to the psychotic range of symptoms (Berger, 1987; Pack, 1987). Nevertheless, psychotropic drugs always should be used cautiously with these patients. Minor tranquilizers should be avoided because they are addictive. Major tranquilizers can be helpful with some clients in small doses but often have serious side affects. Although SSRIs are used frequently today in treating depression, certain classes of antidepressants, for example, the tricyclics, although effective with those who have mood disorders, are highly lethal when used with other substances or as part of a suicide attempt. Moreover, some sedating antidepressants often are abused. The mood-stabilizing drug lithium is quite toxic when combined with alcohol. Noncompliance with drug regimens as well as abuse are common, because clients with borderline disorders tend to use drugs as a way of acting out their intense feelings. Prescribed medications also have multiple meanings, some helpful, others not, beyond their specific utility. For example, they can be seen as an unwanted intrusion, a transitional object, a sign of caring, a magical substance that instills hope, or an indication that there is no hope (Meissner, 1988).

The Role of Psychiatric Hospitalization

Many patients with borderline disorders are admitted to psychiatric hospitals following suicide attempts or other forms of self-destructive behavior or psychotic episodes. Hospital treatment is usually short term and focuses on resolving the immediate crises leading to the need for hospitalization (Friedman, 1973; Nurnberg & Suh, 1978). For many substance abusers with borderline disorders, a phase of inpatient treatment may be essential for them to begin their recovery process (Chernus, 1985; Evans & Sullivan, 2000). When treatment is short-term, a multifaceted, active approach with partialized goals is necessary. Family must be involved in the treatment from the beginning, not only as part of the problem but as part of the solution. Medication for target symptoms may be utilized as part of a holistic approach. Since these clients typically are admitted to hospitals at times of crisis, when they are extremely agitated, impulsive, or disorganized, the short-term model emphasizes the control function of the setting (Nurnberg & Suh, 1978); disruptive behavior is minimized via the provision of a firm, highly structured, unified, and predictable atmosphere in which clients must meet all rules and expectations. In order to provide "optimal holding," it is equally important for staff to relate empathically to, rather than distance themselves from, a client's sense of panic and dire aloneness.

Important requirements of clinical staff include the ability to (1) refrain from retaliating with anger in response to a client's provocative and attacking behavior, (2) refrain from giving too much, to the point of exhaustion or frustration, and (3) refrain from withholding and withdrawing in the face of a client's overwhelming demands. In order to provide a therapeutic holding environment, staff must understand the treatment philosophy that guides their work and have ample opportunity for open communication, sharing and examination of their work. Furthermore, they must receive support in managing their intense reactions to clients, and help in recognizing and dealing with clients' needs and primitive defenses (e.g., splitting and projective identification). When staff–client interactions seem too "real," countertransference acting out occurs. For example, staff may become polarized and fight about their perceptions and management of a client, resulting in a therapeutic stalemate. Staff–client meetings, rounds, and team meetings that embody an atmosphere of openness and acceptance can provide opportunities for all those involved to share their impressions and to plan individualized treatment strategies.

Education about substance abuse should be provided to staff, and treatment planning should embody the principles that have been discussed so far. Discharge planning is paramount, often requiring creativity, advocacy, systems negotiation skills, and persistence. Clients and families need to be involved in this process; indeed, much of the groundwork can be done by family members. Linkages to community resources, such as AA, vocational training, or outpatient settings, generally should be made prior to the time the client leaves the hospital. Lastly, ample time should be allocated to discuss reactions to the plan and specific services.

Couple and Family Treatment

There are many instances in which therapeutic success with individuals who have borderline disorders necessitates work with the family system (Goldstein, 1983, 1990). In addition to showing interlocking pathology, family members typically experience shame, guilt, low self-esteem, frustration, fatigue, helplessness, and hopelessness that escalate their sometimes angry and demanding behavior. An approach that is sensitive to the family's personal needs and defenses and that respects their need for information and their rights as consumers will lessen their more extreme reactions and lead to a therapeutic alliance (Anderson, Hogarty, & Reiss, 1980; Goldstein, 1981b, 1997). Family members of a client with a borderline disorder require a therapeutic holding environment that helps them to contain their anxiety and to become true collaborators in the treatment process. Preventing power struggles, maintaining accessibility, providing information, and involving family members in decision-making processes—all of these efforts facilitate their engagement. Although many families may require treatment of their own, they may be threatened by such efforts and, without the necessary support, will resist and act out, often undermining the primary client's recovery.

Group Treatment

Arguing that unstructured groups mobilize regression and stimulate volatility and defensiveness in individuals with borderline disorders, most clinicians have cautioned against the use of intensive group therapy with this population (Horowitz, 1980; Kernberg, 1984). Supportive, structured, and task-oriented groups, however, can be used effectively with many of these patients to promote ego functioning and interpersonal relationships. Task-oriented groups can provide opportunities for the exercise of autonomy and the expansion of ego and social functioning.

12-Step Programs

Although many therapists have tended to polarize the philosophies of 12-step programs and psychotherapy, the participation of substance abusers with borderline disorders in such programs generally is a necessary but not sufficient part of their recovery. When treatment is in an inpatient setting, it is easy to mandate attendance at such meetings. When treatment is in an outpatient basis, however, it may take longer to motivate these patients to make the commitment to attending such a program. Furthermore, there are some aspects of 12-step programs that are difficult for many patients with borderline disorders. For example, because they live in the moment, lack trust and a sense of continuity with others, are often out of control, and have trouble dealing with their feeling, AA's and NA's focus on relinquishing control, trusting in a Higher Power, and conducting a moral inventory may stimulate regressive and overwhelming feelings (Evans & Sullivan, 1990). These individuals may need help in translating some of the steps to match where they are at, and in "taking what works for them and leaving the rest." The clinician who works with clients who attend 12-step programs must be knowledgeable about, and comfortable with, these programs, and able to help clients integrate the generally compatible but sometimes conflicting foci of the two approaches (Winegar, Stephens, & Varney, 1987). For example, in early stages of sobriety, clients may get the message from 12-step programs that they are not to dwell on their feelings, and so they then question the therapist's efforts to explore emotionally laden issues. The therapist needs to know when it is supportive of clients to minimize or suppress such exploration in order to promote their sense of control and ability to take action, and when it is necessary to help them to get in touch with, verbalize, and get validation for their feelings so as not to become overwhelmed by them.

CONCLUSION

Borderline pathology is common among those who are chemically depend-ent and both the borderline disorder and the substance abuse need to be addressed in the treatment process. After describing the main characteris-tics and causes of borderline pathology, this chapter discussed the assess-ment of individuals who are thought to have both a borderline disorder and chemical dependency. It then described the elements of an integrated treatment approach that can be applied differentially with this population, according to each client's needs and particular problems. The need for inte-grated and individualized treatment challenges mental health and sub-stance abuse professionals and staff to overcome some of the barriers to integrated service delivery that currently exist and to experiment with cre-ative solutions when working with this vexing population.

REFERENCES

Adler, G. (1985). *Borderline psychopathology and its treatment.* New York: Aronson.

Akiskal, H. S. (1981). Subaffective disorders: dysthymic, cyclothymic and bipolar II disorders in the borderline realm. *Psychiatric Clinics of North America, 4,* 25–46.

American Psychiatric Association. (1994). *Diagnostic and statistical manual of men-tal disorders* (4th ed.). Washington, DC: Author.

Anderson, C., Hogarty, G. E., & Reiss, D. J. (1980). Family treatment of adult schizo-phrenic patients: A psychoeducational approach. *Schizophrenia Bulletin, 6,* 490–505.

Attia, P. R. (1988). Dual diagnosis: Definition and treatment. *Alcoholism Treatment Quarterly, 5,* 53–63.

Bacal, H. A. (1985). Optimal responsiveness and the therapeutic process. In A. Goldberg (Ed.), *Progress in self-psychology* (Vol. 1, pp. 202–227). New York: Guilford Press.

Bentley, K. J., & Walsh, J. F. (2001). *The social worker and psychotropic medication* (2nd ed.). Belmont, CA: Brooks/Cole.

Berger, P. A. (1987). Pharmacological treatment for borderline personality disorder. *Bulletin of the Menninger Clinic, 51,* 277–284.

Blanck, G., & Blanck, R. (1974). *Ego psychology in theory and practice.* New York: Columbia University Press.

Blanck, G., & Blanck, R. (1979). *Ego psychology II: Psychoanalytic developmental psychology.* New York: Columbia University Press.

Blume, S. (1989). Dual diagnosis: Psychoactive substance dependence and the per-sonality disorders. *Journal of Psychoactive Drugs, 21,* 139–144.

Brandchaft, B., & Stolorow, R. D. (1984). The borderline concept: Pathological char-acter or iatrogenic myth. In J. Lichtenberg, M. Bornstein, & D. Silver (Eds.), *Empathy II* (pp. 333–358). Hillsdale, NJ: Analytic Press.

Brown, V., Ridgely, M., Pepper, B., Levine, I., & Ryglewicz, H. (1989). The dual crisis: Mental illness and substance abuse. *American Psychologist, 44,* 565–569.

Buie, D. H., & Adler, G. (1982). The definitive treatment of the borderline personality. *International Journal of Psychoanalytic Psychotherapy, 9,* 51–87.

Chernus, L. A. (1985). Clinical issues in alcoholism treatment. *Social Casework: The Journal of Contemporary Social Work, 66,* 67–75.

Corwin, M. D. (1996). Early intervention strategies with borderline clients. *Families in Society: The Journal of Contemporary Human Services, 77,* 40–49.

Dirksen, J. J. L., & Hendriks, G. A. J. (1991). Psychoactive substance dependence and borderline personality disorder. In G. M. Schippers & S. M. M. Lammers (Eds.), *Contributions to the psychology of addiction* (pp. 139–155). Amsterdam: Swets & Zeitlinger.

Dulit, R. A., Fyer, M. R., Haas, G. L., Suillivan, T., & Frances, A. J. (1990). Substance use in borderline personality disorder. *American Journal of Psychiatry, 147,* 1002–1007.

Dungee-Anderson, D. (1992). Self-nurturing: A cognitive behavioral treatment approach for the borderline client. *Clinical Social Work Journal, 20,* 295–312.

Evans, K., & Sullivan, J. M. (2000). *Dual diagnosis: Counseling the mentally ill substance abuser* (2nd ed.). New York: Guilford Press.

Fewell, C. H., & Bissell, L. (1978). The alcohol-denial syndrome: An alcohol focussed approach. *Social Casework, 59,* 6–13.

Friedman, H. (1973). Some problems of inpatient management with borderline patients. *American Journal of Psychiatry, 126,* 47–52.

Goldstein, E. G. (1981a). The family characteristics of borderline patients. Paper presented at the 58th annual meeting of the American Orthopsychiatric Association, New York.

Goldstein, E. G. (1981b). Promoting competence in families of psychiatric patients. In A. Maluccio (Ed.), *Building competence in clients: A new/old approach to social work intervention* (pp. 317–342). New York: Free Press.

Goldstein, E. G. (1983). Clinical and ecological approaches to the borderline client. *Social Casework: The Journal of Contemporary Social Work, 64,* 353–362.

Goldstein, E. G. (1990). *Borderline disorders: Clinical models and techniques.* New York: Guilford Press.

Goldstein, E. G. (1994). Self-disclosure in treatment: What therapists do and don't talk about. *Clinical Social Work Journal, 22,* 417–433.

Goldstein, E. G. (1995). *Ego psychology and social work practice* (2nd ed.). New York: Free Press.

Goldstein, E. G. (1997). Countertransference reactions to borderline couples. In M. F. Solomon & J. P. Siegel (Eds.), *Countertransference in couples therapy* (pp. 72–86). New York: Norton.

Grinker, R. R., Werble, B., & Drye, R. (1968). *The borderline syndrome.* New York: Basic Books.

Gunderson, J. G., & Chu, J. A. (1993). Treatment implications of past trauma in borderline personality disorder. *Harvard Review of Psychiatry, 1,* 75–81.

Gunderson, J. G., Kerr, J., & Englund, D. W. (1980). The families of borderlines: A comparative study. *Archives of General Psychiatry, 37,* 27–33.

Hatzitaskos, P., Soldatos, C, R., Kokkevi, A., & Stefanis, C. N. (1999). Substance abuse patterns and their association with psychopathology and type of hostility in male patients with borderline and antisocial personality disorder. *Comprehensive Psychiatry, 40,* 278–282.

Heller, N. R., & Northcut, T. B. (1996). Utilizing cognitive-behavioral techniques in psychodynamic practice with clients diagnosed as borderline. *Clinical Social Work Journal, 24,* 203–215.

Herman, J. L. (1992). *Trauma and recovery.* New York: Basic Books.

Herman, J. L., Perry, J. C., & van der Kolk, B. (1989). Childhood trauma in borderline personality disorder. *American Journal of Psychiatry, 146,* 490–495.

Horowitz, L. (1980). Group psychotherapy for borderline and narcissistic patients. *Bulletin of the Menninger Clinic, 44,* 181–200.

Kernberg, O. F. (1975). *Borderline conditions and pathological narcissism.* New York: Aronson.

Kernberg, O. F. (1984). *Severe personality disorders.* New Haven, CT: Yale University Press.

Kiesler, C., Simpkins, C., & Morton, T. (1991). Prevalence of dual diagnosis of mental and substance abuse disorders in general hospitals. *Hospital and Community Psychiatry, 42,* 400–405.

Klein, D. F. (1977). Psychopharmacological treatment and delineation of borderline disorders. In P. Hartocollis (Ed.), *Borderline personality disorders* (pp. 365–384). New York: International Universities Press.

Kohut, H. (1971). *The analysis of the self.* New York: International Universities Press.

Kohut, H. (1977). *The restoration of the self.* New York: International Universities Press.

Kohut, H. (1984). *How does analysis cure?* Chicago: University of Chicago Press.

Kroll, J. (1988). *The challenge of the borderline patient.* New York: Norton.

Kroll, J. (1993). *PTSD/borderlines in therapy.* New York: Norton.

Levin, J. D. (1987). *Treatment of alcoholism and other addictions: A self-psychology approach.* New York: Aronson.

Levinson, V., & Straussner, S. L. A. (1978). Social workers as "enablers" in the treatment of alcoholics. *Social Casework, 59,* 14–20.

Linehan, M. M. (1993). *Cognitive-behavioral treatment of borderline personality disorder.* New York: Guilford Press.

Masterson, J. F. (1972). *Treatment of the borderline adolescent.* New York: Wiley-Interscience.

Masterson, J. F. (1976). *Treatment of the borderline adult.* New York: Brunner/-Mazel.

Masterson, J. F., & Rinsley, D. (1975). The borderline syndrome: The role of the mother in the genesis and psychic structure of the borderline personality. *International Journal of Psychoanalysis, 56,* 163-1-77.

Meissner, W. W. (1988). *Treatment of patients in the borderline spectrum.* Northvale, NJ: Aronson.

Minkoff, K. (1989). An integrated treatment model for dual diagnosis and addiction. *Hospital and Community Psychiatry, 40,* 1031–1036.

Morgenstern, J., Langenbucher, J., Labouvie, E., & Miller, K. J. (1997). *Journal of Abnormal Psychology, 106,* 74–84.

Mulinski, P. (1989). Dual diagnosis in alcoholic clients: Clinical implications. *Social Casework: The Journal of Contemporary Social Work, 70,* 333–339.

Nurnberg, H. G., & Suh, R. (1978). Time-limited treatment of hospitalized border-line patients: Considerations. *Comprehensive Psychiatry, 19,* 419–431.

Osher, F., & Kofoed, L. (1989). Treatment of patients with psychiatric and psychoactive substance abuse disorders. *Hospital and Community Psychiatry, 40,* 1025–1030.

Pack, A. (1987). The role of psychopharmacology in the treatment of borderline patients. In J. S. Grotstein, M. F. Solomon, & J. A. Lang (Eds.), *The borderline patient* (Vol. 2, pp. 177–186). Hillsdale, NJ: Analytic Press.

Ridgeley, M., Goldman, H., & Willenbring, M. (1990). Barriers to the care of persons with dual diagnoses: Organizational and financing issues. *Schizophrenia Bulletin, 16,* 123–132.

Schwartzman, G. (1984). Narcissistic transferences: Implications for the treatment of couples. *Dynamic Psychotherapy, 2,* 5–14.

Shapiro, E. R., Shapiro, R. L., Zinner, J., & Berkowitz, D. (1977). The borderline ego and the working alliance: Implications for family and individual treatment. *International Journal of Psychoanalysis, 58,* 77–87.

Slipp, S. (Ed.). (1988). *The technique and practice of object relations family therapy.* Northvale, NJ: Aronson.

Solomon, M. F. (1985). Treatment of narcissistic and borderline disorders in marital therapy: Suggestions toward an enhanced therapeutic approach. *Clinical Social Work Journal, 13,* 141–156.

Stewart, R. H., Peters, T. C., Marsh, S., & Peters, M. J. (1975). An object relations approach with couples, families, and children. *Family Process, 14,* 161–172.

Wallace, J. (1978). Working with the preferred defense structure of the recovering alcoholic. In S. Zimberg, J. Wallace, & S. B. Blume (Eds.), *Practical approaches to alcoholism therapy* (pp. 19–29). New York: Plenum Press.

Wallen, M., & Weiner, H. (1989). Impediments to effective treatment of the dually diagnosed patient. *Journal of Psychoactive Drugs, 21,* 161–168.

Walsh, F. (1977). Family study 1976: 14 new borderline cases. In R. R. Grinker & B. Werble (Eds.), *The borderline patient* (pp. 158–177). New York: Aronson.

Weick, A., Rapp, C., Sullivan, W. P., & Kisthardt, W. (1989). A strengths perspective for social work practice. *Social Work, 34,* 350–354.

Wells, M., & Glickauf-Hughes, C. (1986). Techniques to develop object constancy with borderline clients. *Psychotherapy, 23,* 460–468.

Wheeler, B. K., & Walton, E. (1987). Personality disturbances of adult incest victims. *Social Casework: The Journal of Contemporary Social Work, 68,* 597–602.

Winegar, N., Stephens, T. A., & Varney, E. D. (1987). Alcoholics Anonymous and the alcoholic defense structure. *Social Casework: The Journal of Contemporary Social Work, 68,* 223–228.

Wolf, E. S. (1988). *Treating the self: Elements of clinical self psychology.* New York: Guilford Press.

Zweben, J., & Smith, D. (1989). Considerations in using psychotropic medication with dual diagnosis patients in recovery. *Journal of Psychoactive Drugs, 21,* 221–228.

CHAPTER 18

Treatment of Gay, Lesbian, and Bisexual Substance Abusers

Evan Senreich
Elena Vairo

A 38-year-old married man who lives with his wife and three children consumes approximately 10 cans of beers a day. He has anonymous sex with other men in a public restroom about twice a week.

A 40-year-old woman in a 20-year monogamous sexual relationship with another woman has recently been fired from her job due to the consequences of her escalating alcohol and cocaine usage.

A 17-year-old male who smokes about five joints of marijuana daily feels confused about his sexual orientation. He has had sex with both males and females and does not know how he feels about these experiences. His peers make fun of him, regularly calling him "fag" and "homo."

A 52-year-old married woman with one teenage child abuses alcohol, Xanax, and Valium. She has homoerotic fantasies but has never had sex with a woman.

A 34-year-old male has a history of prostituting himself with other men in order to support his crack addiction. Before he became substance dependent, he only felt attracted to women. Now he feels confused about his sexual orientation and is experiencing a great deal of shame about having prostituted himself.

It is not clear which of the above individuals identify as gay, lesbian, bisexual, or heterosexual, particularly without an in-depth exploration of each person's subjective view of his or her sexuality. However, each of these five people is in need of substance abuse treatment. Regardless of how these individuals identify themselves, their homosexual behaviors and/or desires must be taken into account during their treatment, because these issues may have a significant impact on the recovery process.

Although categorizing specific sexual acts as homosexual or heterosexual is a straightforward matter, conceptualizing people's sexual orientation as gay, lesbian, or bisexual is much more complex. If substance abuse clinicians are not cognizant of the wide range of homosexual experiences and simplistically label their clients, they will potentially miss a significant number of issues that impact on their clients' recovery. Furthermore, they may push clients into gay-specific treatment modalities that may not best serve them at the time. The purpose of this chapter is to identify and highlight assessment and treatment issues that may arise when homosexuality is a part of a recovering person's life.

IDENTIFYING THE POPULATION

Studies of the prevalence of homosexuality and bisexuality in the United States point to the amorphousness of the concept of sexual orientation. In an often cited 1948 study by Kinsey, Pomeroy, and Martin, although only 4% of male respondents reported they were exclusively homosexual throughout their lives, 37% reported some homosexual experience to the point of orgasm. Kinsey and colleagues also found that women had fewer homosexual experiences in their lives than men, with only 13% of female respondents stating that they had had a homosexual experience resulting in orgasm (Kinsey, Pomeroy, Martin, & Gebhard, 1953).

Although most recent studies indicate that Kinsey's figures were biased and inflated, they still confirm that a polarized "straight" and "gay" view of sexual orientation does not reflect reality. For example, the National Health and Social Life Survey conducted in the early 1990s (Laumann, Gagnon, Michael, & Michaels, 1994) found that 10% of male and 9% of female respondents reported either homosexual behavior, desire, or identity since age 18. However, only 46% of men and 37% of women who had engaged in homosexual behavior, and only 32% of men and 17% of women who currently felt same-sex desire, identified themselves as homosexual, bisexual, gay, or lesbian. Furthermore, these studies indicated that sexual orientation is not a static entity but can change over time. In fact, there is a debate in the field whether a gay or lesbian identity is an actual innate, "essential" human phenomenon, or whether it is a contemporary social construct that came about as a reaction to the intense stigma and oppression of people who engage in homosexual behavior (Broido, 2000; Stein, 1998).

THE SCOPE OF SUBSTANCE ABUSE PROBLEMS AMONG GAY, LESBIAN, AND BISEXUAL INDIVIDUALS

A considerable number of studies over the last three decades have attempted to survey problem drinking and alcoholism among lesbian women and gay men. However, there is a great deal of controversy concerning the results of this research. Based on these studies, the common perception has been that gay men and women are a high-risk group for alcoholism, with a problem drinking rate of about 30% of the homosexual population (Bickelhaupt, 1995; Finnegan & McNally, 1987; van Wormer, Wells, & Boes, 2000; Warn, 1997; Zehner & Lewis, 1984). This rate is three times higher than that of the general population (Alexander, 1997; Cabaj, 1996b). However, many researchers are now disputing this common perception, as more recent studies do not confirm such high rates. Weinberg (1994) refers to the common perception that one-third of gay men are alcohol dependent or abusers as "part of the mythology of gay alcohol studies" (p. 2).

There are serious methodological problems in many of the older surveys. For example, the three earliest studies (Fitfield, 1975; Lohrenz, Connelly, Coyne, & Spare, 1978; Saghir & Robins, 1973), which took place prior to 1980, obtained at least part of their samples in gay bars. One of these (Fitfield, 1975), which is widely cited in the literature, was based on a sample from gay bar patrons and bartenders, as well as a small number of people in recovery from alcohol problems. The comprehensive McKirnan and Peterson (1989) study also chose approximately 5% of its respondents from gay bars. The Morales and Graves Study (1983) included prisoners. Bux (1996), in carefully reviewing much of the literature, came to four conclusions:

1. Gay men and lesbian women are less likely to abstain from alcohol than heterosexuals individuals.
2. Gay men appear to have little increased risk of alcoholism over heterosexual men.
3. Lesbian women appear to be at higher risk than heterosexual women for alcohol abuse, and match both heterosexual and gay men in heavy and problematic drinking.
4. Gay men appear to have reduced their consumption of alcohol prior to the mid-1990s.

Another trend noted by various researchers is that in contrast to the heterosexual population that tends to drink less with increasing age, gay men and lesbian women tend to maintain prior levels of alcohol consumption as they grow older (Bradford, Ryan, & Rothblum, 1994; McKirnan & Peterson, 1989; van Wormer et al., 2000).

Research concerning the use of substances other than alcohol among gay men and lesbian women is even more inconclusive. Studies (Kelly, 1991; McKirnan & Peterson, 1989; Morales & Graves, 1983; Skinner & Otis, 1996) indicate that gay people regularly use a variety of substances at rates higher than the general population. However, it does appear that the patterns of drug use resemble that of alcohol usage. For example, McKirnan and Peterson (1989) found that although the rate at which gay men and women abstained from marijuana and cocaine use was far lower than that of the general population, there was no significant difference in heavy usage of these substances between gay and heterosexual men. Heavy marijuana and cocaine use among lesbian women far exceeded that of heterosexual women, but was similar to that of heterosexual and gay men. Finally, as noted above regarding alcohol consumption, usage of drugs by older gay men and women did not decrease as much as usage among the older heterosexual population.

Certain drugs appear to have particularly high usage in the gay male community. Amyl nitrite and its relatives ("poppers") have been used heavily by gay men (McKirnan & Peterson, 1989; Sigell, Kapp, Fusaro, Nelson, & Falck, 1978, Woody et al., 1999). In fact, over the years, studies have found that amyl nitrite and chemically related inhalants were the third most commonly used class of substances among gay men after alcohol and marijuana (Kelly, 1991; Morales & Graves, 1983). The use of methamphetamine has increased dramatically in recent years among gay men and some groups of lesbian women (SAMHSA, 2001). After many years as a destructive substance of abuse among the gay male population of San Francisco and Los Angeles, methamphetamine has more recently become widespread among white gay men in New York City (Jacobs, 2004). Ecstasy (MDMA), Special K (ketamine), and GHB (gamma hydroxybutyrate, a sedative/hypnotic) have also become frequent substances of abuse in urban gay environments (Nelson & Morrison, 2001; SAMHSA, 2001).

In conclusion, it is a simplistic myth that gay men and lesbian women are a particularly high-risk group for alcohol and other substance dependence. However, moderate and recreational alcohol and other drug usage bordering on substance abuse appears to be more frequent among gay men and women, and all clinicians need to be attuned to the possibility that their gay or lesbian clients may use substances in a problematic way.

THE ASSESSMENT OF GAY, LESBIAN, AND BISEXUAL CLIENTS

In every treatment setting, the first step in the assessment process involves discovering what brought the client into treatment at that particular point in time. Regardless of the client's sexual orientation, when the presenting problem involves substance abuse issues, it is natural and appropriate to begin assessment with an exploration of the client's alcohol and other drug use, as well as the impact it has had on his or her life. A thorough clinical assessment, however, should go beyond questions about the use of substances and capture a feel for the total person. While stereotyping is certainly discouraged, it behooves the clinician to understand how issues of sexual orientation contribute to the client's alcohol and other drug use, as well as how these issues might impact on recovery efforts. Since issues pertaining to homosexuality may take weeks or months to surface, the assessment of sexual orientation ought to be approached as a dynamic and open-ended process that evolves as the client and clinician establish a working relationship.

First and foremost, clinicians working with gay, lesbian, and bisexual clients who are abusing substances must be knowledgeable about chemical dependency treatment. In addition, clinicians need to be aware of the following significant issues when assessing clients who have a history of homosexual desires, behavior, and/or identity: They include the impact of homophobia, the "coming out" process, the role of the gay bar, the need for gender-specific treatment of lesbian clients, the impact of sexual objectification on gay male clients, specific issues of bisexual clients, the impact of homosexual prostitution, the impact of homosexuality in prison, family dynamics, and issues related to HIV infection.

Assessing the Impact of Homophobia

Finnegan and McNally (1987) define homophobia as "an intense, irrational fear and dread of homosexuality and homosexuals" (p. 32). They furthermore state that "homophobia permeates American culture like the air we breathe; thus it is virtually impossible for any of us to grow up without becoming homophobic. Everyone—both gay and non-gay—seems to be homophobic to some degree" (pp. 32–33). In the United States, homosexual people have been viewed as sinners, moral degenerates, sick, insane, ludicrous, worthy of ridicule, subversives, predators, and criminals. It is certainly true that since the advent of the gay rights movement over 30 years ago, conditions have vastly improved. However, even with the profound improvement in recognizing the basic human rights of gay people, and with the presence of openly gay men and women in everyday life, homosexual and bisexual individuals are still subject to both overt and subtle social and legal oppression. For example, in a study of the prevalence of victimization of gay men and lesbian women, Otis and Skinner (1996) found that 43.7% of the gay men in their sample reported they received threats or verbal abuse in the prior 2 years, of which 81% were attributed by the respondents to their sexual orientation. Of the lesbian women in the study, 40.6% reported they received such threats or verbal abuse, of which 57.1% were attributed to their sexual orientation. Furthermore, Nystrom (1997), in a study of mental health issues of gay men and lesbian women, found that 14.2% of the respondents reported they were denied employment and 9.1% reported they were denied housing due to their sexual orientation.

An important consequence of this societal or "external" homophobia is "internalized homophobia," a term that "refers to the phenomenon of gays and lesbians absorbing the fears and prejudices of the society and turning these fears and prejudices within" (van Wormer et al., 2000, p. 31). Thus, gay and bisexual people often experience deep feelings of shame and self-loathing in regard to their homosexuality (Allen & Oleson, 1999). Many writers attribute the phenomenon of gay substance abuse, at least partly, to the shame-inducing, isolating, and self-alienating effects of internalized homophobia (Cabaj, 1996b; Finnegan & McNally, 1987; Rathbone-McCuan & Stokke, 1997; Warn, 1997). However, Bux (1996) notes that there is little empirical support at this time for a correlation between internalized homophobia and alcoholism. Weinberg (1994), who conducted an in-depth qualitative and quantitative study of 46 gay men and their drinking behaviors, noted that the men whose lives were most affected by drinking had the most negative views of their homosexuality. However, it was Weinberg's conclusion that due to the isolating, self-destructive effects of heavy alcohol consumption, "alienation is a result, rather than a cause, of pathological drinking" (Weinberg, 1994, p. 148).

During the assessment process, it is important for the clinician to be sensitive to the effects of both external and internal homophobia in the client. Homophobia pervades our society to such an extent that it is difficult for both client and clinician to grasp its full impact. Clients may not be aware of how it has affected them or how they have tried to cope with it. The clinician must evaluate any overt current and historical exposure to homophobia in the client's life, and should remain vigilant to indirect or subtle forms of this oppression as the client reveals more about him- or herself. The clinician should determine how the client deals with external homophobia, how it has been internalized, and whether substance use is part of that coping system.

Clinicians also must be sensitive to the double stigma of racism and homophobia experienced by gay and lesbian substance abusers from racial and ethnic minority groups. Some may experience marginalization by both the ethnic group with which they identify and by the predominantly white European American homosexual milieu, and may feel alienated from both worlds (Green, 1994; Icard & Traunstein, 1987; Marsiglia, 1998; Martinez, 1998). Furthermore, many African American men who reject a gay or bisexual identity, but secretly have sex with other men, have recently adopted an identity known as "being on the down low" (Denizet-Lewis, 2003). The strength of clients' identification and/or alienation in regard to both their ethnicity and their sexual orientation must be carefully assessed in determining available social supports for the recovery process, and in determining suitable referrals. Clinicians also need to be sensitive to possible extreme degrees of internalized homophobia in immigrant gay people who may have been raised in cultures that have far more oppressive homophobia than the United States (Carballo-Dieguez, 1998).

The group that is perhaps the most negatively affected by homophobia is gay and bisexual adolescents. These youths are still dependent on their families and may live with the threat or reality of rejection, ridicule, punishment, and/or physical abuse from their parents and siblings. Furthermore, there is the threat or reality of derision, ostracism, and violence from adolescent peers, who are often more homophobic than adults (D'Augelli, 1996). Such abuse is often experienced in isolation due to the lack of knowledge of other gay and bisexual people. The literature is replete with statistics regarding substance abuse, school-related problems, running away, homelessness, conflicts with the law, prostitution, and especially suicidality among gay and bisexual adolescents (Saulnier, 1998; Savin-Williams, 1994). In addition to its other destructive effects, substance abuse has been particularly identified as a high risk factor for suicide attempts in gay and bisexual youth (Hammelman, 1993; Hartstein, 1996). Clinicians therefore need to be vigilant in assessing not only issues of substance abuse but also family rejection, taunting by peers, and suicidality in the gay and bisexual teenagers who are their clients.

ASSESSING THE "COMING-OUT" PROCESS

Clinicians assessing a substance-abusing client must understand the concept of "coming out" as a significant life-cycle issue for gay men and lesbian women. Morris (1997), for example, states that "coming out is arguably the most significant event in the lives of lesbian women" (p. 2). Many gay men would agree with this comment as well. However, a precise definition of this term, which is the shortened version of the expression "coming out of the closet" is elusive. It means different things to different people, and refers to a wide array of events and internal cognitive and emotional processes. Generally, when a self-identified gay man or lesbian woman refers to the period in his life when he or she "came out," he or she is referring to an internal process of self-identification as gay or lesbian and/or a set of external actions that solidified the individual's gay or lesbian identity. The term might refer to the first time a person participated in same-gender sex. It could be the person's realization that he or she is attracted to people of the same sex and telling friends or family about it without yet engaging in homosexual behavior. It could be a man who has been engaging in anonymous gay sex for a considerable period of time while living an overtly heterosexual existence, finally accepting that he is gay and deciding to meet men in gay bars. It could be a woman in a monogamous relationship with another woman, accepting after a period of time that she is a lesbian. It could be a teenager realizing he is gay and attending a gay organization for the first time. It is important to understand the client's usage of the term *coming out* as this special period in his or her life. The term is also used by gay men and women to refer to telling others openly that one is gay; for example, "coming out at work," "coming out to friends," and "coming out to family."

There are several theoretical stage models of the process of coming out in the literature, but they have a tendency to be unrealistically linear and insensitive to unique variations in sexual identity (Fassinger, 1991). When assessing gay and lesbian substance abusers, it is important to explore the relationship of the particular client to the coming-out process. Some clients may not have come out yet, some may be in the process of coming out, and others may have come out years ago and have a firmly established gay identity. Clinicians must carefully evaluate how recovery will be affected by the presence or absence of a coming-out process, and be aware that this assessment may change during the course of treatment.

An important issue in assessment is how to help the client come out to staff. Clients may not reveal their sexual orientation during the intake process due to previous life experiences of homophobia, internalized shame about their homosexuality, previous homophobic experiences from treating professionals, fears regarding lack of confidentiality, and/or denial about the significance of their own homosexuality in recovery. Furthermore, staff may make assumptions that clients are heterosexual. It therefore falls to the clinician to take the lead in providing an atmosphere in which discussion of sexual orientation can unfold. A positive step toward normalizing homosexuality for clients is to include questions about sexual orientation in the initial assessment (Lipton, 1996). This kind of normative questioning sends a message that the clinician is nonjudgmental and comfortable with all sexual orientations (Finnegan & McNally, 1987), whereas not asking about same-gender sexual issues reinforces the client's anxiety, shame, and secrecy. Gender-neutral language should be used when referring to significant others until a client's sexual orientation becomes clear (Kominars & Kominars, 1996). This careful wording indicates to the gay or bisexual client that the clinician does not assume heterosexuality. Assurances of confidentiality and statements that all responses, including those related to sexual behavior, are highly acceptable also enhance the "coming out in assessment" process. Furthermore, if gay and bisexual issues are treated positively in the program as a whole, the client will feel encouraged to reveal his or her sexual orientation issues. For example, highly visible signs and literature concerning gay and lesbian issues may help the client feel more comfortable in revealing his or her homosexuality during the assessment process.

Assessing the Role of the Gay Bar

Long before the advent of the modern gay liberation movement, the gay bar functioned as a social center of gay and lesbian life. "The gay bar has historically been the protected place where homosexual persons could meet, socialize, be the dominant culture, make sexual contacts, start relationships, hold hands, dance, belong—all the things nongays can integrate into the totality of their lives and therefore take for granted" (Blume, 1985, pp. 79–80). Before the 1970s, it was one of the few reasonably safe, comfortable, nonanonymous locations where gay people could gather and converse. In large cities that have recognized gay and lesbian populations, there are now many alternatives to gay bars. However, the gay bar remains an integral part of gay life, although more so for gay men than women (Blume, 1985). Furthermore, in smaller cities, the gay bar may still be the only place for gay people to meet. In discussing the importance of alcohol in many gay men's lives, Weinberg (1994) believes that "reference group theory" is the most likely explanation: "People drink because their friends drink, and they regulate their drinking in terms of the unstated norms of their group" (p. 146). In addition to the gay bar, in the 1990s, there has been a proliferation of gay and "gay friendly" dance clubs in the large cities, particularly for gay men, and this has brought on an epidemic of "club drug" usage, which includes Ecstasy (MDMA), methamphetamine, Special K (Ketamine), cocaine, GHB, and other drugs. Clinicians need to assess both the impact of the gay bars and clubs on the client's substance abuse as well as the important function of the gay bar in the client's social and sexual life.

Assessing the Need for Gender-Specific Treatment of Lesbian Women

Lesbian women not only experience the profound effects of homophobia in their lives, but also have to deal with a male-dominated society in which women are relegated to a lower social, economic, and political status. When a gay woman is being assessed in a mixed-gender substance abuse program or in a program that has a majority of men, the clinician must carefully evaluate her feelings about being treated in such an environment. As there are very few lesbian-only treatment tracks, clinicians must carefully explore whether a lesbian woman would feel more comfortable in women's groups, mixed gay male and lesbian groups, or in generic groups. The clinician must not assume that lesbian women are comfortable being in treatment with gay men. Gay women's issues are actually more similar to those of heterosexual women, just as gay men's issues are more similar to those of heterosexual men. However, lesbian women also may feel quite alienated in women's programs that are not sensitive to gay clients (Rathbone-McCuan & Stokke, 1997).

Assessing the Impact of Sexual Objectification on Gay Male Clients

A high prevalence of sexual objectification takes place in gay male social life. In the same way that heterosexual men objectify women, homosexual men often objectify each other. Particularly in larger urban areas, gay men place a great deal of emphasis on male physicality, sexuality, and body image. For many gay men, keeping attractive and in shape is an important self-esteem issue, and negative self-image issues can develop as a result of feeling physically inferior (Warn, 1997). Youthful attractiveness and self-worth can become synonymous in this sexually charged environment, and this dynamic needs to be carefully explored. Clinicians should assess if their clients "cruise" for sex partners in bars, clubs, on the street, or in anonymous sex situations in order to affirm a tenuous sense of self-worth through validation of physical attractiveness (Cohler & Galatzer-Levy, 1996). The use of alcohol and other drugs as a way to self-medicate when looking for sex partners is an important assessment factor. Furthermore, although studies indicate that older gay men are as well adjusted as their heterosexual and younger gay counterparts (Berger, 1985; Berger & Kelly, 1996), clinicians need to be sensitive to possible feelings of loss regarding sexual attractiveness and evaluate any accompanying damage to self-esteem as a recovery issue for this subgroup.

Clinicians must not necessarily assess the faster, looser sexual behaviors of some of their gay male clients as pathological. The sexual mores of gay males in urban environments are different from those of heterosexual men, and this should be respected. Clinicians may be too quick to label a gay man a sex addict or sexually compulsive when he talks about multiple sex partners or anonymous sexual experiences. The meaning of the sexual behavior and how the client affectively experiences it are most important. Warn (1997) discusses the need to differentiate between compulsive sex that feels driven and unsatisfying and casual sex that is pleasurable. For gay men who are substance abusers, it is extremely important to discern whether promiscuous behavior is an integral part of the chemical dependency problem, or unrelated to it. Some gay clients whose substance abuse and sexual behaviors are interwoven will not be able to continue their sexual behaviors and maintain abstinence from alcohol and other drugs. Others can abstain from substance use without substantially changing their sexual patterns, or by finding "cruising" environments that provide less temptation to use substances. Most importantly, the clinician needs to quickly determine whether the client is practicing safer sex for the prevention of HIV and other sexually transmitted diseases. If the client is at risk, safer sex education needs to begin immediately during the assessment process.

Assessing Bisexual Clients

Assessment issues of bisexual clients differ from those of gay and lesbian clients. As noted previously, most people who have functioned bisexually or who have sexual desires for both genders do not identify themselves as bisexual or gay. Most bisexual individuals do not have a defined self-concept with which to identify, as gay people do. Although it is easier for bisexual people to "pass" or maintain a public persona as "straight" (Matteson, 1996) and thus fit into the heterosexual world, there are difficulties that bisexual men and women face that do not apply to gay men and lesbian women. Bisexual people are caught between two sexual identities in a society that has created a false dichotomy of sexual orientations. These individuals may struggle for years with identity questions—"Am I straight or am I gay?"—in a society that does not acknowledge the validity of bisexuality. They therefore often hide their homosexuality from heterosexual people, and yet do not really fit into the gay world. In fact, bisexual individuals are often rejected by gay people as being "closet cases" who cannot admit they are really gay. Bisexual people thus have little support in their own bisexual coming-out process, and few groups and organizations are available to help them. Furthermore, if they are open about their bisexuality, many heterosexual and gay people may be hesitant to begin a serious sexual relationship with them, knowing that they are also attracted to the other gender. A thorough assessment of a bisexual substance abuser must include an evaluation of how these issues of alienation and lack of validation affect the person's use of substances.

Assessing the Impact of Homosexual Prostitution

During the assessment process, clinicians often fail to address the reality that many men who are addicted to cocaine, crack cocaine, or heroin resort to homosexual prostitution in order to support their habit, and that this reality may have significant ramifications in recovery. Morse, Simon, and Burchfiel (1999) reported that 79% of the male prostitutes they interviewed reported using two different substances at least twice a week, and 43% used two substances daily. The vast majority of substance-abusing male prostitutes do not identify themselves as homosexual. In a study of male street prostitutes in Atlanta (Boles & Elifson, 1994), it was found that 46% identified as heterosexual, 36% as bisexual, and 18% as homosexual. Over three-quarters of the male prostitute sample were cocaine users, over half were crack cocaine users, and more than half were IV drug users. During the assessment process, gay men are more apt to discuss their history of prostitution than are heterosexual and bisexual men. For heterosexually identified men, their history of prostitution may be a source of great shame, self-loathing, and sexual identity confusion, and they are apt to keep this experience a secret in recovery—which unwittingly enhances the potential for relapse. Clinicians should ask their male client, in a sensitive, nonjudgmental way, whether he has engaged in prostitution in order to support his addiction, and then explore his current emotional reactions to having engaged in this behavior.

Assessing the Impact of Homosexuality in Prison

Many clients in substance abuse treatment, particularly those in long-term residential programs, have a history of incarceration. One study in a California prison found that 55% of its heterosexual sample had engaged in homosexuality while in prison. Furthermore, 14% of all male prisoners in the sample had been sexually victimized (Wooden & Parker, 1982). Cahill (2000) states that between 9 and 22% of the entire prison population has been raped. Although homosexuality is present in women's prisons, it is generally less violent and less traumatic than in men's prisons (Lockwood, 1980). Homosexual encounters in men's prisons, when coerced through either violence or persuasion, may result in subsequent emotional turmoil (Long, 1993). Clinicians whose clients have a history of incarceration must be aware that these clients may have engaged in homosexual behavior in prison, with possibly complicated emotional reactions to those experiences, including posttraumatic stress disorder. If the client is too filled with shame and self-loathing to deal with this issue, he may continue medicating himself through the use of substances. It is therefore important to explore whether clients with a history of incarceration had sexual experiences in prison. Because clients may initially keep this part of their history a secret, the assessment of the impact of sexual experiences in prison is an ongoing process.

Family Assessment Dynamics

Family assessment with gay, lesbian, and bisexual substance abusers must include nontraditional family models. Nardi (1982) identifies three family subsystems that apply to gay men and women. These are the family of origin, the "extended family" of close friends, and the primary relationship with a significant other. A fourth subsystem he does not mention is that of the children of the gay person or those of his or her significant other.

Assessment of the family of origin includes the issues of the client's family role, codependency, and possible parental substance abuse. In addition, the impact of the client's homosexuality on the relationship with his or her family and how it will affect recovery, particularly if it is a source of tension and secrecy, needs to be explored.

When assessing the extended family of friends, clinicians must be very aware of the heightened importance of friendship for gay men and women. Close friends often serve as the primary family of support for gay people and may fill a much more important role than close friends of heterosexual people. Regarding gay men, Nardi (1999) states: "Friendship networks are the avenues through which gay social worlds are constructed, the sites upon which gay men's identities and communities are formed and where the quotidian dimensions of our lives are carried out" (p. 13).

When assessing the relationship between the gay client and his or her significant other, heterosexual relationship models must not be used. Homosexual relationships are qualitatively different from their heterosexual counterparts in a number of ways. There is far more role flexibility in gay relationships because traditional male–female marriage roles do not apply. Furthermore, particularly for gay men, sexual monogamy is not a norm in many gay relationships, even though the individuals in the relationship are very committed to each other (Shernoff, 1995). Kominars and Kominars (1996) state that less than half of gay male couples are monogamous, whereas 75–85% of lesbian couples are monogamous. The relationships of bisexual men and women also may be sexually nonexclusive, either with same-gender or opposite-gender partners. When working with gay clients who have significant others, the clinician must thoroughly assess both the role of the partner in maintaining the substance abuse and in supporting recovery. The clinician also needs to assess for domestic violence, just as he or she would when working with a heterosexual client. It is estimated that domestic violence happens at the same rate in gay and lesbian relationships as in heterosexual ones; the range of abuse may include threats, intimidation, and physical abuse. Partner abuse often accompanies substance abuse (Browning, Reynolds, & Dworkin, 1991; Shannon & Woods, 1991). However, each issue must be assessed in its own right, because recovery from substance abuse does not necessarily mean that partner abuse will cease.

Because many gay clients, particularly women, are parents, the clinician must assess how the substance abuse is affecting the children of the client, as well as the children of the significant other.

Assessing HIV Issues

HIV is highly prevalent among substance abusers, and it is the responsibility of the assessing clinician to have a thorough understanding of the prevention, etiology, transmission, course, and treatment of this disease. Clinicians need to understand that the AIDS epidemic has been devastating for the gay community, and that a vast portion of the gay male population was wiped out beginning in the early 1980s. Few gay men over 40 years of age in an urban environment have not lost a friend to AIDS, and many have lost most of their friends, lovers, and acquaintances. Some are themselves HIV positive, and are struggling with this potentially deadly chronic condition while also mourning those who have died. Many HIV-negative men who have seen their extended family of friends succumb to AIDS suffer from "survivor guilt" and "faced with such feelings, seek to alleviate them by actively trying to get infected with AIDS" (Alexander, 1997, p. 232). Obstacles to recovery for clients trying to numb themselves from the pain of grief, traumatic stress, and/ or survivor's guilt, must be assessed.

In determining a client's potential for infection, it must be remembered that homosexuality, per se, is not a high-risk behavior for HIV. Anal sex is the primary transmission route of the HIV virus in gay and bisexual men, with the receptive partner particularly at risk. If a gay male client prefers engaging in this sex act, he is aware he is putting himself at risk whenever he has sex with a partner, particularly without a condom. Substance abuse lowers a person's inhibitions and thus increases the risk of unsafe sex (Cabaj, 1997; Holmes & Hodge, 1997; Ostrow et al., 1993; Pohl, 1995). Furthermore, HIV-positive gay and bisexual men are more likely to place others at risk through unsafe sexual practices when using alcohol or amyl nitrate (Robins, Dew, Kingsley, & Becker, 1997).

It is important to note that African Americans and Hispanic Americans are disproportionately HIV positive (Kuszelewicz & Lloyd, 1995). In a study conducted in New York, 33% of the young black gay men were infected with HIV, in comparison to 2% of young white gay men (Steinhauer, 2001). Both homeless gay and bisexual youths who engage in prostitution (Campbell & Peck, 1995) and adult male prostitutes (Boles & Elifson, 1994) are high risk for both HIV infection and substance abuse. When assessing lesbian substance abusers, one must remember that they are at risk for HIV infection as well, primarily through IV drug use or sex with an HIV-positive man for reasons such as personal choice, need for money, coercion, or sperm donation (Glassman, 1995).

Case Example

The following case description is an illustration of how inadequate assessment of sexual orientation issues may lead to subsequent treatment failure:

> Daryl, a 35-year-old crack-dependent African American male entered a long-term residential substance abuse treatment program that utilized a therapeutic community model. He had graduated from this program 2 years before but relapsed after 14 months. Before entering treatment, he had lived with his girlfriend of 5 years, their 1-year-old son, and her 7-year-old daughter from a different man. Daryl breezed through the first stages of treatment, as he was familiar with the therapeutic community model. In the "reentry phase," which involved his leaving the facility daily to work as a truck driver, he experienced his first relapse. He was confronted in group settings and grounded for a month after his urine tested positive for cocaine in a random screen. Daryl was assigned to a social worker for intensive individual work dealing with the relapse. After a month, he obtained another job as a driver. Two months later, he tested positive for cocaine again. In order to avoid confrontation, grounding, and possible discharge, Daryl "split" treatment and returned to his girlfriend.
>
> Soon after Daryl left, his social worker was facilitating a men's group in which Daryl had been a member. When the worker brought up Daryl's relapse and departure, a number of the men giggled and made homophobic gestures to each other. When the worker inquired about the laughter, the group avoided answering. The worker continued pressing the issue until one member mockingly answered, "Of course Daryl relapsed—he was too busy checking out boys to worry about his recovery." Normally the group was very sympathetic toward people who relapsed, so the social worker became upset about the group's flippant, uncaring responses toward Daryl. Furthermore, he was surprised by the revelation of Daryl's homosexuality and disappointed by his own ignorance about the client's sexual orientation. He confronted the group about their homophobic reaction. Unbeknown to both Daryl and the group, the social worker himself was gay.

In this vignette, although the clinician was himself gay, it did not occur to him to assess sexual orientation issues when working with Daryl, because the client lived with his girlfriend, presented as a stereotypically heterosexual truck driver, and "passed" as heterosexual to the treatment staff. Thus by adhering to stereotypes, the worker completely missed a major issue in the client's life that probably contributed to Daryl's multiple relapses. Furthermore, although clients are routinely asked during the intake assessment in this therapeutic community whether they are gay, bisexual, or heterosexual, the issue is not explored in depth with an awareness of the complexity of sexual orientation. Thus clients uncomfortable with their homosexuality can easily respond with a cursory "heterosexual." In addition, assessment of sexual orientation needs to be an ongoing issue, not one that is forgotten after intake.

This case description also demonstrates the atmosphere of homophobia that can pervade treatment programs, and how clients may need to hide the issue to feel safe. Although Daryl had been through two long-term treatment episodes, he had never mentioned his bisexuality or homosexuality to the treatment staff. Although his peers knew of this issue and may have even mocked him about it, no one brought up his bisexuality in any of the many therapy and encounter groups. Homophobia may have rendered his sexual orientation a taboo subject. Given that this particular therapeutic community had a small number of openly gay clients, this case example also shows that clients with bisexual issues may experience a lack of support in treatment settings, feeling alienated from both the heterosexual and gay populations. Furthermore, the possibility of Daryl having engaged in homosexuality in prison was never assessed, even though he had indicated that he had a history of incarceration. The possibility of his having ever engaged in prostitution to support his habit was never explored either. Finally, because Daryl was perceived by the program counselors as a non-IV drug user in an ongoing heterosexual relationship, his risk of currently engaging in unsafe sexual practices in regard to HIV was not discussed.

If any member of the treatment staff had attempted to assess any of the aforementioned issues related to homosexuality in depth in a normalizing way, Daryl may have been able to reveal and process issues around sexual orientation and internalized homophobia. Perhaps the outcome of Daryl's treatment would have been more favorable.

TREATMENT OF GAY, LESBIAN, AND BISEXUAL CLIENTS

Substance abuse treatment for people who have a history of homosexual behavior, desire, and/or identity must take into account that each person's experience of his or her sexual orientation is unique. Counselors need to respect each client's individuality and must not act on preformed judgments about what gay people need in the recovery process. That being said, the following treatment recommendations may be considered when working with this population.

"Gay-Affirmative" Treatment

In the treatment of gay, lesbian, and bisexual substance abusers, practitioners must be "gay affirmative," which means that in the treatment room, the client's homosexuality is fully accepted, not merely tolerated. A gay-affirmative substance abuse clinician appreciates both homosexuality and bisexuality as valid and rich orientations and views the oppression and stigma of homosexual behaviors, desires, and identities as pathological (Davies, 1996). Homosexuality is not to be viewed as second best to heterosexuality, but on an equal plane. Treatment must be gay affirmative in order to counter the effects of external and internal homophobia. Kominars (1995) points out how internalized homophobia is a major relapse trigger that must be dealt with in recovery. Anger, fear, guilt, and isolation are all consequences of internalized homophobia and obstacles to maintaining abstinence. Developing the self-esteem to work though the impact of homophobia becomes a necessary part of the recovery process. Eliciting feelings pertaining to homophobia may bring up powerful emotions and associations. Therefore, clinicians need to be sensitive to the client's tolerance for this exploration and should not press too quickly, particularly when abstinence is still tenuous (Cabaj, 1995).

Providing gay-affirmative treatment means that gay, lesbian, and bisexual clients feel welcome in the treatment environment. Literature and postings in the facility should address the needs of this population. Homophobic remarks and attitudes of clients in treatment must be countered and explored. Staff should be knowledgeable about homosexual issues and aware of sober gay activities and programs in the community. Practitioners in detox and rehab settings need to be aware of outpatient gay and lesbian treatment tracks in the community and explore with the client whether he or she would want to be referred to such programs.

Treatment of Ethnic and Racial Minorities

If gay and bisexual clients from ethnic and racial minority groups express feelings of alienation and/or poor self-image in regard to their ethnicities, as well as negative feelings about their sexual orientation, treatment ought to include strengthening self-concept in regard to both identities. Clinicians need to be aware that such clients may feel different from their peers in gay-specific treatment programs and 12-step meetings, as well as in settings where their ethnic or minority group is in attendance. In large cities, there may be 12-step meetings for gay men and women, with a large percentage of racial and ethnic minorities present. However, in communities that do not offer these options, clinicians need to offer more ongoing support and allow clients to verbalize their feelings of alienation so that they can utilize available resources more effectively.

Coming Out as a Treatment Issue

Coming out may be a significant issue for some gay, lesbian, and bisexual clients in substance abuse treatment. For many, the coming-out process can be supportive of recovery as clients work through issues of se-crecy and shame and develop a positive sense of self. However, the anxiety engendered by this major life transition, along with potentially negative responses from others, could trigger relapse. Clinicians must be attuned to the full range of responses that the coming-out process may elicit. Moreover, for some clients, coming out may not necessarily be part of recovery, and this choice should be respected as well. The client in substance abuse treatment should not be pushed to tell peers, friends, family, or work associates that he or she is gay, particularly if the client is not ready to deal with the possible difficult consequences. In addition, clinicians need to respect that the coming-out process for bisexual indi-viduals is usually more difficult, complicated, and lengthier than for gay and lesbian people, and that many functionally bisexual people never identify as bisexual (Reynolds & Hanjorgiris, 2000) and thus really never come out.

The Role of the Gay Bar in Relapse Prevention

Due to the significant social role of the gay bar, clinicians need to be care-ful in prohibiting clients in treatment from going to them as a relapse pre-vention measure, since this may alienate individuals from treatment. Finnegan and McNally (1987) state that "for many gays, that's like telling them, their social life is over—that they can no longer go to what is often the only place available to meet other gays in a relatively safe atmosphere" (pp. 66–67). On the other hand, some clinicians may mistakenly minimize the danger a client faces in going to gay bars or clubs, rationalizing that it is "just a part of gay life." The clinician may underestimate the relapse potential of frequenting these settings, and may unwittingly collude with the client by not confronting him or her about this behavior and exploring social alternatives to the gay bar.

Utilizing a Feminist Perspective in Treating Lesbian Women

A dictionary definition of feminism is "the theory of the political, eco-nomic, and social equality of the sexes" (*Merriam-Webster*, 2000, p. 428). In substance abuse treatment, feminism may empower the lesbian woman who feels "less than" as a female and as a homosexual. Further-more, there is a mutuality with other women inherent in feminism that is very helpful in recovery: Feminism "depends on the premise that women can consciously and collectively change their social place" (Humm, 1992, p. 1). Clinicians should take advantage of this concept of collec-tive empowerment when working with gay substance-abusing women. Heyward (1992) emphasizes that for lesbian women, healing from addiction is a process of liberation from oppression in a context of "mutual relation."

Clinicians need to recognize that many of the current treatment models were developed by men for men. For example, many gay women may feel alienated by the reliance on the concept of powerlessness that pervades 12-step recovery programs, because they have felt powerless living in a male-dominated society their entire lives (Rathbone-McCuan & Stokke, 1997). Nevertheless, many women have been helped by lesbian-specific 12-step meetings, as well as by gay mixed-gender meetings and women's meetings. Furthermore, many male-oriented substance abuse treatment programs stress personal responsibility and autonomy in recovery, with dependence on others viewed as codependence, a form of addictive emotional behavior. This view can be antithetical to a woman's way of interacting with the world. Using a relational model of substance abuse treatment (Byington, 1997), with its emphasis on connection, can be more beneficial for lesbian women.

Mitigating Sexual Objectification as a Treatment Goal for Gay Men

When treating gay men whose self-worth is negatively affected by issues of physical attractiveness and sexual objectification, a goal of recovery work would be to help them broaden their self-concept and enhance their self-esteem by facilitating their identification and appreciation of aspects of self apart from how successful they are in the sexual arena. Furthermore, diminishing the client's sexual objectification of others may reduce social isolation by enhancing the depth and meaningfulness of relationships. Through individual and group therapy, clinicians can encourage clients to explore and reflect on the multidimensionality of human interactions. In addition, 12-step programs can be helpful in creating a more balanced perspective by focusing on issues of spirituality.

Treating Bisexual Clients

Bisexual clients may experience alienation in substance abuse treatment, because they do not wish to identify and be identified with the openly gay and lesbian clients, and yet they fear they may not be accepted by the heterosexual clients if they reveal their bisexuality. Thus bisexual clients may be more secretive in treatment than gay and lesbian clients, particularly in urban environments where gay and lesbian clients feel safer to express themselves. In gay-affirmative substance abuse treatment it is very important to normalize the bisexuality of these clients and help them appreciate their desire to have sexual relations with both genders.

Dealing with Homosexual Prison Experiences and Male Prostitution

As indicated previously, men in treatment are often loathe to reveal past experiences of sex in prison and male prostitution. Therefore, it may fall to the clinician to raise these topics in both individual and group settings in a fashion that is normalizing and accepting. In addition, practitioners need to take proactive steps in confronting uncomfortable reactions to these subjects in group settings, where laughter and mocking comments may greet the person revealing these experiences. The topic of sex in prison can often be more easily addressed in groups specifically designed for clients who have a history of incarceration. However, clients who have been victimized in prison may still be reluctant to share this information with peers. Male clients who have been exclusively heterosexual before engaging in prostitution or homosexuality in prison may experience significant sexual orientation confusion and shame, particularly if they are currently feeling homosexual desires that did not previously exist. Clinicians need to deal with these possible responses in a way that respects the individuality of each client's experiences. Treatment should include normalizing feelings and diminishing the client's sense of shame and self-loathing.

Family Treatment

When working with the family of origin of gay or bisexual substance abusers, many potentially volatile issues concerning sexual orientation may emerge. The substance-abusing client may be hiding his or her sexual orientation from parents and siblings, and treatment may or may not involve coming out to them. The family may blame the substance abuse on the client's homosexuality, or vice versa. Parents of the gay client may experience a great deal of guilt about their offspring's homosexuality. In such cases, education about both substance abuse and homosexuality should be integrated into treatment.

When alcohol and other drugs are a significant element in the social life of the client's network of friends, involving the "extended family" in treatment may be a necessity. However, if substance abuse is an entrenched norm of the client's circle of friends, treatment may need to support limiting contact with them and/or finding alternative friendships. In this instance, clinicians should have knowledge of different social and activity groups in the gay community, in order to encourage the client to make new friends who are sober. If the client's significant other abuses substances, treatment may include couple therapy. In addition, helping the client to maintain abstinence while his or her partner is still using substances is a crucial treatment goal, and may involve the client leaving the partner. Even when the significant other is not abusing substances, it is advisable to include him or her in treatment when appropriate.

HIV Issues in Treatment

Safer sex education and monitoring clients' high-risk behaviors in regard to HIV transmission are essential parts of treatment. If the substance abuser is HIV positive, the clinician must be aware of the possibility of relapse due to feelings of hopelessness engendered by such a diagnosis, or by changes in health status. The clinician needs to emphasize repeatedly that maintaining abstinence may result in improved health and a longer life. In addition, when working with clients who have lost friends and lovers to AIDS, facilitating grief work is often an important part of recovery for them.

Spirituality in Treatment

The concept of spirituality holds a powerful position in the history of recovery from alcohol and other drug addictions, and is a vital part of 12-step programs. Many gay and bisexual people in recovery associate spirituality with organized religion. Because most Western Judeo-Christian religious institutions have espoused homophobic attitudes that reject anyone who is not functionally heterosexual or asexual, these gay or bisexual men and women feel very alienated from discussions of spiritual concepts. The emphasis in Alcoholic Anonymous (AA) to recognize and surrender to a "Higher Power" may feel repulsive to someone who has fought for years to free him- or herself from the clutches of homophobic religious teachings. However, in noting the importance of a sense of spirituality for gay people, Davidson (2000) contends that affirming goodness, cultivating a sense of community, and connecting with God or a creator can promote positive self-esteem and a sense of belonging. Kus (1992) believes it is important to create a distinction between spirituality and religion when working with gay substance abusers in recovery. Clinicians need to recognize the importance of encouraging substance-abusing gay clients to attend specialized gay or lesbian 12-step meetings. At these meetings, many gay people may feel more able to separate spirituality from their previous homophobic religious experiences and develop a support system for creating a sense of spirituality in recovery that is consonant with gay experience (Kus & Latcovich, 1995). Furthermore, spiritual practice can help people deal with the mass destruction of the AIDS epidemic (Davidson, 2000). However, if the client still does not want to include 12-step programs in his or her recovery, even after exploring his or her resistance, then alternative venues of support need to be found.

Clients should not be automatically referred to gay AA or NA meetings without first exploring their feelings about such referrals. Some may have substantial issues of homophobia and may not be ready to attend gay meetings, whereas others may wish to attend such meetings but may be distracted by sexual tension if people are "cruising" there (Warn, 1997). Moreover, gay-identified female clients may quickly become enmeshed romantically with other women at the meetings (Rathbone-McKuan & Stokke, 1997). The predominately gay membership of a meeting also may bring up the same feelings of lack of self-worth and isolation that some have experienced when they are trying to connect to others in gay bars or other gay meeting places, particularly if the gay meeting has cliques and is not particularly welcoming to new members. Therefore, clinicians need to explore if general AA or NA meetings might be more therapeutic for some gay and bisexual clients in early recovery.

Case Example

The following vignette demonstrates a number of the treatment issues presented in this chapter.

> Angela, a 26-year-old white Roman Catholic female, was referred to an outpatient alcoholism treatment program by an emergency room social worker after sustaining a head injury. She told the emergency room staff that she had fallen down in the bathroom, hitting her head on the sink, after consuming a pint of vodka. After being questioned, she revealed that she drank daily. It was noted that she exhibited many of the signs of alcohol dependence.
>
> During the intake process at the treatment program, Angela discussed how she had been working in a club as an exotic dancer for the past 4 years. She stated that this type of job was the only way she could maintain a comfortable lifestyle, as she had dropped out of high school in 11th grade and had few marketable skills. Since dancing seminude in public clashed with the Roman Catholic values of her upbringing, she began to consume alcohol in order to lower her inhibitions. Furthermore, the manager of the club encouraged her to snort cocaine to enhance the duration of her performance. She used approximately a gram of cocaine each night that she worked. During the intake process, Angela stated that she was heterosexual. She revealed that she had had two relationships with men that lasted over a year. She was currently single and sharing an apartment with another female dancer from the club.
>
> After being diagnosed with alcohol and cocaine dependence, Angela was assigned to a female individual counselor, a mixed-gender early recovery group, and a women's recovery group. She had difficulty maintaining abstinence during the first few months of treatment

while working at the club. However, Angela subsequently quit her job and focused on her sobriety. She developed a close working relationship with her individual counselor and made good use of her groups, particularly the women's group. However, she felt uncomfortable at AA meetings and only attended sporadically. Seven months into treatment, Angela missed a session of her women's group. The following day, she arrived at the program for her individual session with dark glasses and a black eye. Trusting her counselor, Angela revealed that she had been beaten by her substance-abusing female roommate, who was actually her lover. She told the counselor that after feeling attracted to women for several years, this was her first lesbian relationship. Furthermore, Angela discussed how she was ashamed of her homosexual feelings and had not talked about them with anybody in her life.

The counselor became quite concerned about Angela being battered and the shame she was feeling about her sexual orientation. During the next couple of weeks, the counselor further explored the domestic violence and offered Angela resources, including safe housing. In addition, the counselor told Angela about support groups and AA meetings at a local gay community center, as well as a group for victims of domestic violence. However, Angela adamantly declined to use any of these services, stating that she only wanted to discuss her homosexuality with the counselor and not with others. The counselor agreed to respect the client's wishes, thinking that if she pressed the issue too quickly, Angela might flee treatment. Two months later, a new member of the women's group casually mentioned that she was gay. Angela witnessed how the other clients readily accepted the new member. This observation, coupled with the work she had been doing with her individual counselor, set the stage for Angela to disclose to the group that she too was gay. Her peers were very supportive of her coming out to them. The other lesbian group member and a heterosexual group member ended up accompanying Angela to her first gay and lesbian AA meeting. Over time, with the support of her new network of friends from the treatment program and AA, Angela decided she could no longer tolerate her lover's substance abuse. With the encouragement of the counselor, Angela asked her partner to attend a couple's session with her at the treatment program. When her lover declined her request, Angela made a decision to leave her.

In this case example, the counselor's acceptance of Angela's homosexuality and the role modeling by another group member helped to counteract Angela's internalized homophobia and enable her to come out to the women's group and utilize gay resources in the community. The counselor's decision to respect Angela's initial wish to work exclusively in individual sessions on the issue of sexual orientation enabled Angela to explore the difficult issues of shame and fear about her homosexuality. The counselor was aware that coming out can be an anxiety-producing process and that this client needed to proceed cautiously in her early phases of recovery. Angela's involvement in the women's group was also very helpful in her recovery, as she felt more able to reveal deeper feelings in a same-sex group. Although it did not materialize, the therapist's encouraging of Angela to bring her lover to a session was therapeutically sound and actually clarified for Angela the need to leave the relationship, because it was not supportive of her recovery.

TRANSFERENCE, COUNTERTRANSFERENCE, AND SELF-DISCLOSURE

Effective assessment and treatment of gay, lesbian, and bisexual substance-abusing clients requires that the clinician be aware of his or her feelings and attitudes concerning homosexuality. A clinician whose homophobic attitudes are unresolved or unmanageable should not work with this population, because his or her negative attitudes will inevitably be communicated to the client, regardless of good intentions (Cabaj, 1996a; DeCrescenzo, 1985). It takes critical self-examination on the part of the clinician to monitor his or her own homophobia, which may otherwise contaminate the treatment process. Indeed a shallow, politically correct acceptance of homosexuality may actually be more detrimental than blatant rejection, because the latter is more easily recognizable and therefore more readily challenged. Furthermore, it is important to recognize that gay, lesbian, and bisexual clinicians are not exempt from the need to conduct such an honest self-assessment, as they, too, were raised in a homophobic culture (Mallon, 1998).

Even clinicians who are comfortable with gay and lesbian clients may have certain negative biases when working with bisexual individuals, such as believing that they are "psychologically or emotionally damaged, are developmentally immature, or have a borderline personality disorder, with changing sexual behavior manifesting as a symptom of poor impulse control or acting-out behavior" (SAMHSA, 2001, p. xix). Practitioners working with bisexual clients must explore and challenge such preconceived myths.

Clinicians, whether gay, bisexual, or heterosexual, may wonder if and when they should disclose their sexual orientation to gay or bisexual clients. Because there are no definitive answers to this clinically complex issue; this decision must be made on a case-by-case basis, and must always be guided by what is right for the client and not by the clinician's personal agenda (Gabriel & Monaco, 1995; Mallon, 1998; Sophie, 1988).

Some clients know from the start that they would prefer to work with a gay clinician and may initially request that information. Other clients may be well into treatment before they openly speculate about their clinician's sexual orientation, at which point they may pose the question directly. Still others may hint at wanting to inquire about the clinician's sexual orientation, but do not ask directly. Regardless of the timing, a clinician's unwillingness to directly answer such a question is likely to provoke suspicion and anger in the client and may destroy the treatment process, even when handled skillfully (Gabriel & Monaco, 1995). On the other hand, if the client only drops hints about wanting to know the clinician's sexual orientation, it may indicate ambivalence about obtaining this information. In such a case, the clinician should avoid immediate self-disclosure and explore in depth whether the client really wants this information and whether it would help or hinder treatment (Sophie, 1988). If the clinician is gay or bisexual, disclosing his or her sexual identity can provide a positive role model and may enhance the recovery process (Cabaj, 1996a; Finnegan & McNally, 1987; Mallon, 1998; Morrow, 2000). On the other hand, an unsolicited or premature disclosure may dissuade the client from sharing negative thoughts and feelings about his or her sexual orientation and thereby impede the work. Gay clinicians, furthermore, must be careful not to overidentify with gay clients or confuse boundaries and roles by becoming a mentor, advisor, or a friend (Cabaj, 1996a; Morrow, 2000).

For some gay or bisexual clients with strong homophobic feelings, having an identified heterosexual clinician who is gay affirming can be more therapeutic than working with an identified gay clinician, because they may respond more to positive validation of their homosexuality from a clinician who is "straight" (Ubell & Sumberg, 1992). However, regardless of the sexual orientation of the clinician, his or her acceptance of gay men and women, empathy for their oppression, ethics, integrity, knowledge, warmth, competence, and willingness to learn are what matter the most (Marmor, 1996).

CONCLUSION

Clinicians must have knowledge of the significant issues that may affect gay, lesbian, and bisexual substance abusers, as discussed in this chapter. When working with this population, assessing and treating the client's substance abuse needs to be the primary focus. For maximum effectiveness, a gay-affirmative perspective is necessary. Although the relationship between issues of homophobia and substance abuse in gay and bisexual populations is not clear, clinicians must be cognizant of the damaging effects of this oppression both for the client and the clinician. Most importantly, the clinician must view all clients with a history of homosexual behaviors, desires, and identities as unique and not hold onto "cookie-cutter" quasi-therapeutic concepts about the needs of gay, lesbian, and bisexual substance abusers. Knowledge of the general issues of this population, a strong focus on recovery from alcohol and other drugs, a gay-affirmative approach, and respect for each client's individuality create a healthy recipe for working with gay, lesbian, and bisexual substance abusers.

REFERENCES

Alexander, C. J. (1997). *Growth and intimacy for gay men*. New York: Haworth Press.

Allen, D. J., & Oleson, T. (1999). Shame and internalized homophobia in gay men. *Journal of Homosexuality, 37*, 33–43.

Berger, R. M. (1985). Rewriting a bad script: Older lesbians and gays. In H. Hidalgo, T. L. Peterson, & N. J. Woodman (Eds.), *Lesbian and gay issues: A resource manual for social workers* (pp. 53–59). Silver Spring, MD: National Association of Social Workers.

Berger, R. M., & Kelly, J. J. (1996). Gay men and lesbians grown older. In R. P. Cabaj & T. S. Stein (Eds.), *Textbook of homosexuality and mental health* (pp. 305–316). Washington, DC: American Psychiatric Association Press.

Bickelhaupt, E. E. (1995). Alcoholism and drug abuse in gay and lesbian persons: A review of incidence studies. In R. J. Kus (Ed.), *Addiction and recovery in gay and lesbian persons* (pp. 5–14). New York: Harrington Park Press.

Blume, E. S. (1985). Substance abuse (of being queer, magic pills, and social lubricants). In H. Hidalgo, T. L. Peterson, & N. J. Woodman (Eds.), *Lesbian and gay issues: A resource manual for social workers* (pp. 79–87). Silver Spring, MD: National Association of Social Workers.

Boles, J., & Elifson, K. W. (1994). Sexual identity and HIV: The male prostitute. *Journal of Sex Research, 31*, 39–46.

Bradford, J., Ryan, C., & Rothblum, E. (1994). National lesbian health care survey: Implications for mental health care. *Journal of Consulting and Clinical Psychology, 62*, 228–242.

Broido, E. M. (2000). Constructing identity: The nature and meaning of lesbian, gay, and bisexual identities. In R. M. Perez, K. A. DeBord, & K. J. Bieschke (Eds.), *Handbook of counseling and psychotherapy with lesbian, gay, and bisexual clients* (pp. 13–33). Washington, DC: American Psychological Association.

Browning, C., Reynolds, A. L., & Dworkin, S. H. (1991). Affirmative psychotherapy for lesbian women. *The Counseling Psychologist, 19*, 177–196.

Bux, D. A. (1996). The epidemiology of problem drinking in gay men and lesbians: A critical review. *Clinical Psychology Review, 16*, 277–298.

Byington, D. B. (1997). Applying relational theory to addiction treatment. In S. L. A. Straussner & E. Zelvin (Eds.), *Gender and addictions* (pp. 31–46). Northvale, NJ: Aronson.

Cabaj, R. P. (1995). Sexual orientation and the Addictions. *Journal of Gay and Lesbian Psychotherapy, 2*, 97–117.

Cabaj, R. P. (1996a). Sexual orientation of the therapist. In R. P. Cabaj & T. S. Stein

(Eds.), *Textbook of homosexuality and mental health* (pp. 513–524). Washington, DC: American Psychiatric Association Press.

Cabaj, R. P. (1996b). Substance abuse in gay men, lesbians, and bisexuals. In R. P. Cabaj & T. S. Stein (Eds.), *Textbook of homosexuality and mental health* (pp. 783–799). Washington, DC: American Psychiatric Association Press.

Cabaj, R. P. (1997). Gays, lesbians, and bisexuals. In J. H. Lowinson, P. Ruiz, R. Millman, & J. Langrod (Eds.), *Substance abuse: A comprehensive textbook* (pp. 725–731). Baltimore: Williams and Wilkins.

Cahill, T. (2000). Stop prison rape. *Fortune News, 34,* 18–19.

Campbell, C. A., & Peck, M. D. (1995). Issues in HIV/AIDS service delivery to high risk youth. *Journal of Gay and Lesbian Social Services, 2,* 159–177.

Carballo-Dieguez, A. (1998). The challenge of staying HIV-negative for Latin American immigrants. *Journal of Gay and Lesbian Social Services, 8,* 61–82.

Cohler, B. J., & Galatzer-Levy, R. (1996) Self psychology and homosexuality: Sexual orientation and maintenance of personal integrity. In R. P. Cabaj & T. S. Stein (Eds.), *Textbook of homosexuality and mental health* (pp. 207–223). Washington, DC: American Psychiatric Association Press.

D'Augelli, A. R. (1996). Lesbian, gay, and bisexual development during adolescence and young adulthood. In R. P. Cabaj & T. S. Stein (Eds.), *Textbook of homosexuality and mental health* (pp. 267–288). Washington, DC: American Psychiatric Association Press.

Davidson, M. G. (2000). Religion and spirituality. In R. M. Perez, K. A. DeBord, & K. J. Bieschke (Eds.), *Handbook of counseling and psychotherapy with lesbian, gay, and bisexual clients* (pp. 409–433). Washington, DC: American Psychological Association.

Davies, D. (1996). Towards a model of gay affirmative therapy. In D. Davies & C. Neal (Eds.), *Pink therapy* (pp. 24–40). Buckingham, UK: Open University.

DeCrescenzo, T. A. (1985). Homophobia: A study of the attitudes of mental health professionals toward homosexuality. In R. Schoenberg & R. S. Goldberg, with D. A. Shore (Eds.), *With compassion toward some: Homosexuality and social work in America* (pp. 115–136). New York: Harrington Park Press.

Denizet-Lewis, B. (2003, August 3). Double lives on the down low. *The New York Times Magazine,* pp. 28–33, 48, 52–53.

Fassinger, R. E. (1991). The hidden minority: Issues and challenges in working with lesbian women and gay men. *The Counseling Psychologist, 19,* 157–176.

Finnegan, D. G., & McNally, E. B. (1987). *Dual identities: Counseling chemically dependent gay men and lesbians.* Center City, MN: Hazelden Foundation.

Fitfield, H. L. (1975). *On my way to nowhere: Alienated, isolated, and drunk.* Los Angeles: Gay Community Services Center.

Gabriel, M. A., & Monaco, G. W. (1995). Revisiting the question of self-disclosure: The lesbian therapist's dilemma. In J. M. Glassgold & S. Iasenza (Eds.), *Lesbians and psychoanalysis* (pp. 161–172). New York: Free Press.

Glassman, C. (1995). Lesbians and HIV disease. *Journal of Gay and Lesbian Social Services, 2,* 61–74.

Greene, B. (1994). Ethnic-minority lesbians and gay men: mental health and treatment issues. *Journal of Consulting and Clinical Psychology, 62,* 243–251.

Hammelman, T. L. (1993). Gay and lesbian youth: Contributing factors to serious attempts or considerations of suicide. *Journal of Gay and Lesbian Psychotherapy,* 2, 77–89.

Hartstein, N. B. (1996). Suicide risk in lesbian, gay, and bisexual youth. In R. P. Cabaj & T. S. Stein (Eds.), *Textbook of homosexuality and mental health* (pp. 819–837). Washington, DC: American Psychiatric Association Press.

Heyward, C. (1992). Healing addiction and homophobia: Reflections on empowerment and liberation. In D. L. Weinstein (Ed.), *Lesbians and gay men: Chemical dependency treatment issues* (pp. 5–18). New York: Haworth Press.

Holmes, K. A., & Hodge, R. H. (1997). Gay and Lesbian People. In J. Philleo & F. L. Brisbane (Eds.), *Cultural competence in substance abuse prevention* (pp. 153–174). Washington, DC: NASW Press.

Humm, M. (1992). History of feminism in Britain and America. In M. Humm (Ed.), *Modern feminisms* (pp. 1–7). New York: Columbia University Press.

Icard, L., & Traunstein, D. M. (1987). Black, gay, alcoholic men: Their character and treatment. *Social Casework, 68,* 267–272.

Jacobs, A. (2004, January 12). The beast in the bathhouse. *New York Times,* pp. B1, B5.

Kelly, J. (1991). *San Francisco lesbian, gay, and bisexual alcohol and other drugs needs assessment study: Vol. 1.* Sacramento, CA: EMT Associates.

Kinsey, A. C., Pomeroy W. B., & Martin, C. E. (1948). *Sexual behavior in the human male.* Philadelphia: Saunders.

Kinsey, A. C., Pomeroy W. B., Martin, C. E., & Gebhard, P. H. (1953). *Sexual behavior in the human female.* Philadelphia: Saunders.

Kominars, S. B. (1995). Homophobia: The heart of darkness. In R. J. Kus (Ed.), *Addiction and recovery in gay and lesbian persons* (pp. 29–39). New York: Harrington Park Press.

Kominars, S. B., & Kominars, K. D. (1996). *Accepting Ourselves and Others.* Center City, MN: Hazelden Foundation.

Kus, R. J. (1992). Spirituality in everyday life: Experiences of gay men of Alcoholics Anonymous. In D. L. Weinstein (Ed.), *Lesbians and gay men: Chemical dependency treatment issues* (pp. 49–66). New York: Haworth Press.

Kus, R. J., & Latcovich, M. A. (1995). Special interest groups in Alcoholics Anonymous: A focus on gay men's groups. In R. J. Kus (Ed.), *Addiction and recovery in gay and lesbian persons* (pp. 67–82). New York: Haworth Press.

Kuszelewicz, M. A., & Lloyd, G. A. (1995). Lesbians and gays of color and HIV/AIDS: A literature review, 1988–1993. *Journal of Gay and Lesbian Social Services, 2,* 107–119.

Laumann, E. O., Gagnon, J. H., Michael R. T., & Michaels, S. (1994). *The social organization of sexuality: Sexual practices in the United States.* Chicago: University of Chicago Press.

Lipton, B. (1996). Opening doors: Responding to the mental health needs of gay and bisexual college students. In M. Shernoff (Ed.), *Human services for gay people: Clinical and community practice* (pp. 7–24). New York: Haworth Press.

Lockwood, D. (1980). *Prison sexual violence.* New York: Elsevier.

Lohrenz, L. J., Connelly, J. C., Coyne, L., & Spare, K. E. (1978). Alcohol problems in several midwestern homosexual communities. *Journal of Studies on Alcohol, 39,* 1959–1963.

Long, G. T. (1993). Homosexual relationships in a unique setting: The male prison. In

L. Diamant (Ed.), *Homosexual issues in the workplace* (pp. 143–170). Washington, DC: Taylor & Francis.

Mallon, G. P. (1998). Knowledge for practice with gay and lesbian persons. In G. P. Mallon (Ed.), *Foundations of social work practice with lesbian and gay persons* (pp. 1–30). New York: Haworth Press.

Marmor, J. (1996). Nongay therapists working with gay men and lesbians: A personal reflection. In R. P. Cabaj & T. S. Stein (Eds.), *Textbook of homosexuality and mental health* (pp. 539–545). Washington, DC: American Psychiatric Association Press.

Marsiglia, F. F. (1998). Homosexuality and Latinos/as: Towards an integration of identities. *Journal of Gay and Lesbian Social Services, 8,* 113–125.

Martinez, D. G. (1998). *Mujer, Latina, lesbiana*: Notes on the multidimensionality of economic and sociopolitical injustice. *Journal of Gay and Lesbian Social Services, 8,* 99–112.

Matteson, D. R. (1996). Psychotherapy with bisexual individuals. In R. P. Cabaj & T. S. Stein (Eds.), *Textbook of homosexuality and mental health* (pp. 433–450). Washington, DC: American Psychiatric Association Press.

McKirnan, D. J., & Peterson, P. L. (1989). Alcohol and drug use among homosexual men and women: Epidemiology and population characteristics. *Addictive Behaviors, 14,* 545–553.

Merriam-Webster's Collegiate Dictionary (10th ed.). (2000). Springfield, MA: Merriam Webster.

Morales, E. S., & Graves, M. A. (1983). *Substance abuse: Patterns and barriers to treatment for gay men and lesbians in San Francisco.* San Francisco: San Francisco Prevention Resources Center.

Morris, J. F. (1997). Lesbian coming out as a multidimensional process. *Journal of Homosexuality, 33,* 1–22.

Morrow, S. L. (2000). First do no harm: Therapist issues in psychotherapy with lesbian, gay, and bisexual clients. In R. M. Perez, K. A. DeBord, & K. J Bieschke (Eds.), *Handbook of counseling and psychotherapy with lesbian, gay, and bisexual clients* (pp. 137–156). Washington, DC: American Psychological Association.

Morse, E. V., Simon, P. M., & Burchfiel, K. E. (1999). Social environment and male sex work in the United States. In P. Aggleton (Ed.), *Men who sell sex: International perspectives on male prostitution and HIV/AIDS* (pp. 83–101). Philadelphia: Temple University.

Nardi, P. M. (1982). Alcohol treatment and the non-traditional "family" structures of gays and lesbians. *Journal of Alcohol and Drug Education, 27,* 83–89.

Nardi, P. M. (1999). *Gay men's friendships.* Chicago: University of Chicago.

Nelson, B., & Morrison, D. (2001, January 16). How Ecstasy works: Studies suggest the "hug drug" disrupts nerve cell function, perhaps for life. *Newsday,* pp. C3, C6.

Nystrom, N. (1997, February). *Mental health experiences of gay men and lesbians.* Paper presented at the meeting of the American Association for the Advancement of Science symposium "Assessing Health Needs of Gay Men and Lesbians," Houston, TX.

Ostrow, D. G., Beltran, E. D., Joseph, J. G., DiFrancesco, W., Wesch, J., & Chmiel, J.

S. (1993). Recreational drugs and sexual behavior in the Chicago MACS/CCS cohort of homosexually active men. *Journal of Substance Abuse, 5,* 311–325.

Otis, M. D., & Skinner, W. F. (1996). The prevalence of victimization and its effect on mental well-being among lesbian and gay people. *Journal of Homosexuality, 30,* 93–121.

Pohl, M. I. (1995). Chemical dependency and HIV infection. *Journal of Gay and Lesbian Social Services, 2,* 15–28.

Rathbone-McCuan, E., & Stokke, D. L. (1997). Lesbian women and substance abuse. In S. L. A. Straussner & E. Zelvin (Eds.), *Gender and addictions* (pp. 167–196). Northvale, NJ: Aronson.

Reynolds, A. L., & Hanjorgiris, W. F. (2000). Coming out: Lesbian, gay, and bisexual identity development. In R. M. Perez, K. A. DeBord, & K. J. Bieschke (Eds.), *Handbook of counseling and psychotherapy with lesbian, gay, and bisexual clients* (pp. 35–55). Washington, DC: American Psychological Association.

Robins, A. G., Dew, M. A., Kingsley, L. A., & Becker, J. T. (1997). Do homosexual and bisexual men who place others at potential risk for HIV have unique psychosocial profiles? *AIDS Education and Prevention, 9,* 239–251.

Saghir, M. T., & Robins, E. (1973). *Male and female homosexuality: A Comprehensive investigation.* Baltimore: Williams & Wilkins.

SAMHSA (Substance Abuse and Mental Health Services Administration). (2001). *A provider's introduction to substance abuse treatment for lesbian, gay, bisexual, and transgender individuals.* Rockville, MD: U.S. Department of Health and Human Services.

Saulnier, C. F. (1998). Prevalence of suicide attempts and suicidal ideation among lesbian and gay youth. *Journal of Gay and Lesbian Social Services, 8,* 51–68.

Savin-Williams, R. C. (1994). Verbal and physical abuse as stressors in the lives of lesbian, gay male, and bisexual youths: Association with school problems, running away, substance abuse, prostitution, and suicide. *Journal of Consulting and Clinical Psychology, 62,* 261–269.

Shannon, J. W., & Woods, W. J. (1991). Affirmative psychotherapy for gay men. *The Counseling Psychologist, 19,* 197–215.

Shernoff, M. (1995). Male couples and their relationship styles. *Journal of Gay and Lesbian Social Services, 2,* 43–57.

Sigell, L. T., Kapp, F. T., Fusaro, G. A., Nelson, E. D., & Falck, R. S. (1978). Popping and snorting volatile nitrites: A current fad for getting high. *American Journal of Psychiatry, 135,* 1216–1218.

Skinner, W. F., & Otis, M. D. (1996). Drug and alcohol use among lesbian and gay people in a Southern U.S. sample: Epidemiological, comparative, and methodological findings from the Trilogy Project. *Journal of Homosexuality, 30,* 59–92.

Sophie, J. (1988). Internalized homophobia and lesbian identity. In E. Coleman (Ed.), *Foundations of social work practice with lesbian and gay persons* (pp. 1–30). New York: Haworth Press.

Stein, T. S. (1998). Social construction and essentialism: Theoretical and clinical considerations relevant to psychotherapy. *Journal of Gay and Lesbian Psychotherapy, 2,* 29–49.

Steinhauer, J. (2001, February 11). Undeterred by a monster: Secrecy and stigma keep AIDS risk high for gay black men. *The New York Times,* pp. 37, 40.

Ubell, V., & Sumberg, D. (1992). Heterosexual therapists treating homosexual addicted clients. In D. L. Weinstein (Ed.), *Lesbians and gay men: Chemical dependency treatment issues* (pp. 19–33). New York: Haworth Press.

van Wormer, K., Wells, J., & Boes, M. (2000). *Social work with lesbians, gays, and bisexuals*. Boston: Allyn & Bacon.

Warn, D. J. (1997). Recovery issues of substance abusing gay men. In S. L. A. Straussner & E. Zelvin (Eds.), *Gender and addictions* (pp. 385–410). Northvale, NJ: Aronson.

Weinberg, T. S. (1994). *Gay men, drinking, and alcoholism*. Carbondale: Southern Illinois University Press.

Wooden, W. S., & Parker, J. (1982). *Men behind bars*. New York: Plenum Press.

Woody, G. E., Donnell, D., Seage, G. R., Metzger, D., Marmor, M., & Koblin, B. A. (1999). Non-injection substance use correlates with risky sex among men having sex with men: Data from HIVNET. *Drug and Alcohol Dependence, 53,* 197–205.

Zehner, M. A., & Lewis, J. (1985). Homosexuality and Alcoholism: Social and Developmental Perspectives. In R. Schoenberg & R. S. Goldberg (Eds.), *With compassion toward some: Homosexuality and social work in America* (pp. 75–89). New York: Harrington Park Press.

CHAPTER 19

Substance Abuse in Homeless Persons

Shelley Scheffler

Homelessness, to some, represents not having a permanent place to live; to others it is a state of being due to deviant individuals, and to still others it is the result of a failing society. With these varying views notwithstanding, the number of homeless persons has increased within the past 15–20 years. Currently, there are higher rates of women, children, and severely and persistently mentally ill individuals among the homeless population. It is important to note that, consistently through time, alcohol and other substance abuse has been coupled with homelessness both as the cause and the consequence (Baumohl, 1996).

According to the Stewart B. McKinney Act (1994),

> a person is considered homeless who lacks a fixed regular and adequate night time residence and has a primary night time residency that is: a supervised publicly or privately operated shelter designed to provide temporary living accommodations; an institution that provides a temporary residence for individuals intended to be institutionalized, or a public or private place not designed for, or ordinarily used as a regular sleeping accommodation for human beings. (National Coalition for the Homeless, 1999a, p. 6)

This chapter focuses on the prevalence, etiology, and treatment of substance abuse in homeless individuals. More specifically, the role of the social worker and the application of innovative approaches are highlighted.

THE HISTORICAL CONNECTION BETWEEN HOMELESSNESS AND SUBSTANCE ABUSE

Homelessness in the United States can be traced back to the settlement of the Western frontier, where unattached men, often cowboys and loggers, went to find work. Once the frontier was developed, job opportunities were reduced and many of these men took to the road. They came to be called "hobos," a name applied to those who wandered and worked, as opposed to "tramps," who wandered but did not work. Life on the road was often romanticized, and hobos were depicted as individuals who were not willing to comply with prevailing social norms. The economic depression of 1873 created widespread unemployment and its concomitant, homelessness. Run-down areas that provided cheap shelter to meet the needs of the poor came to be known as "skid row," a term taken from an area in Seattle filled with saloons, brothels, flophouses, and other facilities designed to meet the needs of homeless men. Studies of these areas show that alcohol played a major role in the lives of the inhabitants and often served as the context for social interaction (Garrett, 1989).

The economic prosperity of the 1920s saw a decline in homelessness, only to be followed by the devastating Great Depression, which created widespread poverty and an increased transient population. The United States pulled out of the Depression in the late 1930s. The prevailing view was that "those who remained homeless in the economic boom years and after World War II tended to be middle-aged male alcoholics and persons with deep emotional and psychological problems" (Leepson, 1982, p. 802).

Until the 1960s, consuming alcoholic beverages in public was a criminal offense, and "alcoholics" were considered "morally degenerate" rather than sick and in need of treatment. Often they were thrown in jail; the stereotype of the homeless person as alcoholic prevailed. In the 1960s alcoholism was decriminalized and designated a disease requiring specialized medical treatment. Although the homeless alcoholic person was no longer jailed for drinking, the stereotyping of homelessness as an alcohol-driven state was not diffused (Stark, 1992). At the same time that alcoholism was being defined as a disease, the Mental Health Act of 1964 paved the way for the deinstitutionalization of mentally ill people. Poor planning for the return of psychiatrically impaired individuals to the community contributed to a new group of people among the homeless population, not only those with mental illness, but a subgroup with co-occurring substance use disorders and mental illness.

CHARACTERISTICS OF HOMELESSNESS

A survey conducted in 1999 by the National Law Center on Homelessness and Poverty estimated that there are 700,000 people homeless on any given night, and up to 2 million people who experience homelessness during 1 year (National Coalition for the Homeless, 1999b). The U.S. Conference of Mayors conducted a study to determine the makeup of the homeless population. They found that among urban homeless people, 45% were single men, 38% were families, 25% were children under the age of 18, and 14% were single women (U.S. Conference of Mayors, 1998). Almost half (49%) of the homeless population was African American, greatly overrepresenting their numbers in the United States; 32% was Caucasian, 12% was Hispanic, 4% was Native American, and 3% was Asian. Of those surveyed, 46% cited domestic violence as a primary cause of homelessness. Research done by Koegal and associates (Koegal, Melamid, & Burman, 1996) found that 20–25% of the single-adult homeless population suffers from some form of severe and persistent mental illness. However, only 5% of the estimated 4 million people with a serious mental illness are homeless at any given point in time (Task Force on Homelessness and Severe Mental Illness, 1992).

Studies indicate that the lifetime prevalence of drug and/or alcohol abuse in homeless persons ranges between 30–60% (Toro, 1998; Toro et al., 1999) and that rates of alcohol, drug, and mental disorders are much higher in homeless groups than in the general population (Fischer & Breakey, 1991). A study of the relationship between alcoholism and homelessness found that the rates of alcoholism were as much as nine times higher than the general population, and about 10–20% higher among those in shelters than on the streets (U.S. Department of Housing and Urban Welfare, 1989). Of the 50,000 estimated homeless persons in New York City (NYC) in 1994, approximately half was estimated to be in need of chemical dependency treatment (Appel, 1995).

From the 1980s to 1990s, shifts in the economy and social systems contributed to an increase in the number of women, children, adolescents, and severely and persistently mentally ill people among the homeless population. Impacted by the shortages of low-income housing, changes in Social Security income eligibility, and welfare reform, young African American and Hispanic people became at higher risk for homelessness. In addition, serious health conditions such as HIV/AIDS, tuberculosis, and hepatitis C were major compounding factors in this vulnerable group. At the same time, alcohol, most frequently identified as the drug of choice by the homeless, was combined with the use of crack. The high-level addictiveness of crack cocaine resulted in a widespread use that created a new path to homelessness. For example, a survey of random urine samples collected in a NYC homeless shelter showed that 64% were positive for crack cocaine (Jencks, 1994).

Studies of homeless adults report that one-third to one-half have some form of physical illness that ranges from acute to chronic medical problems (Bassuk & Rosenberg, 1988). Reports on the prevalence of HIV infection show that there are higher rates in the homeless than the housed population, and that more people living on the street are infected than those who live in shelters. One study of homeless adults found that 9% of the population was HIV positive (Zolopa et al., 1994); another study of homeless psychiatric patients living in a shelter found a 19% prevalence rate (Susser, Valencia, & Conover, 1993). Hepatitis C, a serious blood-borne infection, also is reported to be rapidly increasing among the homeless population, particularly among drug-injecting users or HIV-infected individuals (HCH Clinicians' Network, 1999).

According to reports one-third of the homeless population is chronically mentally ill. Studies of homelessness among severely mentally ill adults show higher rates of alcohol and other drug abuse, greater symptom severity, and poorer family relationships than among those who were never homeless (Caton et al., 1994). The federally funded PATH program, which has served 127,231 homeless people, found that for those with reported diagnoses, 44% had schizophrenia or other psychotic disorders, 28% had affective disorders, and nearly half had co-occurring alcohol or other substance abuse problems (U.S. Department of Health and Human Services, 1996).

Throughout the history of homelessness, there has been a marked absence of literature on homeless women. The limited studies done in the 1960s and 1970s found that although fewer in number, homeless women were similar to their male counterparts and were frequently characterized as isolated, emotionally disturbed, alcoholic, and plagued with numerous health problems (Lam, 1987). Since the mid-1980s there has been a significant increase in the number of women who are homeless; currently, women comprise one-fifth of the homeless population. No longer characterized as "bag ladies" or "isolated alcoholics," their homeless status is primarily attributed to the feminization of poverty, domestic violence, and psychological and substance use disorders (Deming, McGoff-Yost, & Strozier, 2002; Rosencheck, Bassuck, & Salomon, 1999).

Researchers have explored the extent to which alcohol problems are an antecedent to homelessness. In a study comparing homeless individuals who drank heavily with those who did not, the results showed no significant difference in patterns of disaffiliation between the two groups and did not establish alcohol as the causative factor of homelessness (Garrett & Schutt, 1987). Another study by Caslyn and Morse (1991) found that the length of time spent homeless and the degree of transience were not predictive of alcohol problems, though there was a significant correlation with stress. This study did not clarify whether the high levels of stress existing prior to homelessness overwhelm an individual's adaptive coping ability, subsequently leading to drinking as a form of self-medication, or whether a preexisting drinking problem precipitates life crises that ultimately result in homelessness. One study compared homeless and never-homeless women and found that lifetime drug abuse was a risk factor for homelessness and that heroin and cocaine abuse were more common among homeless than never-homeless women (Caton et al., 2000).

A consistent trend throughout the research on homelessness shows that this population is more likely to have spent time in their youth in a foster care situation and/or have had other types of adverse childhood experiences, such as physical or sexual abuse (Koegal et al., 1995; Susser, Lin, Conover, & Struening, 1991). A study of homelessness, mental illness, and substance abuse found that many respondents grew up in families that lacked one or both parents, and even when parents were present, a majority of fathers and other family members are reported to be substance abusers and/or had psychiatric problems (Rahav et al., 1995).

Overall, research shows homelessness as both an effect and cause of substance abuse and serious mental and physical health problems. On one hand, substance abusers are more likely to become homeless than non-abusers; on the other hand, poverty and harsh living conditions may contribute to the risk for alcohol and drug abuse.

THEORIES OF HOMELESSNESS

Theories of homelessness vary, attributing homelessness to the person, the society, or social and economic factors. Social Darwinism, with its notion of "worthy" and "unworthy" poor (Blau, 1987) has had an ongoing and insidious influence in this country. The theory of homelessness due to personal choice or the personality of the individual originated in the 19th century and was based on the concept of "faulty constitution" (Jahiel, 1992). The influence of these beliefs is evident in the continuing stigmatization of substance abusers, the current limitations in eligibility requirements for Social Security benefits, and the stringent regulations for substance abusers in the Welfare reform movement. Within this framework, homeless persons with alcohol and other substance abuse problems are blamed for their homelessness, and access to benefits and services for the poor is tightly regulated.

Viewed from a social context, homelessness is seen as preceded by instances of marginal subsistence, losses, and failures (Jahiel, 1992). Commonly occurring among vulnerable people who are poor and whose early childhood experience left them ill prepared to take their place in a competitive world, the homeless population is frequently composed of single males from minority groups, with little education and few occupational skills, and with minimal possibility of obtaining help from friends and family who often are no better situated (Koegal, Burnam, & Baumohl, 1996). A related theory discusses the homeless population from the perspective of the "underclass"; that is, living in shelters and on the street may be part of the adaptive repertoire of an individual who may not be educated, is incapable of earning a decent living, and has different values from the prevailing society (Miller, 1996).

A structural view of homelessness proposes that there is a defect in the prevailing economic and social systems, and that homelessness is the end result when people are not able to pay for housing. In this view, homelessness is attributed to lack of employment, changes in public assistance benefits, and decreases in affordable housing, and is coupled with vulnerable individual characteristics, such as mental illness, substance abuse, minority status, or domestic violence.

THE IMPACT OF HOMELESSNESS

To further our understanding of homelessness, it is important to identify the impact of being without a home on the day-to-day functioning of an individual. Clearly, the absence of a stable environment that reflects an individual's "persona" has certain implications and consequences for psychosocial functioning (Jahiel, 1992). For most adult individuals and families, a home provides protection from the elements; a consistent place to eat, sleep, wash, and keep clothing clean; a place for possessions; a personal space and control over entry; accessibility by phone or mail; the opportunity to belong to a community; and personal dignity. Frequently, the loss of these protective factors quickly debilitates those with compromised or vulnerable coping skills. For example, homeless substance abusers use drugs and alcohol in public places. By doing so they open themselves to negative feedback and the withdrawal of public empathy, because they are judged by their behavior, not by the factors that may have precipitated or exacerbated their substance use disorder. It is not uncommon for an individual to transfer some of the needs that a home fills to the home they know, whether it is the street or the shelter. Social interactions among homeless persons are often based on the need for affiliation and protection of their sense of self. An example can be seen in the case of Ruth.

> Ruth is a 53-year-old white female who became homeless 10 years ago when her sister, with whom she lived, died. Together they had managed to keep a shabby one-room apartment, which Ruth found she could not do by herself and so entered the shelter system. Ruth has a 19-year-old son in a residential psychiatric facility. Although she speaks about him often, she does not know exactly where he is and has made no request for help in finding him. She drinks daily, frequently appearing to be drunk in the late afternoon, though she vehemently denies any drinking problem.
>
> Ruth describes her early childhood as very happy. She states that she attended an exclusive residential school with children whose parents were connected to the United Nations. She does not speak about

her parents, emphasizing instead the privilege she had of attending such a school. It is believed that, in reality, it was a home for abandoned children.

Ruth's daily life consists of doing laundry, ironing clothes, and participating in the shelter work program. She assists the supervisor with processing time sheets and answering phones. She has gained recognition because of her extreme efficiency, on which she prides herself. Her drinking begins primarily late in the day, and she can function until early afternoon. Because this is not a regular paying job, the supervisor tolerates her lateness and absenteeism. In the midst of shelter residents who often have either severe psychiatric problems or negative, hostile attitudes, she is seen as a high-functioning, valued resident. During her stay in the shelter, Ruth has refused offers to help her get a job or alternate housing, although she repeatedly talks about her wish to get a decent apartment in a decent neighborhood. At one point, she briefly became involved with an on-site case management program at the shelter, but quickly left when the social worker addressed her drinking problem.

The case of Ruth highlights many factors associated with alcohol and drug problems among the homeless population. Ruth experienced early loss of her family, although the reasons are unknown, and grew up in an institution. Prior to becoming homeless, she lived in poverty with her sister. Unable to sustain herself in the community after the loss of her sister, and burdened with all the stress and failure related to having a son with psychiatric problems, she came to the shelter. Within this context, normal needs for affiliation and affirmation were transferred to her existing environment and, from her view, met by the shelter staff, who became her social support network. These relationships helped her preserve her view of herself as a "worker" and therefore different from the other homeless women, and at the same time avoid facing her problem with alcohol.

Social interactions between homeless individuals are often focused on lengths of time being without a home. Individuals who are recently homeless or whose homelessness is sporadic focus on getting out of the shelter or off the streets. Their talk is usually about getting a job, an apartment, or other activities that will move them out of their homeless condition. The chronic homeless tend to focus on forming friendships and establishing their identities based on behavior related to homelessness, such as mastery at panhandling, getting food, and other skills needed for survival. Quick convivial relationships are formed around the sharing of meager resources, though at the same time there often is a distrust of peers and social bonds. Snow and Anderson (1993), in their study of homelessness, found that many homeless street people create an explanation of their homelessness that exempts them from personal responsibility and keeps the door open for positive change. For the homeless who use and abuse alcohol, interactions frequently revolve around survival activities and the procurement and consumption of alcohol. Commonly called "bottle gangs," these homeless individuals base their social interactions within the context of their alcohol use.

COMPREHENSIVE CARE FOR SUBSTANCE-ABUSING HOMELESS PERSONS

Helping homeless individuals requires a comprehensive approach along a continuum of care. Though we may not be able to accurately assess whether homelessness is the precipitating factor for substance abuse, or vice versa, we do know that the challenges to this group to recover and improve their lives is multifaceted. Studies of homeless persons that measured their hierarchy of needs reported that permanent housing, financial security, and employment were the highest on the list, followed by medical, mental health, and substance abuse treatment, and improving family and social contacts (e.g., Morse, 1999).

Jahiel (1992) proposes a three-pronged approach to caring for the homeless population. One prong attends to their immediate needs, which includes providing shelter, meals, mental health or substance abuse treatment, protection, and education aimed at improving the safety and quality of homeless life. Such services must be readily available, accessible, and acceptable to the recipients. The second prong includes services such as procurement of housing, income, and protected work, offered within the context and needs of homeless people. The third prong focuses on prevention and includes providing education and training for persons at risk, early treatment for mental disorders and substance abuse, prevention of housing or job displacement, raising wages, extending unemployment payments, and increasing the availability of low-income housing

Moving out of a state of homelessness is not a simple matter. In our affluent culture, it is often difficult to understand the extensive assistance necessary to prepare an individual for this transition. For instance, housing requires proof of identity as well as sufficient funds for security and the first month's rent. Landlords will not rent to those who present themselves shabbily dressed, unclean, or smelling of alcohol. To obtain work, a person needs adequate clothing, a way to clean him- or herself, and transportation. Sufficient funds for the initial period of work are needed until the first paycheck arrives. Telephone numbers and addresses are often necessary to receive information from a potential employer or landlord. These resources are not readily available to the homeless, nor are they easily obtained. Moreover, the adaptive strategies necessary to maintain oneself on the street or in the shelter are often skills that are not readily transferable to mainstream life.

The Priorities of Substance-Abusing Homeless Persons

Although there are many interpretations of the term *homelessness,* they all include the absence of housing. Therefore, getting housing first, before tackling other issues, is important in the process of reconnecting the homeless person to mainstream society. Growing research shows that meeting basic needs first is critical in approaching any of the other issues a homeless person or family may have. Wright, Rubin, and Devine (1998) assert that treatment for alcohol, drug, and mental health issues is rarely effective when it does not address the more fundamental issues of poverty, housing, welfare, and employment. In turn, treatment may be most effective when combined with the provision of housing. Sosin, Bruni, and Reidy (1995) found housing to be a major incentive for homeless people to remain in substance abuse treatment. Low-demand settings that seek to minimize barriers to access, impose few requirements, and expect motivation to be the result of the service, rather than a prerequisite for it, have the best prospects of facilitating and maintaining treatment involvement, particularly during the first phase of engagement (Burman et al., 1995). Oakley and Dennis (1996) found that housing stability is essential for successful substance abuse treatment and/or recovery that is combined with supportive services and meaningful daily activities in the community. Despite the evidence that positive treatment outcomes are associated with the provision of housing, substance abuse remains a major barrier to homeless persons seeking entry into housing programs (Burman et al., 1995).

INTERVENTIONS

The combination of substance abuse and homelessness is a multidetermined problem that requires comprehensive care. For many individuals with below-living wage incomes, the onset or exacerbation of an addictive disorder may be the catalyst to homelessness, and homelessness among those individuals with alcohol and other substance use disorders is frequently prolonged by the debilitating effects of their drug and alcohol use. Often, homeless individuals use alcohol and drugs as an immediate and available respite from their stressful living situations. However, by doing so, they frequently enter a vicious cycle whereby substance abuse interferes with actions that would move them from homelessness, and this failure contributes to their need to return to substance use for relief. There are many homeless substance abusers who wish to recover but need extensive help in overcoming barriers to treatment systems (National Coalition for the Homeless, 1999b).

Traditional substance abuse services are not usually prepared to deal with the issues that accompany people who are homeless. The needs of the substance-abusing homeless population cannot be successfully addressed within the narrow scope of recovery, with the presumption that once abstinence is achieved all the other pieces of the life puzzle will fall nicely into place. Not discounting the fact that the chances of lifestyle improvement certainly increase with sobriety, the solution to homelessness does not lie solely with the individual. Over the past 20 years, low-cost housing options have been significantly reduced due to economic and political trends. Therefore, even when a person is motivated toward recovery, the return to normal functioning is a challenging task once he or she has become homeless.

Intervening with homeless substance abusers requires a careful integration of case management services and substance abuse treatment within a strengths-based practice approach. As noted previously, we can no longer plainly say that homelessness is solely the result of addictive behavior. In a world where access to economic opportunities, education, and social and family support is limited by many factors, it is vital that we intervene with the homeless substance abuser in the context of the reality of his or her world.

Case Management Services

The need for self-esteem, physical and material well-being, and relief from psychic pain are factors that need to be addressed in efforts to successfully motivate and treat homeless substance abusers. A nationwide survey of services to the homeless found that exemplary programs have shifted their emphasis from detoxification and staff-intensive residential recovery program activities to housing and other support services aimed at the extensive needs of the homeless alcoholic person (Wittman, 1989).

Outreach and engagement efforts are sometimes critical in beginning the reconnecting process, especially for individuals who have been homeless for long periods of time and are experiencing severe mental illness and/or chronic substance abuse (Barrow, Hellman, Lovell, Plapinger, & Struening, 1991). The components of the continuum of care model proposed by the U.S. Department of Housing and Urban Development (1998) include outreach and assessment, immediate shelter, transitional housing with supportive services, and permanent housing. Social work skills are an essential part of this approach, which is often instituted by a team of professionals and consumers.

Case management assessments need to pay special attention to the client's current living situation including questions related to sleeping location, sources of food, support systems, presence of mental illness, use of alcohol and other drugs, exposure to violence or abuse, the cause of homelessness and plans for getting out of the homeless situation (Usatine, Gelberg, Smith, & Lesser, 1994). Of course, this assessment needs to be conducted within a culturally sensitive approach that does not overwhelm the person or disregard the presenting request for help.

Knowledge of homelessness and substance abuse need to be integrated with essential case management functions, which include (1) engaging clients who are often mistrusting of service delivery systems; (2) the ability to conduct psychosocial assessments and develop individualized service plans; (3) competence in crisis intervention and suicide assessment and prevention; and (4) networking abilities that develop linkages with local services and resources that can provide food, emergency shelter, housing, substance abuse treatment services, medical and psychiatric treatment, and all other services relevant to this population. Case management services also include monitoring clients' progress and needs, and the willingness to advocate for equity and appropriate services (Morse, 1999).

Initial approaches to the homeless substance abuser frequently require extensive outreach efforts. Mobile vans, drop-in centers, and strategically positioned outreach workers are often the essential ingredient in motivating an individual toward treatment, as exemplified in the following case.

John, a 27-year-old African American, had watched social workers from the municipal outreach program interview men at the local delicatessen, a daytime hangout for homeless people. One day he approached a worker to find out why he was there. The worker told him about the services available through his agency and offered him a cup of coffee. John told him that he had been without an apartment for the past 2 years, and although he and his buddy would rent a room whenever they got money, recently they both were living in the subway. John said that his friend smoked crack and that lately he was acting crazy; without provocation he was starting fights on the street, using drugs openly, and basically jeopardizing their tenuous existence. John stated he was worried and wanted to know if he could get help for him.

The worker recognized the possibility that John was not only talking about his friend but also himself. He told John about different resources in the community that would provide food, clothing, and shelter, as well as treatment. The worker offered to show him where to go, but John refused. Recognizing John's ambivalence, the worker did not push his offer; instead, he began to stop by to visit him when he was in the neighborhood. John was showing the apparent strain of living in the subway and seemed to welcome the worker's interest. The worker began talking about the difficulty John was having in getting help for his friend, and if it were not possible to obtain this help, to consider taking better care of himself. In their discussions, John admitted to smoking crack but stated that it was not a serious problem.

With the onset of the winter and the arrest of his friend, John seemed more willing to accept help for himself. The worker referred him to one of the smaller men's missions and made an appointment to see him the following week at the home office of the outreach team. John did well at the mission; he significantly reduced his drug use and kept his appointments with the social worker. After several weeks, the worker introduced the idea of a drug treatment program for John. Initially John refused, stating that he saw his primary problem as the need for money (this need was being addressed via an application for public assistance). As John began to trust the worker, he grew more open to the worker's recommendation that he attend an outpatient day treatment drug program that offered both educational and vocational services as well as housing assistance.

In this case, outreach performed in a known and nonthreatening setting helped John engage in the process of getting his needs met and becoming more motivated for treatment. The social worker's sensitivity and willingness to help with the client's stated priorities set the stage for an eventual exploration of treatment options.

Harm Reduction

Total abstinence has been the traditional goal of substance abuse services. However, not all substance abusers are able to achieve this goal, and therefore many forgo any of the benefits treatment provides. Harm reduction strategies serve to reduce the adverse effects of substance abuse until such time as the person is willing and able to enter the recovery process (Marlatt, Tucker, Donovan, & Vuchinich, 1997). Distributing bleach kits for cleaning needles, needle exchange programs, and methadone maintenance programs are all viable treatment options in the efforts to reduce drug seeking behavior and its concomitants such as drug dealing and criminal acts, and in helping individuals avoid HIV and other health hazards of street drug use.

Following the introduction of the harm reduction approach during the 1980s came other models of substance abuse treatment that approached recovery as a fluid process and emphasized the individualization of interventions. Treatment models such as motivational interviewing and the stages of change, strengths-based practice, solution-focused brief therapy, and cognitive-behavioral therapy shift the view of a "one-size-fits-all" recovery process to one that addresses the needs and priorities of individuals while emphasizing their strengths and abilities. These approaches have particular relevance to helping homeless substance abusers.

Strengths-Based Practice Approach

An important feature in working with homeless substance abusers is the ability to assess them within the framework of their functioning. In substance abuse treatment, a common question used to help people in recovery shift their negative view of life is to ask "Is the glass half empty or half full?" Yet often treatment providers themselves mirror the failure to see the positive. Assessment and treatment tend to be problem oriented, emphasizing the "half empty" without recognizing the incredible strengths needed to survive extremely adverse conditions, whether it be homelessness or the sequelae of substance abuse. The strengths-based perspective emphasizes the power of the self to heal with the help of the environment (Saleebey, 1992). Applying this model helps clinicians appreciate clients' coping abilities and identify their strengths. Together, worker and client have the opportunity to develop a plan based on hopefulness and possibilities.

Solution-Focused Brief Therapy

The model of solution-focused therapy helps clients engage their own unique resources and strengths in solving their problems. When used with the substance-abusing homeless client, it promotes the evaluation of existing skills and the process of change. Often, homeless people are reluctant to enter treatment because the distance from where they are to where they feel they are expected to be seems too great. In solution-focused treatment the worker collaborates with the client in developing solution-building activities that utilize *existing resources*. If a client is hungry, the solution is to eat, and the plan may be to go to soup kitchens, food pantries, etc. This treatment approach emphasizes negotiating treatment goals that are (1) small, specific, and measurable; (2) described situationally; (3) stated in interactional and interpersonal terms; (4) focused on the presence rather than the absence of something; and (5) realistic and immediately achievable within the context of the client's life.

Using the concept of exceptions—those periods of time when the client does *not* experience the problem or complaint for which he or she is seeking treatment—helps worker and client identify potential solutions for the client's problems (Berg & Reuss, 1998; de Shazer, 1991). The technique of identifying exceptions is applicable to substance abuse treatment, in that it is rare for any addiction to progress without periods of reduction in use or attempts at abstinence.

> Felipe is a 35-year-old Hispanic man with an 18-year history of drug and alcohol abuse. He had been living with his girlfriend for the past 3 years in her apartment and had a low-paying but steady job. When they separated, he went to live with his mother who resides in a federally funded housing project for seniors. Neighbors complained about Felipe's behavior while under the influence of drugs and alcohol, and his mother received a letter warning her about illegally housing people not on her lease. Frightened of being evicted, she asked Felipe to leave,

permitting him to shower and eat there occasionally. Unable to get to work regularly, he then lost his job.

Felipe had been raised by his mother and her boyfriend and had never met his biological father. He is the third of four children and reports a good relationship with two of his sisters; he does not know the whereabouts of his older brother. He left school after the completing the 11th grade and was attending a GED program until the recent changes in his life occurred. From the time that Felipe left school, he has managed to care for himself by working at low-paying jobs; his longest period of employment was 4 years. Felipe began using crack cocaine at age 17, and heroin and alcohol at 19. However, from his view he has always been able to function while using, and has had periods of abstinence until recently. Prior to the breakup of his relationship with his girlfriend, she had asked him to go into drug treatment, but he had refused.

Being homeless, jobless, withdrawing from drugs, and without any money, Felipe began sleeping in the train station, trying to avoid being bothered by the police. He met other homeless men, who shared drugs, alcohol, and information about surviving on the streets with him. They told him about a mobile medical van that parked outside the train station on a regular basis and offered free services. Feeling desperate and sick, Felipe went there for help. After a preliminary medical exam, the worker gave him a sandwich and coffee, talked to him about drug treatment, and gave him a referral to an outpatient methadone maintenance program.

In the initial phase of treatment, while Felipe was being brought to a stabilizing dose of methadone, the social worker helped him develop realizable treatment goals. His priorities were housing and employment. Recognizing that permanent housing was not an immediate option, going to a shelter seemed the most viable short-term alternative. In this case, the worker addressed the client's priorities and worked with him in developing a plan that emphasized options and choices within a realistic framework. Felipe would live in a shelter while he continued looking for a place to live. From his view, returning to stable housing was the first step in his recovery process. Using the concept of exceptions in this solution-based treatment, Felipe was asked to identify times in his life when he had maintained an apartment, a job, a relationship, and reduced his drug and alcohol abuse. The worker used this approach to build motivation and help Felipe recognize the strengths he already possessed that would help him recover from his substance abuse problems.

This case example highlights the shift away from classical approaches to treating substance abusers, where the demand for abstinence transcends all other needs. Traditionally, "hitting bottom" is seen as a prerequisite to the recovery process, a window of opportunity for motivating abstinence and recovery. Although such an approach may work for some, for many homeless individuals, the "bottom" is so deep they are not able to use it as a steppingstone upward. Solution-focused treatment emphasizes small, achievable goals based on clients' needs and drawing upon their existing strengths. Such an approach helps promote positive feelings in the completion of doable tasks and the incremental accomplishments.

Stages of Change and Motivational Interviewing

The stages of change model (Prochaska & DiClimente, 1986) offers a framework with which to assess clients' readiness to change. As indicated by Hanson and El-Bassel in Chapter 2, five fluid stages form the recovery process. A precontemplation phase describes individuals who do not see their substance abuse as a problem and therefore are not ready to enter the stages of change that treatment requires. Assessment within this model promotes the age-old social work theory of "starting where the client is at." The stages of change assessment is the guide for selecting strategies from motivational interviewing, an approach that is designed to engage and enhance the client's intrinsic motivation to change. One of the many important features of this model is that it moves away from the traditional labeling of clients as "resistant" when they are not committed to change, and instead uses various techniques to build motivation. Five basic motivational principles underlying this approach support the idea that motivation for change occurs when individuals perceive a discrepancy between where they are and where they want to be (Miller & Rollnick, 1991), as demonstrated in the following case example.

> Mary, 35 years old, is the white mother of two children ages 5 and 6. She has an 18-year history of drug abuse and has been in and out of treatment facilities, with intermittent periods of recovery for up to 3 years. Mary has a high school education and has worked as a secretary during her drug-free periods. Four years ago she met Michael, a crack dealer in her neighborhood. He moved into her apartment with her two children (from a previous relationship) and stayed there until his incarceration for drug dealing 6 months ago.
>
> Mary attributes her current crack addiction to fear that Michael would leave her unless she was using drugs with him. At the time he was arrested their rent was 6 months in arrears and Mary and her children were evicted. She tried to survive on the street by panhandling to feed her children, but a neighbor notified the child welfare authorities. The children were removed and placed in foster care, and Mary was mandated to treatment as part of the plan to have her children returned to her care.
>
> Although she complied by applying for admission to an outpatient program, without her children, she had a difficult time conceptualizing recovery for herself. Never having been separated from them,

she was convinced that she would never get them back. Homeless and without any resources, Mary began exchanging sex for drugs and a place to stay.

Mary met with a worker at the drug treatment program, who referred her to a shelter for temporary housing. Once her immediate needs were addressed, the next step was to help her feel motivated to participate in a recovery process. Using the stages of change model, Mary was assessed as being in the contemplative stage. She knew that her drug use was a problem but felt unable to stop.

Within an empathic framework, the worker assisted Mary in exploring the positives and negatives of her addiction. The positive aspects for Mary were that she did not feel nervous and overwhelmed when she was using, and that using drugs was something that she and Michael had shared. The main negative aspect was that her children would not be returned until she stopped using. Yet she was unsure that she could even handle her children without Michael and drugs. Mary was not ready to identify her high-risk drug-seeking behavior as negative; instead, she saw it as a need based on her impoverished circumstances. The worker used problem-solving techniques to help Mary identify other ways to address her nervousness and feelings of being overwhelmed. She also reframed Mary's ambivalent statements, supporting her strengths in caring for her children and her stated wish to have them returned. These techniques were used to increase Mary's motivation where she was at: within the contemplative stage of recovery.

WORKERS' ROLES AND EXPECTATIONS

Workers find that it is often difficult to engage homeless substance abusers because of their distrust of authority and wariness of service providers. In addition, the lifestyle of homeless individuals is often incompatible with the structure and requirements of treatment services. When homeless people do come for help, it is rarely a simple case; extensive intervention and creativity in connecting them to different services are usually required (McMurray-Avila, 1997).

Working with this population requires great flexibility on many levels. The worker may need to make referrals for entitlements or locate a nearby soup kitchen to meet the needs of the client. At the same time, the worker needs to address the problems of substance abuse and often has to work with a client who may be physically repulsive due to lack of clean clothing and bathing facilities. It is important that workers have patience in approaching clients and realize that it may take an extraordinary amount of time to build a working relationship. Prognosis is often poor, and it is important to keep expectations based in reality.

The plight of the homeless population often taps into some of the deeper, darker fears that we, as humans, all carry within ourselves. The fear of being alone in the world, without shelter, friends or family, or the ability to alter our situation often underlies clinicians' reluctance to become involved with helping homeless clients. Such countertransference reactions also may impact clinicians' ability to continue this kind of work for any length of time.

Supervision and staff support can often mediate some of the stress from working with this population. It is important for workers to be able to identify countertransference issues as they arise and to articulate them in a supportive and understanding environment. Seasoned workers, by sharing their experiences, can help newer workers prepare for some of the uncomfortable feelings that occur in working with this population. In addition, balancing caseloads with both motivated and difficult clients helps to prevent burnout.

The positive aspect of working with this population is that some do recover and return to a reasonably normal life. Being part of the process of helping someone who is coming from the depths of desperation can be an inspiring experience. In working with a group whose needs are so great, any intervention, even one as small as getting a client a meal, immediately alleviates some of his or her misery.

CONCLUSION

The issue of loss has always been a part of the progression of substance abuse, whether it is loss of family, friends, work, or material goods. Among these many losses today is the possible loss of a permanent place to live. Given current economic and social factors, once a person has become homeless, the options for returning to a reasonable place to live have become increasingly limited. It is critical that social workers are aware of the impact that becoming and being homeless creates and begin to intervene in meaningful ways. Workers need to explore interventions that are appropriate for helping homeless persons and that recognize the importance of prioritizing needs and individualizing treatment. Recent trends in substance abuse treatment view recovery as a dynamic process and are more compatible with the challenges of homelessness. Integrating case management services and substance abuse treatment along a continuum of care is essential in enhancing recovery opportunities for the homeless substance abuser. Models of treatment such as solution-based therapy and motivational interviewing embrace the notion of starting where the client is at, emphasize the need for active integration of clients in their own treatment, and promote an individualized approach to recovery. These views of substance abuse reflect the values and skills of the social work profession and appropriately address the needs of the homeless substance-abusing population.

REFERENCES

Appel, P. W. (1995). *New York state transient survey: Final report*. Albany, NY: Office of Alcoholism and Substance Abuse Services.

Barrow, S. M., Hellman, F., Lovell, A. M., Plapinger, J. D., & Struening, E. L. (1991). Evaluating outreach services: Lessons from a study of five programs. In N. Cohen (Ed.), *Psychiatric outreach to the mentally ill (New Directions for Mental Health Services*, Vol. 52, pp. 29–45). San Francisco: Jossey-Bass.

Bassuk, E. L., & Rosenberg, L. (1988). Why does family homelessness occur? A case-control study. *American Journal of Public Health, 78*(7), 783–788.

Baumohl, J. (Ed.). (1996). *Homelessness in America*. New York: Oryx Press.

Berg, I. K., & Reuss, N. H. (1998). *Solutions step by step: A substance abuse treatment manual*. New York: Norton.

Blau, J. S. (1987). *The homeless of New York: A case study in social welfare policy*. Unpublished doctoral dissertation, Columbia University, New York.

Burman, M. A., Morton, S. C., McGlynn, E. A., Peterson, L. P., Stecher, B. M., Hayes, C., & Vaccaro, J. V. (1995). An experimental evaluation of residential and non-residential treatment for the dually diagnosed homeless adults. *Journal of Addictive Disorders, 14*(4), 111–134.

Caslyn, R. J., & Morse, G. A. (1991). Correlates of problem drinking among homeless men. *Hospital and Community Psychiatry, 42*(7), 721–725.

Caton, C. L. M., Hasin, D., Shrout, P. E., Opler, L. A., Hirshfield, S., Dominguez, B., & Felix, A. (2000). Risk factors for homelessness among indigent urban adults with no history of psychotic illness: A case-control study. *American Journal of Public Health, 90*(2), 258–263.

Caton, C. L. M., Shrout, P. E., Eagle, P. F., Opler, L. A., Felix, A., & Dominguez, B. (1994). Risk factors for homelessness among schizophrenic men: A case-control study. *American Journal of Public Health, 84*, 265–270.

Deming, A. M., McGoff-Yost, K., & Strozier, A. (2002). Homeless addicted women. In S. L. A. Straussner & S. Brown (Eds.), *The handbook of addiction treatment for women* (pp. 451–469). San Francisco: Jossey-Bass.

Garrett, G. R. (1989). Alcohol problems and homelessness: History and research. *Contemporary Drug Problems, 16*, 301–330.

de Shazer, S. (1991). *Putting difference to work*. New York: Norton.

Garrett, G. R., & Schutt, R. K. (1987). The homeless alcoholic: Past and present. In *Homelessness: Critical issues for policy and practice* (pp. 29–32). Boston: Boston Foundation.

HCH Clinicians' Network. (1999, March). Chronic hepatitis C: Silent intruder, insidious threat. *Healing Hands, 3*(2), 32.

Jahiel, R. I. (1992). *Homelessness: A prevention oriented approach*. Baltimore: Johns Hopkins University Press.

Jencks, C. (1994). *The homeless*. Cambridge, MA: Harvard University Press.

Koegel, P., Burnam, M. A., & Baumohl, J. (1996). The causes of homelessness. In J. Baumohl (Ed.), *Homelessness in America* (pp. 24–34). New York: Oryx Press.

Koegal, P., Melamid, E., & Burman, M. A. (1995). Childhood risk factors for homelessness among homeless adults. *American Journal of Public Health, 85*(12), 1642–1649.

Lam, J. (1987). *Homeless women in America: Their social and health characteristics.* Unpublished doctoral dissertation, University of Massachusetts, Amherst.

Leepson, M. (1982). *The homeless: Growing national problem.* Washington, DC: Editorial Research Reports.

Marlatt, G. A., Tucker, J. A., Donovan, D. M., & Vuchinich, R. E. (1997). Help-seeking by substance abusers: The role of harm reduction and behavioral–economic approaches to facilitate treatment entry and retention. *NIDA Research Monograph, 165,* 44–84.

McMurray, A. M. (1997). *Organizing health services for homeless people.* Nashville, TN: National Health Care for the Homeless Council.

Miller, K. (1996). Gimme shelter: The communication of America's homeless. In E. Ray (Ed.), *Communication and disenfranchisement* (pp. 79–94). Mahwah, NJ: Erlbaum.

Miller, W. R., & Rollnick, S. (1991). *Motivational interviewing: Preparing people to change addictive behavior.* New York: Guilford Press.

Morse, G. (1999). A review of case management for people who are homeless: Implications for practice, policy and research. In L. B. Fosburg & D. L. Dennis (Eds.), *Practical lessons: The 1998 National Symposium on Homelessness research* (Vol. 7, pp. 1–34). Washington, DC: U.S. Department of Housing and Urban Development, U.S. Department of Health and Human Services.

National Coalition for the Homeless. (1999a). *Homelessness in America: Unabated and increasing.* Washington, DC: Author.

National Coalition for the Homeless. (1999b). *Who is homeless?* (NCH Fact Sheet #3). Washington, DC: Author.

Oakley, D. A., & Dennis, D. L. (1996). Responding to the needs of homeless people with alcohol, drug and/or mental disorders. In J. Baumohl (Ed.), *Homelessness in America* (pp. 179–186). New York: Oryx Press.

Rahav, M., Rivera, J. J., Nuttbrock, L., Ng-Mak, D., Sturz, E. L., Link, B. G., Struening, E. L., Pepper, B., & Gross, B. (1995). Characteristics and treatment of homeless, mentally ill, chemical abusing men. *Journal of Psychoactive Drugs, 27*(1), 93–103.

Rosencheck, R., Bassuck, E., & Salomon, A. (1999). Special populations of homeless Americans. In L. B. Fosburg & D. L. Dennis (Eds.). *Practical lessons: The 1998 National Symposium on Homelessness research* (Vol. 2, pp. 1–29). Washington, DC: U.S. Department of Housing and Urban Development, U.S. Department of Health and Human Services.

Saleebey, D. (1992). *The strengths perspective in social work practice.* New York: Longman.

Snow, D. A., & Anderson, L. (1993). *Down on their luck: A study of homeless people on the street.* Berkeley & Los Angeles: University of California Press.

Sosin, M., Bruni, M., & Reidy, M. (1995). Paths and impacts in the progressive independence model: A homeless and SA intervention in Chicago. *Journal of Addictive Diseases, 14*(4).

Stark, L. (1992). Barriers to health care for homeless people. In R. Jahiel (Ed.), *Homelessness: A prevention oriented approach.* Baltimore: Johns Hopkins University Press.

Susser, E. S., Lin S. P., Conover, S. A., & Struening, E. L. (1991). Childhood antecedents of homelessness in psychiatric patients. *American Journal of Psychiatry,* *148,* 1026–1030.

Susser, E., Valencia, E., & Canover, S. (1993). Prevalence of HIV infection among psychiatric patients in a New York City men's shelter. *American Journal of Public Health, 83*(4), 568–570.

Task Force on Homelessness and Severe Mental Illness. (1992). *Outcasts on Main Street.* Washington, DC: Interagency Council on Homelessness.

Toro, P. A. (1998). Homelessness. In A. S. Bellack & M. Hersen (Eds.), *Comprehensive clinical psychology. Vol. 9: Applications in diverse populations* (pp. 119–135). New York: Pergamon Press.

Toro, P. A., Wolfe, S. M., Bellavia, C. W., Thomas, D. M., Rowland, L. L., Daeschler, C. V., & McCaskill, P. A. (1999). Obtaining representative samples of homeless persons: A two-city study. *Journal of Community Psychology, 27*(2), 157–178.

Usatine, R. P., Gelberg, L., Smith, M. H., & Lesser, J. (1994). Health care for the homeless: A family medicine perspective. *American Family Physician, 46,* 139–146.

U.S. Conference of Mayors. (1998). *A status report on hunger and homelessness in America's cities.* Washington, DC: Author.

U.S. Department of Health and Human Services. (1996). *Projects for assistance in transition from homelessness.* Rockville, MD: Author.

U.S. Department of Housing and Urban Development. (1998). *The 1998 National Symposium on Homelessness research.* Washington, DC: Author.

U.S. Department of Housing and Urban Welfare. (1989). *Report on the 1988 National Survey of Shelters for the Homeless.* Washington, DC: Author.

Wittman, F. D. (1989). Housing models for alcohol programs serving homeless people. *Contemporary Drug Problems, 16,* 483–504.

Wright, J. D., Rubin, B. A., & Devine, J. A. (1998). *Beside the golden door: Policy, politics and the homeless.* New York: Aldine de Gruyter.

Zolopa, A., Hahn, J., Gorter, R., Miranda, J., Wlodarczyk, D., Peterson, J., Pilote, L., & Moss, A. (1994). HIV and tuberculosis infection in San Francisco's homeless adults. *Journal of the American Medical Association, 272*(6), 455–461.

CHAPTER 20

HIV/AIDS and Intravenous Drug Users

Issues and Treatment Implications

Larry M. Gant
Diane Pincus Strom

Ms. N., a 38-year-old black woman, learned she had HIV when her 3-year-old daughter became sick. Ms. N. had stopped using drugs intravenously some years earlier out of fear of becoming infected. It was a shock to learn she had stopped too late. The child, in fact, subsequently died. A 4-year-old daughter also carries an AIDS diagnosis, and a 7-year-old son is showing early symptoms of HIV infection. An 11-year-old, however, is completely healthy. Ms. N., who is divorced, waits for her own symptoms to develop. For a time, Ms. N. was on a combination drug treatment regimen, but her physician informed her that she was among the 40% of persons living with HIV that does not respond to combination therapy. She also was informed that combination therapy protocols have not been well developed for children and youth. She thus prays to remain healthy long enough to see her children die; otherwise, who will care for them?

C., a 57-year-old Puerto Rican woman, has reluctantly agreed to have her 23-year-old son live with her; in the past he has stolen from her neighbors, and she is not sure he can be trusted. Now, however, he is dying of AIDS. She knows how to care for him because his two older brothers also died of AIDS, and she cared for them.

Human immunodeficiency virus (HIV) and acquired immune deficiency syndrome (AIDS) are both medical diagnoses; however, they reflect broader

443

implications than medical ones alone. HIV/AIDS has a significant impact not only on the person with AIDS but also on his or her significant others and on all of society. Children also may be infected, as Ms. N.'s three younger children are, or left orphaned, as her oldest child may likely be; parents such as C. are caring for their adult sons and daughters as they lay dying; hospital resources are strained, as hospitals and staff struggle with care and treatment issues with a disease that—due to medical innovations in the United States—vacillates between being fatal and manageable, if chronic and expensive. Problems of drug use and treatment, poverty, homelessness, discrimination, and inequitable resource allocation, all long-standing social ills, have been intensified by HIV/AIDS.

There are strong associations between HIV/AIDS and substance abuse, suggesting that the epidemics of HIV/AIDS and substance abuse are "co-occuring." Such observers suggest that it is inappropriate to ignore the larger oppressive social, political, and economic forces that have led to the "ghettoization" of black and Hispanic populations in the inner cities, where there are high levels of drug trafficking, unemployment, poverty, and racism—all of which are building blocks for high rates of addiction and HIV infection. It is within these urban, poor, black and Hispanic communities that HIV/AIDS is most prevalent today (Stine, 1999; Stokes & Peterson, 1998).

Many intravenous drug users living with HIV/AIDS can access a comprehensive range of services provided through the Ryan White Comprehensive AIDS Resources Emergency (CARE) Act of 1990. Nonetheless, because of circumstances directly or indirectly related to their drug use, intravenous drug users with HIV/AIDS often require additional intervention to cope with their medical status and psychosocial situation. This chapter examines the specific needs of intravenous drug users with AIDS or HIV infection and delineates the multiple tasks facing social workers and other professionals concerned with providing services to these individuals.

BACKGROUND AND DEFINITION OF AIDS

In early 1981, unofficial sources reported that homosexual men in Los Angeles and New York were developing a rare form of pneumonia called pneumocystis carinii pneumonia (PCP). By mid-1981 a total of 26 homosexual men were officially recorded as having either PCP or Kaposi's sarcoma (KS), an equally rare form of cancer. One name used for the syndrome at that time was gay-related immune deficiency (GRID); despite this designation, by late 1981 the condition also had been identified in intravenous drug users. The dual necessities of (1) advancing federal legislation and funding and (2) destigmatizing gay men were driving forces that led to the transformation, facilitated by the Centers for Disease Control and Prevention (CDC) of GRID to HTLV-III and ultimately to HIV/AIDS (Shilts, 1987).

Sharing syringes and other equipment for drug injection is a well known route of HIV transmission, yet injection drug use contributes to the epidemic's spread far beyond the circle of those who inject: People who have sex with an intravenous drug user also are at risk for infection through the sexual transmission of HIV. Furthermore, children conceived by mothers who contracted HIV through sharing needles or having sex with an intravenous drug user may become infected in utero or postnatally as well. In 2001, the annual rate (incidence) of AIDS among men ages 25–44 years was five times higher for African American men (1 in 350) than for white men (1 in 8,000), and twice as high as Hispanic men (1 in 800) (CDC, 1998). Researchers from the National Cancer Institute reported data indicating that 1 in 250 white men ages 27–39 may be HIV infected, compared to 1 in 33 African American men and 1 in 85 Hispanic men in the same age group. Over 75% of HIV cases attributed to drug use are African American men.

Although two-thirds (69%) of HIV/AIDS cases attributed to drug use are male, the percentage of women with HIV/AIDS has been rising steadily between 1990 and 2000; indeed, AIDS cases among women and adolescent girls increased by 364% between 1991 and 1997 (American Psychiatric Association, 2000). Heterosexual contact with HIV-infected men is the leading risk category for women (38%); however, 29% of HIV/AIDS cases in women result from their intravenous drug use (CDC, 1998). African American and Hispanic women are disporportionately affected, with AIDS rates 17 and 6 times higher, respectively, than for white women (American Psychiatric Association, 2000). IDU-associated AIDS accounts for a larger proportion of cases in women than men, although the epidemiological reasons are not well understood. Since the epidemic began, 58% of all AIDS cases in women have been attributed to injection drug use or sex with partners who inject drugs, compared with 31% of cases in men.

According to the Centers for Disease Control and Prevention (CDC, 1998, 1999), as many as one-third of the nation's 1.2 million intravenous drug users may be HIV infected. Moreover, many infected persons have had drug-using heterosexual partners, and many infants had one or more parents who used or injected drugs. When these linked populations are considered, drug-use-related transmission accounts for one-third (32%) of people living with HIV disease in the United States.

Noninjection drugs (such as crack cocaine) also contribute to the spread of the epidemic when users trade sex for drugs or money, or when they engage in risky sexual behaviors that they might not engage in when sober. One CDC study of more than 2,000 young adults in three inner-city neighborhoods found that crack smokers were three times more likely to be infected with HIV than nonsmokers (Stine, 1999).

HIV can be transmitted via three routes:

1. Unprotected sexual transmission between infected and uninfected individuals, whether the partners are both male, both female (although somewhat rare), or male and female.
2. Exposure to blood through the sharing of needles by drug users, or through transfusion of blood, plasma, packed cells, platelets, or factor concentrates.
3. Perinatal (vertical) transmission occurring during pregnancy, the birth process, or breastfeeding.

Intravenous drug users are potentially at risk in all categories, in so far as they may share needles, are sexually active, and give birth to infected infants.

CHARACTERISTICS OF INTRAVENOUS DRUG USERS

Theories describing the genesis of addictive behavior and related personality disorders draw from a broad range of models and consider numerous biopsychosocial determinants (Alexander, 1990; Chein, Donald, Lee, & Rosenfeld, 1964; Khantzian, 1980, 1985; Mendelson & Mello, 1995; Vaillant, 1975; Wurmser, 1974; Zinberg, 1975). Although it is not within the scope of this chapter to examine these theories, it should be noted that some of the characteristics frequently associated with addiction may have an impact on intravenous drug users' capacity to (1) cope with an AIDS diagnosis (Caputo, 1985), (2) avail themselves of treatments available for HIV infection, and (3) relate to family, friends, health care professionals, and others involved with their treatment and/or care (Flanagan, 1989). The characteristics discussed below may be particularly salient.

Intolerance of Overwhelming Affect

Intravenous drug users frequently have difficulty tolerating anxiety, sadness, or other intense emotions (Wurmser, 1974). A positive result to an HIV test, naturally anxiety provoking for anyone, may be totally unbearable for intravenous drug users. One way they may deal with this is to refrain from taking the test altogether; another is to increase drug use, despite awareness of how hazardous this may be, as a means of numbing the emotional pain.

W. is a 25-year-old Puerto Rican male intravenous drug users with AIDS. He shared needles with his older brother, who died of AIDS about 1 year prior to W.'s diagnosis. After an initial drug-free period accompanied by good medical compliance, W. resumed IV drug use. He stated that he saw no point in remaining drug free; he was going to die, whatever he might do, so why not live the time he had left free of anxiety?

Use of Maladaptive Defenses

Because of their inability to tolerate painful affects, intravenous drug users frequently employ defense mechanisms that allow them to distort reality and thereby avoid constructively confronting their circumstances. Two such mechanisms are denial and externalization. Denial may keep intravenous drug users from examining their potential risk for HIV infection or lead them to claim that a positive result on an HIV test is a mistake. Whereas denial is used adaptively by many people, particularly when faced with a serious medical condition, intravenous drug users may be able to deny reality almost to the point of delusion.

> R. is a 27-year-old African American woman who claims to have been free of intravenous drugs for the last 6 months. She is hospitalized with fever and complains of recent weight loss. Her husband, whom she has not seen in 5 weeks, is believed to be hospitalized elsewhere with AIDS-related symptoms. R. states that she has not shared needles with him, or anyone else, for the last 2 years. She is certain that she cannot possibly be infected and, in fact, must be suffering from a "virus." She does recall nodding out on many occasions and awakening to find that her husband had used her syringes and admits that he may have used them at other times without her knowledge. Nevertheless, she feels she is not really at risk for infection.

The defense of externalization permits intravenous drug users to absolve themselves of responsibility related to the circumstances of their lives (e.g., HIV status, drug use, living situation) and instead to place the blame on others.

> C. is a 23-year-old white woman who supports her drug habit (heroin and crack) by working as a prostitute. Although she has been an intravenous drug user for some 6 years, she believes that the cause of her HIV infection is the sexual contacts she has had. Her partners are to blame for her situation; she is their victim. She therefore refuses to discontinue prostitution, stating, "Some guy gave this to me—what do I care if I give it to some other guy?"

Avoidance of Emotional Dependence

It is not uncommon for intravenous drug users to have experienced severe disappointments in their relationships with parents, other family members, friends, and lovers. Drugs, on the other hand, are generally more reliable; they are neither rejecting nor critical, and as long as there is money to pay for them, they are available. Drug users are very comfortable with their drugs but they may be apprehensive about emotionally involving themselves with people. This resistance to forming relationships may make it difficult for the social worker or other health care professional to establish a working alliance that can then be used to encourage compliance with medical and psychosocial recommendations.

Borderline and Narcissistic Personality Disorders

Intravenous drug users frequently exhibit characteristics associated with borderline and narcissistic personality structures. Of particular significance is a tendency to engage in impulsive, self-damaging behaviors, inappropriate anger, marked shifts of attitude, affect instability, and chronic feelings of emptiness (American Psychiatric Association, 1994; National Association of Social Workers HIV/AIDS Spectrum Project, 2001a, 2001b). These characteristics frequently lead to countertransference reactions on the part of health care providers and, perhaps, more importantly, may make it difficult for intravenous drug users to accept the treatment that is available to them (CSAT, 2000).

Paucity of Resources

Intravenous drug users often have neither the concrete resources nor the psychosocial stability necessary to cope with day-to-day living, much less with the stress associated with a diagnosis of AIDS. The task of planning for ongoing care is arduous, since family and environmental supports may not exist. As noted, many intravenous drug users living with HIV/AIDS can access a comprehensive range of services provided through the Ryan White Comprehensive AIDS Resources Emergency (CARE) Act of 1990. For the most part, however, lack of drug treatment resources (e.g., available treatment slots, appropriate programs for women with children) and the challenges of integrating drug treatment and HIV/AIDS services continue to be two major reasons for discharge delays, frequent lapse and relapse, and insufficient care (CSAT, 2000; National Association of Social Workers HIV/AIDS Spectrum Project, 2001a, 2001b).

Clearly, intravenous drug users, hampered by many troubling characteristics, are ill equipped to cope with HIV infection and AIDS. It is against this backdrop that the physical, social, and emotional implications of HIV infection and its treatment for intravenous drug users may now be explored.

PHYSICAL MANIFESTATIONS AND IMPLICATIONS

Intravenous drug users are at higher risk than the general population for such diseases as tuberculosis, endocarditis, and pneumonia due to their generally poor physical condition. An HIV-infected intravenous drug user who is asymptomatic for HIV disease itself may have significant other medical problems and physical discomfort. The symptoms of HIV disease and AIDS range in severity and have different impacts on how patients look, how they feel, and how capable they are of functioning.

Appearance

Most early signs of HIV infection are not visible ("asymtomatic") and, in that respect, allow the patient to feel "anonymous." Later symptoms are not as kind. Kaposi's sarcoma, for example, although more frequently found in homosexual men, is also occasionally seen in intravenous drug users and is manifested by skin lesions that are easily noticed. Other skin conditions, such as dermatitis or herpes, are also often evident. Oral thrush, characterized by multiple white nodules in the mouth, is a common symptom. Wasting syndrome, involving significant weight loss, leaves patients severely emaciated and weakened. Patients with these symptoms frequently feel "marked" and are embarrassed to leave their homes for fear of being identified as having AIDS. New treatment protocols and regimens may delay the onset of physical manifestations of these opportunistic infections and the asymptomatic phase. However, after approximately 18 months, symptoms inevitably appear in the majority of persons living with HIV/AIDS (American Psychiatric Association, 2000).

Feeling Sick

As HIV systematically destroys the immune system, patients are more likely to become ill more often and take longer time to recover. The symptoms of HIV infection not only leave patients concerned about their appearance but also cause them to feel seriously ill. They may have to cope with pneumonias that lead to shortness of breath and, in the worst scenarios, are life threatening. Other infections may result in severe headaches, blindness, unending fevers, ongoing weakness, body pain, and enlargement of the lymph nodes. Patients may become completely dependent on others for an aspects of care, including feeding, toileting, bathing, and, in some instances, movement. Dementia is another possible manifestation.

In addition to feeling ill because of AIDS, intravenous drug users may continue to be addicted and thus have severe physical discomfort related to drug cravings. Their ability to tolerate this distress and remain drug free (often with the assistance of methadone or other pharmaceuticals) will ultimately influence the effectiveness of those medical treatments that are available to them.

COPING WITH TREATMENTS

With the advent of protease inhibitors combination therapy (often called "drug cocktails") and highly aggressive AIDS retroviral therapy (HAART), the number of treatments available for reducing viral load (i.e., the amount of HIV in the bloodstream) has exploded (American Psychiatric Association, 2000; CSAT, 2000). There also are an increasing number of treatments for the opportunistic infections (e.g., meningitis, hepatitis, thrush, PCP, and shingles). Although these treatments offer some reduction of HIV replication and infection, they may be as uncomfortable as the symptoms themselves.

Medication regimens are complex and complicated. It is not uncommon for regimens to involve 20–40 pills daily, for indefinite periods. Some medications must be taken three or four times daily; some must be taken with food, whereas others cannot be taken with food. Some medications require water, others milk. Some medications have side effects that leave patients weak and nauseated. Others call for the permanent insertion of catheters. Still others, such as "protease hump" or "protease paunch," are quite visible and can signal AIDS status and treatment use.

Moreover, newer classes of AIDS medications and treatments may interfere with medications for drug treatment (e.g., methadone, LAAM, naltrexone, and bupropion). With the clear exception of methadone, there are not many clinical studies examining the interactions of AIDS medications and those used for drug treatment. There have been several studies of the interactions between methadone and the three common AIDS medications: AZT, Crixivan, and Norvir (American Psychiatric Association, 2000; CSAT, 2000; National Association of Social Workers HIV/AIDS Spectrum Project, 2001b; Stine, 1999). The use of Crixivan and Norvir can increase levels of methadone any where from 30 to 100%, whereas methadone increases the level of AZT from two to three times, making these medications much more potent than otherwise (Positively Aware, 2001). Such increased potency leads to increased side effects; if the doses of AZT are not appropriately adjusted, AZT-related toxicity is dramatically increased and damage to the liver may be accelerated. Alternately, if methadone levels are not reduced in the presence of Crixivan or Norvir, clients can experience respiratory failure, overdose, and coma. On the other hand, if methadone levels are reduced too greatly, withdrawal symptoms may occur (CSAT, 2000).

Need for Medication Adherence

Despite the many overlapping and painful side effects, physicians underscore the importance of adherence to treatment regimes: Clients must keep regular appointments with their physicians and health care teams, take medications on schedule, and follow up on recommendations. This compliance is important for at least two reasons: (1) consistent use—at least 90% adherence rate—is crucial for achieving a reduced viral load, and (2) treatment-resistant strains of HIV can emerge when medication use is interrupted or discontinued without the consultation of a physician. It is important to note that as of January 2001, at least 25% of newly identified cases of HIV/AIDS is completely resistant to current combination drug therapies.

Medication regimens are thus unforgiving. The expectations of extremely high adherence rates may be more than many intravenous drug users feel they are capable of meeting (Carpi, 1987; CSAT, 2000). Effective approaches for addressing adherence issues are discussed later in this chapter.

Need for Behavior Change

Adherence issues go far beyond medical issues. Many AIDS-affected intravenous drug users are challenged by medical and drug treatment professionals to change or modify behaviors that lead to secondary infection (i.e., the infection of others by HIV-infected persons). There is a growing movement to endorse "positive prevention" or "poz prevention" among HIV-infected men. Consistent with notions of harm reduction, positive prevention behaviors may take the form of using protection when having sex (e.g., condoms), abstinence, reducing the number of sex partners, as well as refraining from "people, places, and things" where there are greater opportunities for engaging in behaviors that increase a client's risk for drug relapse or HIV infection.

It comes as no surprise that many HIV-affected male/female may feel unable to meet the expectation that they will change their behavior. Some clients may understand the need for safer sex practices, for example, but be unwilling to change their sexual behaviors for fear of being identified as having AIDS.

> A., a 33-year-old single male intravenous drug user from the Dominican Republic who has been hospitalized on two occasions for AIDS-related infections, continues to date several women but does not practice safer sex. He has expressed fear that were he to suggest that he use condoms, he would immediately be suspected of having AIDS and no one would go out with him. He further states that, were his partner to ask him to use a condom he would do so, but since none of them has asked, he is not responsible should any of them become infected.

It also may be difficult for intravenous drug users to change their patterns of drug use (Friedman, DesJarlais, & Sotheran, 1986). Some patients become frightened by the prospect of infection or illness and may seek drug treatment, or they may be vigilant in their attempts either to use only their own drug paraphernalia or to employ good needle-cleaning technique. Other patients, however, have the opposite reaction and, as discussed earlier, increase their use of drugs to cope with anxiety. The challenges associated with adherence may be increased due to depression, inebriation, homelessness, or even good health. Unfortunately, AIDS-affected intravenous drug users are increasingly identified by medical practitioners as bad risks for HAART or combination therapies, despite the increase in practical and demonstrated strategies for working with these groups.

SOCIOECONOMIC RAMIFICATIONS

The effects of AIDS and HIV infection impinge on aspects of the client's life beyond physical functioning and medical symptomatology. The standard of living may be profoundly affected as well, which is further complicated when drug use is a factor (Christ & Wiener, 1985, Gant, Stewart, & Lynch, 1998).

Financial Implications

Persons with AIDS, like most people who are chronically or terminally ill, experience financial changes that are directly attributable to their illness. These changes, which may include loss of income and insurance coverage from traditional sources of employment, also extend to intravenous drug users, who, although possibly working, are more likely be employed in "off-the-books" jobs. This increasing inability to work is significant to society as well, because, as their conditions deteriorate, persons with AIDS will likely be less eligible for benefits that are, at least in part, supplemented by governmental programs (e.g., Social Security Disability, Medicaid). The cost of treatments (e.g., hospitalizations, medications, special procedures) and services (e.g., counseling, home care, transportation) may also be prohibitive, in terms of both real dollars and labor.

Shifts in Housing Availability

The absence of adequate housing is a common problem for intravenous drug users who do not have a diagnosis of HIV/AIDS; with a diagnosis, independent housing situations are extremely difficult to realize. The cost of maintaining an apartment may be more than these individuals can afford; thus they may live with relatives, share an apartment with other drug users, or move frequently from place to place. These arrangements disintegrate when their physical condition deteriorates, either because they require too much care or because roommates reject them for fear of exposure to the virus. Individuals who do have their own housing face the loss of their homes either because they are unable to pay the rent or because they are forced out by neighbors or landlords once their diagnosis is known. Although such actions are discriminatory and illegal, they nevertheless occur with some frequency.

Housing Opportunities for Persons with AIDS (HOPWA) is one program that is part of the CARE Act. HOPWA provides long-term rental assistance for persons with HIV/AIDS. Typically, HOPWA works with identified housing providers to increase the number of housing opportunities in urban and rural communities, providing vouchers directly to these providers. Additionally, HOPWA provides a range of housing assistance services to persons living with HIV/AIDS, including housekeeping, budgeting, home management, and chore services. However, although HIV/AIDS-affected intravenous drug users can obtain housing opportunities under this program, realities of housing shortages and discrimination due to stereotypes of intravenous drug users as undependable, dangerous, unemployable, "NIMBY" ("not wanted in my backyard"), and "one step from active drug use and selling," while on the decrease, continue to be held by housing providers and prospective neighbors (CSAT, 2000).

Downward shifts in income and housing combined with the increased cost of treatments and services can lead to an overall decrease in standard of living. However, some intravenous drug users report a marked increase in their standard of living as a direct result of their HIV infection. Many are now eligible for income assistance, insurance benefits, and access to an impressive continuum of care that can include primary medical care, mental health treatment, dental care, social support and recreational programs, food, drug treatment, clothing, and shelter. Symptomatic individuals may receive an extensive array of services and resources, allowing them to improve their quality of life for the first time in many years.

D., a 46-year-old Russian immigrant, had been without housing for 8 months. Although he was allowed to eat meals at the home of his aunt, he was not permitted to spend the night there. Each evening he took his pillow to the park and slept on the bench. As it became colder, he also took a blanket and stayed in the alley between two buildings, where he was sheltered from the wind. However, upon receiving a diagnosis of AIDS, he was given a room in a local residence hotel.

EMOTIONAL REACTIONS

AIDS-infected individuals face physical, economic, and interpersonal stressors with their idiosyncratic defense systems, coping skills, personality characteristics, and personal histories. There are, however, several reactions that persons with AIDS may share (Gant et al., 1998; National Association of Social Workers HIV/AIDS Spectrum Project, 2001b; Stine, 1999), as discussed below.

Fears Related to Physical Deterioration, Pain, and Death

Much of the anxiety experienced by persons with AIDS and HIV-infected individuals relates directly to the fear of death. It is also frequently focused on pain. This latter experience is particularly meaningful to intravenous drug users who may have begun their drug use specifically because of their inability to tolerate either physical or emotional discomfort. This intolerance may lead to frequent, seemingly unreasonable, requests for painkillers and other numbing medications.

Fear of Physical Incapacitation

The inability to care for oneself is frightening to most people. Intravenous drug users, who may have been avoiding emotional dependence on others for much of their lives, are especially afraid of this prospect. This fear is compounded by the reality of abandonment and rejection, leaving persons with AIDS fearful that, should they become physically incapacitated, there will be no one to whom they can turn for help.

Feelings of Toxicity to Others

Despite education, discussions with medical professionals, and much evidence to the contrary, HIV-infected individuals may believe they are "toxic" and deserve to be isolated from others.

> L., a 35-year-old black man, had been hospitalized while on a job assignment related to a work program in a low-security prison. He worried that, should he be returned to prison, he would be easily identified as an AIDS patient and the authorities would not permit him to eat in the dining room, play cards, or even talk to other inmates. On the other hand, he felt that they would be correct to treat him in this way; he was, after all, an AIDS patient. During visits from his social worker he would scrub the chair before offering it to her, remind her to be careful not to touch anything in his room, and sit far apart from her so as not to "contaminate" her with his germs.

Obsessive Thinking

HIV-infected individuals may be vigilant in regard to symptoms, blood results, and so forth. This vigilance can include such things as searching the body for evidence of skin lesions, taking an HIV test monthly to confirm the result, and checking T-cell counts on a weekly basis. Some of this behavior may, indeed, be adaptive and alert the patients and medical staff to the early signs of infection. Some practitioners cautiously endorse the use of compulsive behaviors and obsessive thinking as a way to monitor medication adherence. However, if left unchecked, obsessive thinking may lead to a decrease in patients' ability to function.

Self-Blame and Guilt

It is common for patients confronted with a chronic or terminal illness to ask "Why me?" In the case of intravenous drug users with AIDS, the answer is too readily accessible and laden with stigma and guilt: They are surrounded by many who are eager to remind them that they are somehow responsible for their condition. This knowledge is often accompanied by self-blame ("I did this to myself; no one put the needle in my arm but me") and guilt ("I deserve this for how I've lived my life; what did I think was going to happen?"). These feelings may be intensified significantly when they have infected someone else, such as a sexual partner, or, in the case of female intravenous drug users, their children.

Helplessness and Loss of Control

HIV-infected individuals may feel helpless, stripped of the capacity to make any difference whatsoever in the course of their illness. The feeling of losing control can be experienced in regard to relationships, emotions, finances, and other significant parts of their lives as well. It is also frequently accompanied by a sense of hopelessness.

Depression

Depression is a common and expectable response to multiple assaults. Depression accompanies loss, and persons with AIDS face losses on all fronts: loss of physical capacity, loss of friends (either through abandonment or because they, too, have died of the disease), loss of self-esteem, loss of life. Other losses are less obvious; long-term plans (e.g., education, seeing one's children grow) are less secure, and dreams of "someday" may never come to fruition. Uncertainty becomes commonplace.

Rage

Intravenous drug users, because of their poor tolerance of frustration, frequently react with rage when they feel frightened, ignored, or out of control. AIDS, with its accompanying feelings of helplessness and anxiety, may lead to that exact reaction. Intravenous drug users may externalize the rage they feel at themselves, becoming unable to tolerate the health and good fortune of others, as well as the insensitivity they perceive others as displaying toward them.

> S., a homeless 24-year-old Hispanic woman, remained in the hospital for 30 days, awaiting housing and other services. As her condition deteriorated, she became increasingly agitated at the medical staff. Finally, after being told to return to her room one afternoon, she threatened the nurses with spitting into their mouths so that they would know what it is like to have AIDS.

Fear of Exposure

Concern about the reactions of others frequently leads HIV-infected individuals to keep their health status a secret. Perhaps equally powerful is the fear that the high-risk behavior that led to the infection also will be exposed. This possibility may lead individuals to deny the presence of any risk factors or to lie about the factors that may have led to their infection.

> M. is a 19-year-old Cuban American man who feared his father's reaction to his drug use. He told his physicians and family that he had been frequenting prostitutes and that was the only possible source of his HIV infection. His arrest for drug dealing some weeks after discharge was an unfortunately dramatic way for his drug use to be exposed.

IMPACT ON FAMILIES AND SIGNIFICANT OTHERS

Intravenous drug users interact with a large network of friends, lovers, family, drug companions, employers, and so forth. The nature of these relationships inevitably changes as these significant others learn of the person's medical condition. These changes may have both positive and negative effects on patients.

Rejection and Stigmatization

It is not unusual for family members and significant others to fear contagion, feel unable to cope with the patient's deterioration and likely death, or be worried that they will somehow be identified as being similar to the patient. Thus they may avoid the patient or, in some instances, disappear from his or her life altogether (Christ & Wiener, 1985). In the case of intravenous drug users, it is possible that this rejection has less to do with AIDS than with their behavior prior to becoming ill. If patients have been manipulative, demanding, or involved in illegal activity, for example, it is possible that their friends and family separated from them long before HIV infection became a factor.

Families who choose to care for a person with AIDS as his or her condition deteriorates may hide the true nature of the illness for fear that the stigma of AIDS will be focused upon them, leading to loss of jobs, friends, and so forth. This fear of being stigmatized is closely related to feelings of shame and embarrassment concerning both the actual diagnosis and the high-risk behavior that may have been associated with HIV transmission.

> G., a 32-year-old man of Italian descent, had undergone drug treatment and been drug free for 4 years. When he became ill, his parents welcomed him into their home and cared for him devotedly until his death. Throughout this 14-month period, they refused to allow anyone in their home to visit for fear that the symptoms G. was exhibiting would be easily recognizable as AIDS. Subsequent to his death, they told other relatives that he had had cancer.

Tension and Isolation

Relationships may become characterized by an underlying tension, a sensation of "walking on eggshells." Persons with AIDS may feel afraid to express themselves honestly, not wanting to alienate those around them, particularly if they are dependent upon them for care. Family and friends, in their efforts to be "upbeat," may not mention AIDS or ask the patient how he or she is feeling. There also may be an underlying anger at the patient for becoming ill in the first place. These emotions can be so powerful that those involved may be incapable of confronting them.

The combination of the tension and the negative reactions of friends, family, and significant others (indeed, of society in general) may leave persons with AIDS and their families feeling isolated from the outside world, as well as one another, and thus forced to face this terrifying situation on their own.

Support and Caring

The good news is that many families, friends, and lovers remain available to persons with AIDS, providing emotional support and physical care as well as meeting concrete needs, sometimes with a devotion far beyond that which might be expected. It is also common for family members to reappear after many years of separation when they learn that the patient is ill. This may be difficult for patients to accept in some instances, especially if it reawakens old hurts and disagreements. Occasionally patients may feel they do not deserve any familial support.

E., a 36-year-old man of Haitian background, had grown up in a middle-class suburban home; he said he had been loved by his parents, had had a close relationship with his brothers, and had planned to pursue a college education. He blamed himself for his drug use, calling himself a "rebel" as a teenager. He had left home after a blowup with his father 15 years earlier and had never had contact with his parents again. He knew that if they were aware of his situation (i.e., homeless, ill), they would come for him. He felt he did not deserve that response after the way he had behaved, and he would not allow the hospital staff to contact his family.

Alteration of Relationship Patterns

Upon learning they are HIV-infected, intravenous drug users may feel ready to change their lifestyles. In the best of circumstances, this may mean entering a drug treatment program where success might translate into the loss of long-standing friendships with drug-using companions as well as a change in daily activities and patterns of relationships (Friedman et al., 1986). Sexual practices also may change, leading to shifts in relationships with lovers. All these changes may be puzzling to those around intravenous drug users and, in fact, may feel discordant to the person with AIDS themselves.

The many factors involved in maintaining interpersonal relationships—communication, sexuality, history, emotional connectedness—are all affected by the onset of HIV infection. Whether these factors lead to a general deterioration or improvement in these relationships must be evaluated on a case-by-case basis. It is clear, though, that some degree of change always occurs.

CLINICAL INTERVENTIONS

Clinicians working with persons with AIDS and HIV-infected individuals must intervene in several areas (Caputo, 1985; Mantell, Shulman, Belmont, & Spivak, 1989; Novak, 1989): concrete services, counseling, case management and service integration, education, and advocacy.

Concrete Services

As their medical conditions vacillate between wellness and illness, persons with AIDS are likely to have increasing needs for such services as home care, nursing services related to the administration of special treatments, medical equipment (e.g., hospital beds, wheelchairs), and housekeeping assistance. With longer life spans come additional needs—for example, garments for incontinence, several sizes of undergarments for women (whose breast size vary dramatically and unevenly due to combination therapy). Extended use of combination therapy has substantial medical complications, and clients may need primary medical care to address metabolism of fats and organ damage to the heart, liver, kidneys, and pancreas. Intravenous drug users, with their decreased resources, may require additional services, including housing, extended nursing care, and enrollment in income/benefit programs. In many instances intravenous drug users also may require some form of drug treatment, including detoxification, methadone maintenance, or drug-free residential placement. Social workers must be knowledgeable about the services and programs available in the community and facile in negotiating these systems effectively. The identification of case management and/or CARE Act services is crucial.

Counseling

A major component of social work with persons with AIDS and HIV-infected individuals is counseling concerning the impact of the illness on themselves, their families, their significant others, as well as the mechanisms they use to cope with the situation. Counseling may take place in several modalities, including individual, couple, family, and group. Some specific techniques, discussed below, are useful when counseling on an individual basis. In general, intravenous drug users, because of their sense of emptiness, cannot work with a counselor who is nondirective and silent; the counselor must be available as an understanding, motivating, confronting, and active figure.

Encouraging the Expression of Feelings

Family and significant others may be afraid to discuss the implications of an AIDS diagnosis. In their attempts to help the patient feel hopeful (and because of their own inability to deal with such intense material), they may avoid such painful topics as death and planning for those who remain. Persons with AIDS, however, may need a forum in which to safely share their thoughts and feelings about what is happening to them.

Encouraging Participation in Treatment Planning

In service of avoidance or denial, intravenous drug users may defer to the medical team regarding decision making, thus divorcing themselves from their own treatment plans. But it is crucial that they consciously make such decisions as which treatment to try, what services to request, and where to go for treatment, so as to maintain what control they have in the situation and to establish commitment to (and, potentially, compliance with) the plan. Although it is appropriate for social workers or other clinicians to make recommendations (e.g., when patients are unfamiliar with available resources or are not capable of participating fully due to severity of medical or emotional condition), persons with AIDS are more empowered by contributing input in determining the treatments and services they will receive.

Allowing Denial

The tendency of intravenous drug users to use maladaptive denial has been described previously. Nevertheless, there are times when denial is useful. For example, patients may believe that if they alter their lifestyles, they will be cured of the virus. Such denial may be a factor in motivating behavior changes, including decreasing drug use or shifting relationship patterns, thereby promoting a better quality of life. Denial, however, should not be allowed to serve as a rationale for relapse.

Providing Reliable Support

Intravenous drug users, with their histories of disappointing relationships, may find the opportunity (often for the first time in their lives) to feel emotionally supported via their relationships with social workers. This support, in turn, may help them take a chance on behavior changes that they might otherwise deem too risky. Such supportive relationships also permit them to feel safer in a situation in which they are realistically vulnerable and frightened.

Avoiding Overhelping

It is tempting to provide all-encompassing care for intravenous drug users with AIDS or HIV infection. Such individuals may present as helpless and desperately in need of assistance, tapping into social workers' desire to be helpful (Levinson & Straussner, 1978; National Association of Social Workers HIV/AIDS Spectrum Project 2001b). Nevertheless, it is important to encourage clients to do things for themselves, despite the annoyance they may express due to their feelings of powerlessness. Although at times, it may actually be easier to *do* for these clients, in the long run it is more useful to help them feel empowered and thus capable of taking care of themselves. For example, it is better to give a patient coins to make a telephone call rather than make it for him or her.

Life Review

As with many terminally ill patients, persons with AIDS may need to examine the course of their lives—their accomplishments, regrets, joys, sorrows. Social workers can provide patients with opportunities to discuss aspects of their lives, listening for how resolved they are about each issue. Intravenous drug users often feel saddened by how they have lived and what has happened to their relationships; they need opportunities to share what has been good, and to grieve for what has not been good.

Working through Unfinished Business

It is sometimes possible to resolve situations that patients feel uneasy about but are unable to cope with on their own. Social workers can be allies in this process by locating and counseling significant others, assisting with the purchase of a long-desired item, and so forth.

> R., age 46, had not seen his mother for 22 years; he was not even sure she was still alive, but he suspected she continued to reside in Bogata, Columbia. He wanted to see her and apologize for how he had hurt her years earlier—initially by his behavior, later by leaving. The social worker was able to locate her and arrange for her to come to New York, where she and her son were reunited. She remained with him for about 2 weeks. Soon after her departure, R. described himself as feeling peaceful and stated that he could now die without remorse. He did, in fact, die about a week after making that statement.

Maximizing Quality of Life

Whereas some intravenous drug users are overwhelmed by their diagnosis and increase their substance abuse as a means of coping, others can be helped to change their behaviors, relationships, and coping mechanisms. These major changes, in combination with the receipt of concrete benefits, enable them to improve their living situation and thus their entire quality of life.

> P., a 40-year-old white woman, had used intravenous drugs only occasionally but had shared needles at those times. Although aware that she was at risk, she felt she would never get infected. She cared for her three children, ages 10–16, but was not close with them. When she learned she was HIV infected, she abruptly stopped her drug use. She began to spend more time with her children and found that their relationship improved markedly. She tearfully wondered why it had taken so severe a circumstance to bring about this change but was grateful that she had been able to do so.

Addressing Pain Management Issues

For drug-dependent persons with AIDS, pain management is a critical issue. As indicated previously, some intravenous drug users initiated drug use in order to reduce their personal inability to manage their physical and/ or emotional pain. Recent research in pain management reveals a vast continuum of pain experiences, quite different from the typical "pain ladders" taught in medical, social work, and nursing schools.

The use of pain medications by persons in recovery is a complex issue that is exacerbated when dealing with HIV-infected substance users. At the very least, social workers can facilitate an honest dialogue regarding pain and pain management by both clients and service providers.

Addressing Adherence Issues

The social worker's role is vital to promoting adherence to treatment. He or she can provide education and support to clients who are facing the challenges posed by complex treatment regimens. Social workers can help clients by providing clear and accurate information on such topics as dosing (what to take and when to take it), dietary restrictions, medication storage and handling potential side effects, drug interactions, and any other drug information that may affect adherence.

In work with intravenous drug users living with HIV/AIDS and struggling with adherence issues, Welch and Gant (in press) noted that adherence increased when options for discussing practical issues and concerns people had about adherence were provided; the discussions—conducted either in dyads or groups—allowed for ventilation, support, and encouragement. Social workers should consider giving clients permission to be honest about taking their medication, empathizing via honest discussion of the difficulty of adhering to the medication schedule, working to identify number of missed doses and the reasons for them, reinforcing successful adherence strategies, exploring alternative medication regimens, and engaging partners, family, and community in supporting adherence strategies.

CASE MANAGEMENT AND SERVICE INTEGRATION

Case management involves service integration. However, practitioners often experience various challenges to integrating services across HIV/AIDS and substance abuse sectors. Intravenous drug users with HIV/AIDS have the option of accessing substantial resources through CARE Act programs. However, their ability to effect and maintain essential behavioral and psychological changes ultimately depends on access to drug treatment (CSAT, 2000). Providers need to understand the following challenges in providing essential services to drug-dependent persons with AIDS.

Differences in Philosophy and Access to Services

Drug treatment agencies often operate within an abstinence model of care and treatment. This means that clients are expected to be abstinent before receiving other services. However, many HIV/AIDS service and treatment organizations frequently use a risk-reduction or harm-reduction model. This model suggests that abstinence and the active use are endpoints on a continuum of drug use, and that the goal of harm reduction is twofold: (1) to reduce the harm associated with drug consumption, and (2) to provide immediate (to the extent possible) referral to care and treatment services when requested by the client. This means that active drug-using clients may access services without necessarily demonstrating abstinence.

Differences in Level of Available Services

Funding sources impact on the availability of treatment options and opportunities. The United States drug policy allots a substantial amount of money to drug interdiction (i.e., drug search, seizure, and imprisonment) while providing substantially less funding for drug prevention and treatment. This lack of funding translates into oversubscribed treatment programs with far fewer treatment slots than demand warrants. However, with over 12 billion dollars allocated under the CARE Act for HIV/AIDS care and medical treatment from 1990 to 2001, there are enough resources (with the exception of HOPWA) to meet the demand of most HIV/AIDS care and treatment services. Thus intravenous drug users with HIV/AIDS are less likely to be able to access services for substance abuse treatment than for HIV/AIDS.

PROVISION OF EDUCATIONAL SERVICES

Social workers provide a broad range of educational programs to patients, families and significant others, staff members, and other professionals. They also offer preventive programs to the general public, expending particular effort to reach intravenous drug users who are at especially high risk for exposure to the HIV virus. These programs may include information on transmission, prevention, treatment, safer-sex practices, and syringe exchange programs.

In order to be able to provide current information, social workers must be familiar with the various useful curricula addressing substance abuse and HIV/AIDS issues, such as those provided by the National Association of Social Workers HIV/AIDS Spectrum Project, the American Psychological Association's HOPE Program, and the Treatment Improvement

Protocol (TIP) series 37 (i.e., Substance Abuse Treatment for Persons with HIV/AIDS), published by the Center for Substance Abuse Treatment (CSAT) and the Substance Abuse and Mental Health Services Administration (SAMHSA).

ADVOCACY

Social workers need to advocate on behalf of the needs of individual patients and even for an entire group or subgroup of persons with AIDS (e.g., homeless intravenous drug users). Advocacy for this population is particularly important because some drug treatment programs are not HIV friendly, and some HIV programs are not intravenous drug user friendly. Moreover, issues around HIV treatment differ for active users from those who are in recovery or in a drug treatment program. Finally, managing sobriety and a chronic disease may be overwhelming, particularly in early recovery.

COUNTERTRANSFERENCE REACTIONS

Intravenous drug users who are HIV-infected are an exceedingly difficult population with which to work. Patients who present with a combination of drug use (and the personality characteristics associated with that) and a life-threatening medical condition may evoke several reactions in health care staff, including social workers (Cavrell, 1988; Dunkel & Hatfield, 1986). These reactions may be categorized generally as countertransference, a set of conscious and unconscious thoughts, feelings, and beliefs experienced by the clinician in response to the client or an event. Positive countertransference can lead to an idealization of the client or of the therapy conducted with the client. Negative countertransference can lead to an irrational fear and loathing of the client, the client's situation, and to working with him or her.

In working with intravenous drug users with HIV/AIDS, countertransference can emerge from the core issues that define HIV/AIDS: death, disease, sexuality and sexual orientation, racism, and drug use. Countertransference can be a problem, but, with proper supervision, also a valuable source of information and an important therapeutic tool. Among the common countertransference reactions that often determine the course of the therapeutic relationship are the following:

Fear of Contagion

When dealing with an intravenous drug user who has HIV/AIDS, a worker's fear may derive from several sources, but generally it involves irrational ideas concerning contagion. The clinician also may fear the personality traits that characterize intravenous drug users, especially when an intravenous drug user has been threatening in some way or has a criminal history.

Blaming the Victim

Because the high-risk sex- and drug-related behaviors associated with HIV infection and drug use are frowned upon by society at large, it is not unusual for workers to blame persons with AIDS for their own illness, feeling that they somehow "deserve" to be ill because of their deviant behavior.

Rejection

Fear and blaming may culminate rejection of the intravenous drug user. This rejection may be subtle, manifesting itself as a decrease in the frequency of counseling sessions, slowness in processing applications for benefits, and so forth; or it may be quite obvious, as in transferring a patient to another worker or agency (Mantell et al., 1989).

Homophobia and Addictophobia

Ultimately, fear, blaming, and rejection can lead to a phobia of all homosexuals and all drug users. Should such feelings become widespread, they could lead to a decrease in services and staffing for HIV-related treatment programs.

Helplessness and Hopelessness

Clinicians often feel powerless in the face of the HIV virus: They cannot cure their patients of AIDS. This feeling of impotence can lead workers to feel hopeless about the ultimate value of their interventions in the face of the increasing prevalence of HIV infection and the growing numbers of patients needing long-term care.

> F. is an especially talented social worker who had been working with persons with AIDS for about 1 year. Although occasionally tearful when a patient died or when she felt frustrated in her efforts to plan effectively, for the most part she felt competent in, and gratified by, her work. Then, one day, in an intensive care unit visiting a patient of whom she was especially fond, she became overwhelmed with the feeling that no matter how hard she worked, she would be incapable of curing this man's condition. She felt beaten by the virus and was left with a sense of total powerlessness.

Grief

The relationship between a social worker and patient, particularly when it involves issues of death and dying, can be an intense and intimate one. Unresolved grief and loss may cause clinicians to project feelings about a previous client onto a current client. For example, after suffering a number of losses, a clinician may come to expect decline and loss in current clients and thus want to examine feelings related to anticipatory loss when, in fact, such decline may not happen in light of new treatments. If blocked in their own grief, clinicians may avoid their own pain and be unable to be help clients with their pain.

Rage with the Client and/or the Social Service System

Confronted by seriously needy patients, workers must then negotiate a system that does not sufficiently address these patients' concerns. A series of difficult cases can leave workers enraged at no one in particular and may, at times, cause them to overreact to minor slights and insensitivities.

Guilt

Guilt can derive from several sources. First, workers who are healthy, however empathic they may be, cannot really know how it feels to be sick, especially with AIDS. Second, by virtue of being employed as social workers, it is likely that they have financial and other resources that are greater than those of their patients. Third, there are times when the provocative behavior evidenced by some intravenous drug users may be difficult to tolerate, and workers may find themselves reluctant to be helpful. They may feel especially guilty if they have, in fact, acted out those feelings. Fourth, and more subtly, workers may find that they enjoy working with this population and are somehow energized by the excitement of working "on the edge" of life-and-death situations. This pleasure in their work may feel dissonant against the backdrop of death, illness, and poor quality of life (Cavrell, 1988).

Anxiety

Many social workers complain of anxiety, particularly when confronted with seriously ill clients who have minimum resources and multiple needs. Workers may worry about patients' functioning in the community (e.g., whether they are remaining drug free, whether they are engaging in illegal activities) and about their medical condition (e.g., whether they are losing weight). Workers may be concerned about their own job performance in negotiating the numerous obstacles they confront. They also may be anxious about their own serostatus and that of their loved ones.

Depression

The constant exposure to death, illness, the broad range of emotions, their own feelings of powerlessness, and the ominous sense of relentless onslaught make depression a common response. Depression is inevitably experienced in some degree, but it naturally varies depending upon each worker's coping capacity and defense mechanisms.

Culture, Race, Class, and Lifestyle Issues

People in the United States tend to be preoccupied with ethnicity, culture, and social class. Many U.S. citizens have mixed attitudes about people of color; African Americans suffer a particularly disadvantageous and precarious position, given their history of slavery, commercial exploitation, and systematic dehumanization. As a result, stereotypes invoking criminality, sexuality, intellectual inferiority, and illicit behavior are not uncommon. Honest dialogue regarding race, class, and culture is rare, and almost never a part of dialogues between social worker and client. A client's need to discuss experiences of discrimination may not be addressed. Alternately, the worker may overcompensate for inadequately discussed or unresolved issues and insist on a discussion of client experiences of racism or discrimination even when such issues are not perceived as important by the client.

Mixed feelings about sex are common and range from puritanical avoidance to exploited preoccupation. It is rare for social workers or clients to talk about sex in any explicit way, and thus sexual issues critical to personal development, prevention, and behavior change strategies for persons with AIDS may not be addressed. This can be particularly true for clients who have different sexual orientations, different sexual interests, and different sexual practices from the clinician's.

Similarly, most drug use outside of alcohol and smoking tobacco has been criminalized in the United States. Often, drug users engage in other types of criminal activity in order to support their drug use. Workers' attitudes about criminal behavior and substance use, as well as beliefs about responsibility, pleasure, coping, recovery, deviance, and redemption, can affect their capacity to empathize and work effectively with clients.

Denial

Advanced HIV disease can be disfiguring, dehumanizing, and painful. Disease can feel disgusting and overwhelming to those who witness it, and clinicians may feel embarrassed or ashamed of their reactions. Witnessing cognitive incapacitation, physical decline, and other losses and indignities can undermine a clinician's sense of control and lead to anxiety, avoidance, anger, and a host of other reactions.

Overidentification

The risk of overidentification may be high because many HIV/AIDS service providers are members of communities substantially affected by HIV/AIDS as well as substance abuse. There may be a strong likelihood that social workers are themselves addressing recovery issues, living with HIV/AIDS, have friends or family members who are HIV/AIDS affected, or knew someone who died of an AIDS-related illness. Although shared characteristics between the client and the therapist can promote empathy and rapport, the worker also can run the risk of projecting his or her own concerns or issues on the client or join with the client through inappropriate, non-therapeutic, disclosure.

These responses must be addressed lest they become overwhelming and lead to burnout, ultimately forcing the worker to leave the profession. It is therefore crucial that social workers have a forum in which they can express their feelings honestly. Support groups are especially successful in this regard and should be built into our programming. Supervision is another mechanism for receiving support, provided that supervisors are able to create an atmosphere in which workers feel secure enough to discuss these very difficult reactions.

The American Psychological Association recommends that clinicians who work with persons with AIDS follow the strategies listed below as a way of managing their countertransference:

1. Limit the number of clients with HIV and find a good balance of HIV and non-HIV clients.
2. Network with other mental health providers who work with patients who have HIV, using meetings, e-mail, and phone calls.
3. Develop other, nonclinical ways of addressing the HIV/AIDS epidemic—for example, research, training, supervision, etc.
4. Continually clarify one's role and the limits of service with clients.
5. Develop ways of expressing the pain of grief through psychotherapy, community rituals, and the social support of friends and family colleagues.
6. Organize peer supervision and consultation networks.
7. Participate in spiritual rituals and practices.
8. Find inspiration and meaning in one's work with HIV-infected clients.

CONCLUSION

The provision of clinical services to intravenous drug users with AIDS or HIV infection is a formidable task. Confronted with individuals whose difficulties may include a vast array of physical, social, economic, and psychological problems, social workers must intervene with services on all levels while simultaneously dealing with numerous other issues, including their own reactions. And yet, many social workers continue to rise to this challenge by caring for this population with a commitment and fervor that remain admirable and reflect the hope of our profession.

REFERENCES

Alexander, B. K. (1990). Alternatives to the war on drugs. *Journal of Drug Issues, 20*(1), 1–27.

American Psychiatric Association. (1994). *Diagnostic and statistical manual of mental disorders* (4rd ed.). Washington, DC: Author.

American Psychiatric Association. (2000). *Practice guideline for the treatment of patients with HIV/AIDS.* Washington, DC: Author.

Caputo, L. (1985). Dual diagnosis: AIDS and addiction. *Social Work, 30,* 361–364.

Carpi, J. (1987). Treating IV drug users: A difficult task for staff. *AIDS Patient Care, 1,* 21–23.

Cavrell, D. (1988, June). *Managing countertransference: A guide for AIDS health care professionals.* Poster presented at the 4th International Conference on AIDS, Stockholm, Sweden.

CDC (Centers for Disease Control and Prevention and Prevention). (1998). *HIV/AIDS Surveillance Report 1998, 19*(2), 1–43.

CDC (Centers for Disease Control and Prevention). (1989, June). *AIDS surveillance/epidemiology.* Slide presentation available via download: www.cdc.gov/hiv/graphics/surveill.htm.

CDC (Centers for Disease Control and Prevention). (1990, September). *HIV/AIDS Surveillance Report 16*(1), 1–18.

CSAT (Center for Substance Abuse Treatment). (2000). *Substance abuse treatment for persons with HIV/AIDS.* Treatment Improvement Protocol (TIP) series 37. Rockville, MD: Substance Abuse and Mental Health Services Administration.

Chein, I. G., Donald, L., Lee, R. S., & Rosenfeld, E. (1964). Personality and addiction: A dynamic perspective. In I. G. Chein, L. Donald, R. S. Lee, & E. Rosenfeld (Eds.), *The road to H: Narcotics, delinquency, and social policy* (pp. 227–250). New York: Basic Books.

Christ, G. H., & Wiener, L. S. (1985). Psychosocial issues in AIDS. In T. V. DeVita, Jr., S. Herman, & S. Rosenberg (Eds.), *AIDS etiology, diagnosis, treatment and prevention* (pp. 275–297). New York: Lippincott.

Dunkel, J., & Hatfield, S. (1986). Countertransference issues in working with persons with AIDS. *Social Work, 31,* 114-117.

Flanagan, N. (1989). Understanding your IDU patients: It still helps to know the streets. *AIDS Patient Care, 3,* 23-25.

Friedman, S. R., DesJarlais, D. C., & Sotheran, J. L. (1986). AIDS health education for intravenous drug users. *Health Education Quarterly, 13,* 383–393.

Gant, L. M., Stewart, P. A., & Lynch, V. J. (Eds.). (1998). *Social workers speak out on the HIV/AIDS crisis: Voices from and to African-American communities.* Westport, CT: Praeger.

Khantzian, E. J. (1980). An ego/self theory of substance dependence: A contemporary psychoanalytic perspective. In D. J. Lettieri, M. Sayers, & H. W. Pearson (Eds.), *Theories and drug abuse: Selected contemporary perspectives* (pp. 69–83). Rockville, MD: National Institute on Drug Abuse.

Khantzian, E. J. (1985). The self-medication hypothesis of addictive disorders: Focus on heroin and cocaine dependence. *American Journal of Psychiatry, 142,* 1259–1264.

Levinson, V., & Strausssner, S. L. A. (1978). Social workers as "enablers" in the treatment of alcoholics. *Social Casework, 50,* 14–20.

Mantell, J. E., Shulman, L. C., Belmont, M. F., & Spivak, H. B. (1989). Social workers respond to the AIDS epidemic in an acute care hospital. *Health and Social Work, 14,* 41–51.

Mendelson, J. H., & Mello, N. K. (1995). Alcohol, sex and aggression. In J. A. Inciardi & K. McElrath (Eds.), *The American drug scene: An anthology* (pp. 104–136). Los Angeles: Roxbury.

National Association of Social Workers (NASW). (1984, September). *Acquired immune deficiency syndrome.* Washington, DC: Author.

National Association of Social Workers (NASW). (1987a). *New York City chapter position paper on social work practice for people with AIDS, ARC and HIV infection.* New York: New York City Chapter Task Force on AIDS.

National Association of Social Workers (NASW). (1987b, April). *AIDS: A social work response* (proposed revised social policy statement for 1987 delegate assembly of NASW).

National Association of Social Workers (NASW). (1999). *Acquired Immunodeficiency Syndrome and Human Immunodeficiency Virus: A social work response.* Washington, DC: Author.

National Association of Social Workers HIV/AIDS Spectrum Project. (2001a). *Mental health and HIV/AIDS: Social work practice issues.* Washington, DC: Author.

National Association of Social Workers HIV/AIDS Spectrum Project. (2001b). *Substance abuse and HIV/AIDS: Social work practice issues.* Washington, DC: Author.

Novak, C. (1989). Social work services. In P. Blomberg (Ed.), *Comprehensive management of HIV infection: A protocol treatment plan for HIV/ARC/AIDS patients in Northern California* (pp. 228–250). Sacramento, CA: Sacramento AIDS Foundation.

Positively Aware. (2001). *HIV drug guide 2001.* Chicago: Test Positive AIDS Network.

Rubinow, D. R., & Joffe, R. T. (1987). Psychiatric and psychosocial aspects of AIDS.

In S. Broder (Ed.), *AIDS: Modern concepts and therapeutic challenges* (pp. 123–133). New York: Marcel Dekker.

Shilts, R. (1987). *And the band played on.* New York: Penguin.

Stine, G. J. (1999). *AIDS update 1999.* Upper Saddle River, NJ: Prentice-Hall.

Stokes, J. P., & Peterson, J. L. (1998). Homophobia, self-esteem, and risk for HIV among African American men who have sex with men. *AIDS Education and Prevention, 10*(3), 278–292.

Vaillant, G. (1975). Sociopathy as a human process: A viewpoint. *Archives of General Psychiatry, 32,* 178–183.

Welch, L. M., & Gant, L. M. (in press). Voices less heard: HIV-positive African-American women, medication adherence, and self care. *Journal of HIV/AIDS and Social Sciences.*

Wurmser, L. (1974). Psychoanalytic considerations of the etiology of compulsive drug use. *Journal of the American Psychoanalytic Association, 22,* 820–843.

Zinberg, N. E. (1975). Addiction and ego function. *Psychoanalytic Study of the Child, 30,* 567–588.

NOTE

Given the ever-changing state of knowledge regarding HIV/AIDS, existing information can become rapidly outdated. There are literally scores of information access sites on the Internet. Four sites are of particular relevance for persons working with HIV/AIDS-infected drug-using populations:

- The Centers for Disease Control and Prevention and Prevention National AIDS Clearinghouse (*www.cdcnpin.org*), for current demographic information and statistics.
- Join Together Hotline (*www.jointogether.org*), for the latest information on substance abuse and HIV/AIDS issues.
- National Institute on Drug Abuse (NIDA; *www.nida.gov*), for information on drug abuse treatment.
- Health Resources Services Administration (HRSA; *www.hrsa.gov/hab/default.htm*), for CARE Act information by state, city, or region.

PART VI

Looking Toward the Future

CHAPTER 21

Practice and Policy Issues

Shulamith Lala Ashenberg Straussner

Although many of the substances discussed in this book and the problems resulting from their abuse have been around for ages, the field of substance abuse or addictions is constantly evolving: New substances of abuse, new populations, new treatment approaches, and new or changing policies are part and parcel of this field. The previous chapters identified the state of the art of some of the current issues. They addressed the varying perspectives on practice interventions with substance-abusing clients, including the currently "hot topics" of motivational interviewing, harm reduction, and treatment of involuntary and dually diagnosed clients; the changing nature of treatment facilities and new treatment approaches; the need to explore the impact on, and the role of, families of substance abusers; and the special issues of working with clients of different ages (such as adolescents and the increasing population of elderly substance abusers) and of different groups (such as women, homeless persons, those infected with HIV, and those with borderline personality disorders). Where do we go from here?

One of the important current and future issues for the field of addictions treatment, in general, and for social workers, in particular, is the incorporation of *evidence-based practice* (EBP). Social work's focus on interpersonal relationship and the multilevel contextual dynamics inherent in the utilization of the biopsychosocial perspective appear antithetical to the use of randomized controlled trials and the narrow research focus needed to obtain internally valid and reliable outcomes that are core aspects of EBP. What role will social workers play in such studies? How much of EBP will become adopted by social workers, and at what cost to traditional social work skills and values? These are important areas that will need to be addressed in the future.

A related issue is the role of social workers in the development and utilization of the increasing number of standardized screening instruments. Should we integrate instruments such as the Addiction Severity Index into a standard social work intake process? Should more social workers be involved in developing our own screening instruments that focus on environmental and psychosocial issues, which we know play a crucial role in the use and abuse of substances and in maintaining long-term recovery? What is the role of social workers in the growing emphasis on neurobiology and the use of pharmacotherapeutic agents, such as buprenorphine, on one hand, and the use of spirituality and religion on the other? What will social workers need to know about tobacco and smoking cessation in order to provide effective substance abuse treatment? What about the growing problem of gambling addictions? And where do eating disorders fit in?

Relatedly, we need to develop our knowledge base of primary prevention approaches. As the largest group of mental health professionals who are ubiquitous in every social and community setting, social workers need to play a much more crucial role in primary and secondary prevention than they currently do. In order to achieve that goal, *all* social workers must know more about addictions and be comfortable in screening, assessment, motivational interviewing, and referrals of those with potential problems (Straussner & Seinreich, 2002). Where and how such knowledge will be conveyed are questions we still need to answer.

Finally, we need to continue working on refinements to current federal and state drug policies. Issues such as the medicalization and possible decriminalization of marijuana use, the increasing uses of harm reduction approaches, the use of the criminal justice system and its alternatives—all these areas need to be debated within the profession. The important role of social workers as policy developers, advocates, and expert witnesses within the field of addictions needs to be addressed (Phillips & Straussner, 2002). The greatly diminished role of social workers' involvement with families of substance abusers, due to lack of managed care payments for such services, calls for greater advocacy in this area and for greater innovative practices to help families.

Regardless of the nature of the "war on drugs" that politicians advocate for the moment, substance use, abuse, and dependence do not seem likely to diminish in our lifetime. Concrete knowledge of different substances and good clinical skills will always be needed. I hope that the chapters in this second edition have provided the basic knowledge and guidance essential for effective clinical practice with substance-abusing clients and their families, no matter where we work.

REFERENCES

Phillips, N. K., & Straussner, S. L. A. (2002). *Urban social work: An introduction to policy and practice in the cities*. Boston: Allyn & Bacon.

Straussner, S. L. A., & Senreich, E. (2002). Educating social workers to work with individuals affected by substance use disorders. *Substance Abuse, 23*(3, Suppl.), 319–340.

Index

Abandonment, fears of, in borderline disorders, 373–374
Abstinence
  for dual-diagnosis client, 120
  versus harm reduction, 66
  from stimulants, 214–215, 218, 223–225
  treatments based on, 179. *See also* Twelve-step programs
Abuse, in family treatment, 253
ACOSA. *See* Adult children of substance abusers
Acting-out behaviors, 294
Acupuncture, 22–23
  in alcoholism treatment, 178
Addiction, 4
  biochemical/genetic factors in, 11
  criminal histories and, 196
  environmental/sociocultural factors in, 13
  familial factors in, 11
  multifactorial perspective on, 13
  opiate. *See* Opiate addiction
  potential for, 4
  psychological factors in, 11–12
  as self-care effort, 72
  of spouses/partners, 278–279
  theories of, 11–13
Addiction Severity Instrument, 19
Addicts. *See also* Substance abusers; *specific types of substance abusers*

wives of, 265–266. *See also* Families; Partners
Adolescent drug abuse. *See also* Adolescent substance abuse
  of amphetamines, 308
  gateway drugs in, 306–307
  of heroin, 308
  of inhalants, 308
  opiate, 308
  of steroids, 308
Adolescent Drug Involvement Scale, 317
Adolescent Problem Severity Index, 317
Adolescent substance abuse, 305–329
  assessing for, 313–319
    clinician's role in, 317–318
    tools for, 317
  comorbidity with, 315–317
  current trends in, 306–309
  family's role in, 318–319
  laboratory testing for, 318
  prevention of, 309–313
  risk factors for, 309–312
  tools for, laboratory testing, 318
  treatment of, 319–324
    cognitive-behavioral, 323
    family-based, 323–324
    goals for, 321–323
    juvenile justice system in, 320–321
    settings for, 320